The *illustrated* lecture series

Respiratory Medicine

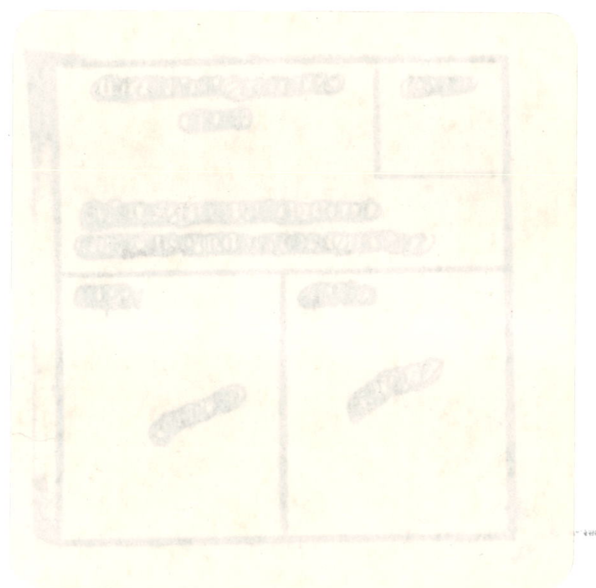

The *illustrated* lecture series

Neurology and Psychiatry	P. N. Plowman
Endocrinology and Metabolic Diseases	P. N. Plowman
Nephrology, Electrolyte Pathophysiology and Poisoning	P. N. Plowman
Haematology and Immunology	P. N. Plowman
Cardiology	T. J. Phillips, P. N. Plowman
Respiratory Medicine	P. N. Plowman
Alimentary Medicine and Tropical Diseases	P. N. Plowman, T. J. Phillips, S. J. Rose

In Preparation

Surgery

Anatomy

Obstetrics and Gynaecology

Pathology

Physiology

Ophthalmology

The *illustrated* lecture series

Respiratory Medicine

P. N. Plowman MA MD (Cantab) MRCP FRCR
Consultant Physician
St Bartholomew's Hospital and Medical College
London EC1   UK

MEDICAL EXAMINATION PUBLISHING COMPANY

Distributors in the United States & Canada:
Medical Examination Publishing Company
A Division of Elsevier Science Publishing Co., Inc.
52 Vanderbilt Avenue, New York, New York 10017

ISBN 0 444 01269 9

Printed in Great Britain

Contents

Contents

Preface

Diseases of the respiratory system was the first subject tackled in the Illustrated Lecture
Series, and it was because the small black and white figures so beautifully illustrated the
text and committed it to memory that we were stimulated to carry on with the whole
series on subjects in internal medicine. It is of course true that the typical chest X-rays,
spirometric tracings, bronchograms etc. of particular conditions lend themselves
particularly well to drawings. However, we also found that the anatomical details, the
clinical stereotypes, the illustrations of clinical procedures etc. could all be well drawn and
that the key phrases in the text could be thereby repeated in diagrammatic form and as
key labels.

This book contains the essentials of respiratory medicine illustrated to a degree never
before attempted and we believe that it comprises a unique teaching text for medical
students and paramedical workers involved with respiratory diseases.

P. N. Plowman

Publisher's Note

Modern medicine is now more interesting and challenging than ever before. Unfortunately, the subject is now so large that it presents a formidable task for students to encompass and for the practising physician to maintain an up-to-date knowledge.

This series of illustrated books represents an entirely new concept which we believe will open up a new method of medical teaching, adding an extra dimension which will keep the reader's interest alive and active throughout the whole syllabus of general medicine.

The most important feature of the book is the linkage and locking of prose with figures in such a way that illustrations (with repeated key phrases) reinforce the comprehension of the text at all stages as one proceeds through the pages. The content of the series also differs from many standard works in that not only does it bring in new sections on subjects such as coma, brain death, blood transfusion reactions, etc. omitted in older texts, but it also recognises that certain diseases (e.g. tertiary syphilis) no longer merit extensive description whilst other subjects (e.g. current successes in oncology) merit a more generous coverage.

This series, when completed and collected together, should comprise a uniquely illustrated textbook for the entire medical curriculum. Although primarily intended for the undergraduate student, these books should also prove substantially helpful to nurses, paramedics and social workers who are academically inclined, and offer a refresher course to the busy practitioner.

We have tried to make academic life for the student easier. We shall welcome criticisms, comments and suggestions from academics, students and other readers since we feel sure that these will help us to improve future editions.

Respiratory Medicine

The Respiratory System

ANATOMY

The respiratory system is commonly divided into upper and lower respiratory tracts (above and below the cricoid cartilage). This division is arbitrary in that an upper respiratory tract infection may spread to cause a bronchitis or pneumonia. The upper respiratory tract includes the nasal passages and sinuses, nasopharynx and larynx.

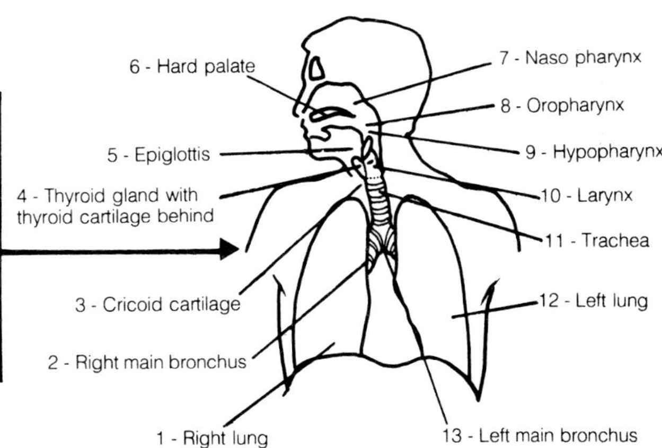

The **mucous membrane** lining the upper respiratory tract is well vascularised and due to its large surface area it acts as a humidifier of inspired air. The lining ciliated columnar cells form a beating carpet membrane and this serves the function of sweeping mucus secretions continuously upwards and also of filtering inspired foreign bodies. The lower respiratory tract is also lined by ciliated columnar epithelium and this again provides an upward transport mechanism for lower respiratory tract secretions, effete pulmonary macrophages and foreign particles.

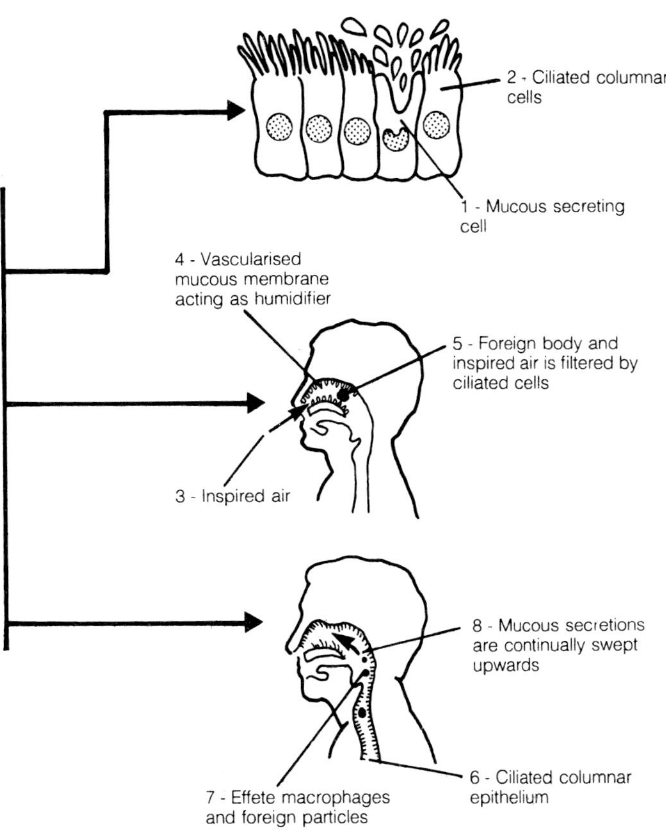

The **trachea** and **major bronchi** are supported by C-shaped cartilaginous hoops, open posteriorly where the cylinder is closed by muscle.

The trachea begins below the cricoid cartilage and bifurcates at the main carina which lies opposite the lower border of the manubrium sterni (the angle of Louis) and posteriorly the 4th/5th thoracic vertebrae. The trachea bifurcates into the right and left main bronchi which enter the lungs to divide into lobar bronchi, to divide in turn, like the branches of a tree, into segmental bronchi of progressively smaller calibre.

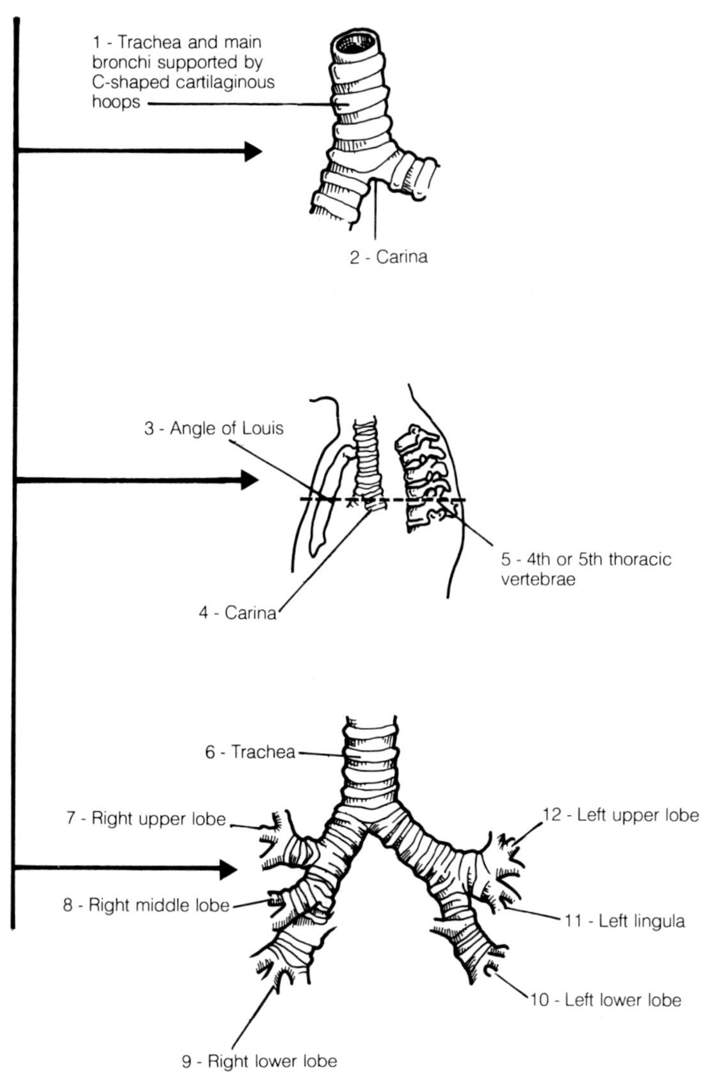

After approximately 16 divisions, the tiny bronchioles without cartilage or mucous glands in their walls (unlike their larger predecessors) become terminal bronchioles which are blind alleys each supplying one acinus – the functional unit of the lung. The terminal bronchiole gives off respiratory bronchioles from which the alveoli (the gas exchanging surfaces) originate.

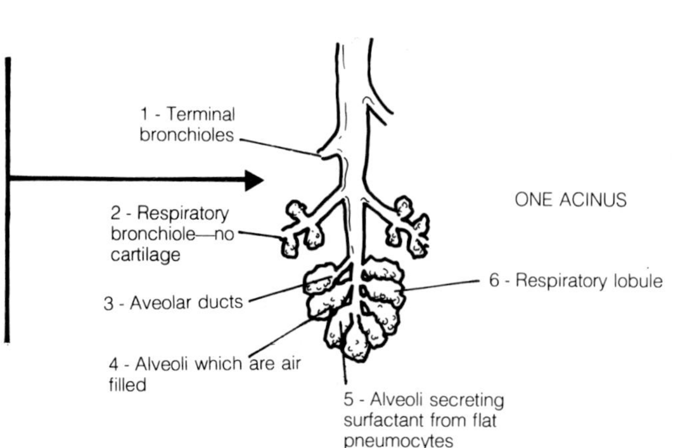

The **alveoli** are air filled sacs lined by flat pneumocytes (whose secretion of low surface tension surfactant keep the alveoli patent) on the lung side and inward of these there is direct contact with pulmonary capillaries. Thus, only a very thin barrier exists between the pulmonary blood stream and inspired air and gas exchange by diffusion is rapidly complete.

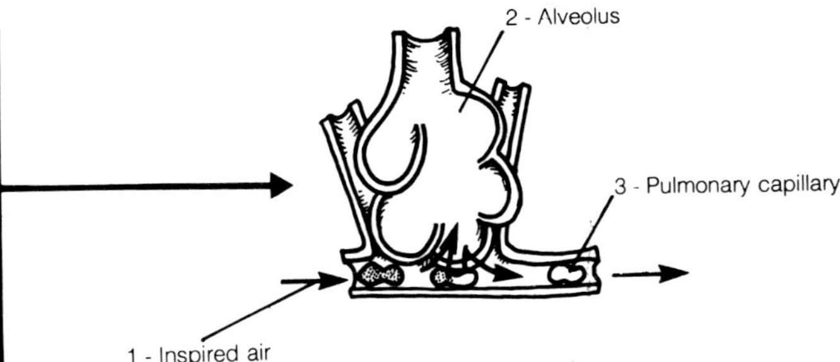

The trachea is palpable in the suprasternal notch where it is normally midline – that is, the clavicular heads of the sternomastoid muscles seem symmetrical either side of the trachea. Significant deviation strongly suggests a major shift in the upper mediastinal structures.

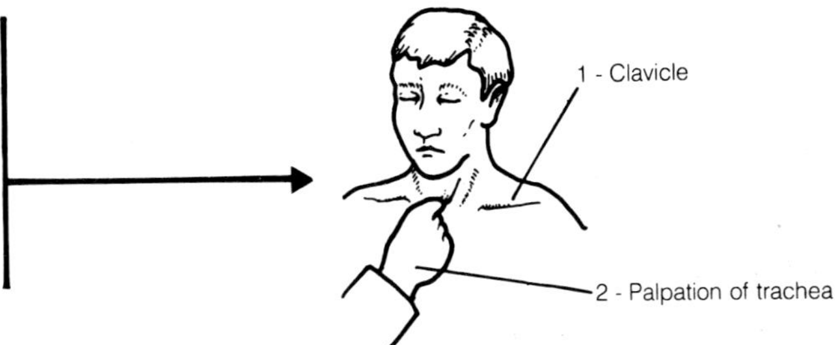

The **right main bronchus** is more vertical than the left: this is of importance as aspirated material, (often the source of bronchopneumonia) is more likely to pass to the right. The right main bronchus first gives off the right upper lobe bronchus from its lateral wall and, continuing as the intermediate bronchus branches anteriorly into a middle lobe bronchus and then proceeds downwards as the right lower lobe bronchus. The **left main bronchus** divides into a left upper lobe bronchus from the lateral wall, which divides itself almost immediately into a large segmental bronchus to that tongue-shaped region in the left lung – the lingula – the homologue of the right middle lobe – and the left upper lobe bronchus itself. After the left main bronchus has divided, it continues downward as the left lower lobe bronchus.

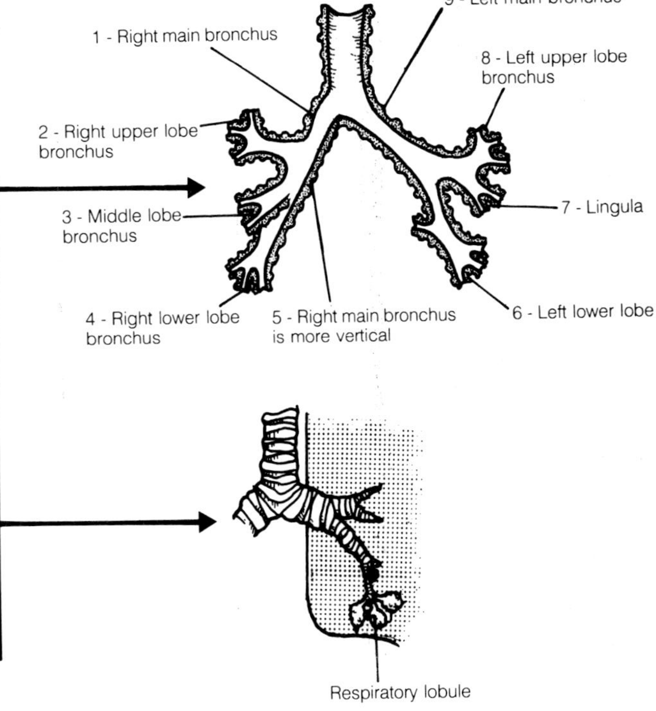

Thus the right lung has three lobes and the left lung two lobes; it is unnecessary for the student to attempt to memorise all the bronchopulmonary segments but some knowledge is valuable and they are exemplified. Segmental lobar collapse due to bronchial occlusion is rare due to collateral air drift at the acinar level; thus one rarely encounters less than lobar collapse. Segmental anatomy is perhaps of most importance in lung infections and to the chest surgeon.

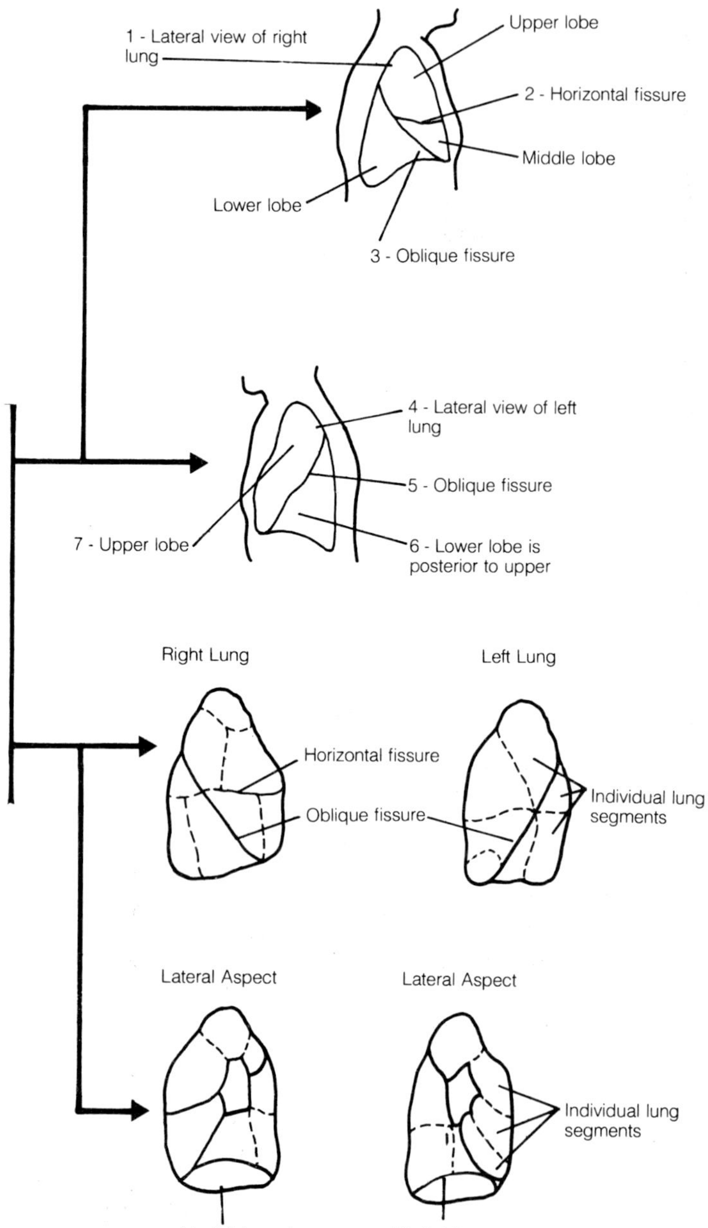

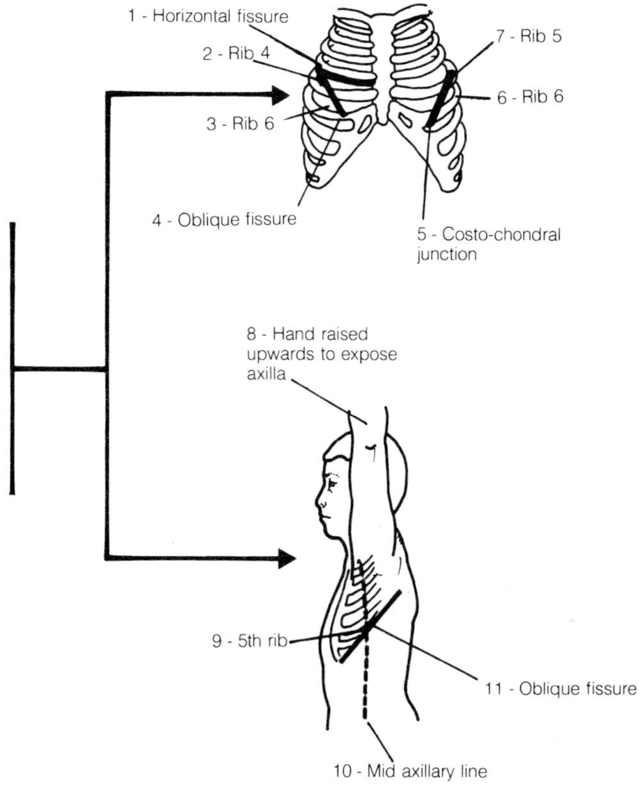

The main lung lobes are separated by **fissures**, the anatomy of which is important. The major or oblique fissures on both right and left sides pass from the junction of the 4th/5th rib with the vertebral column posteriorly, to the sixth costochondral junction anteriorly, crossing the mid-axillary line at approximately the 5th rib level.

A major consequence of this obliquely-angled fissure is that the upper lobes lie anteriorly and the lower lobes tend to lie postero-inferiorly. Physical signs detected when examining the back of the chest (below the apex) more commonly reflect lower lobe pathology.

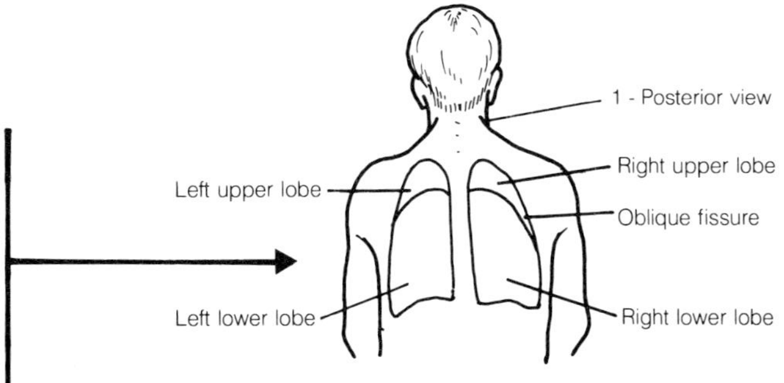

The horizontal fissure divides the right middle lobe from the right upper lobe above. The surface marking of this fissure is from the right fourth costo-chondral junction passing laterally and horizontally to meet the surface marking of the oblique fissure in the mid-axillary line at the level of the fifth rib.

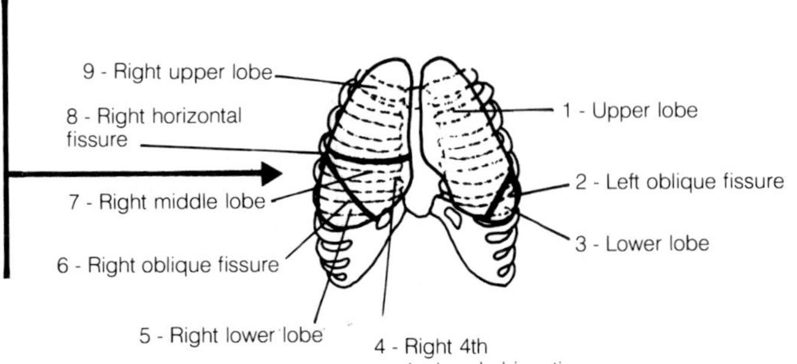

RESPIRATORY FUNCTION

The two main components of respiratory function are ventilation and gas exchange; pulmonary diseases may affect one or both of these separate functions directly or indirectly (e.g. a defect in ventilation may secondarily lead to hypoxaemia and hypercapnia although the gas exchange mechanism is normal).

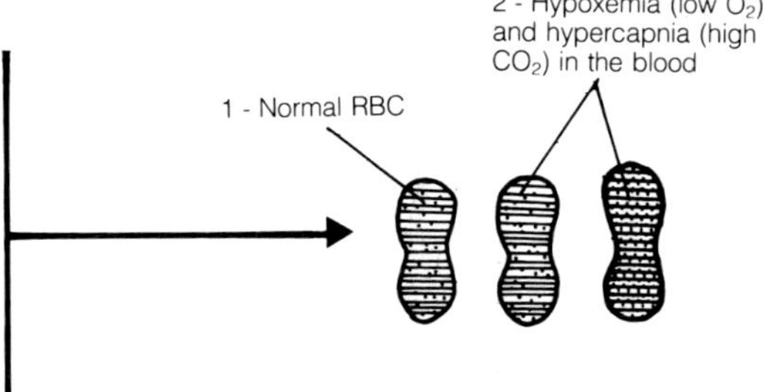

Testing Ventilation – Inspiration occurs when the inspiratory chest muscles and diaphragm contract causing a reduction in intrathoracic pressure. Inspiration thus depends on the nervous system, neuromuscular integrity, normal lung elasticity and space to expand within the chest. During quiet breathing, expiration is a passive recoil process.

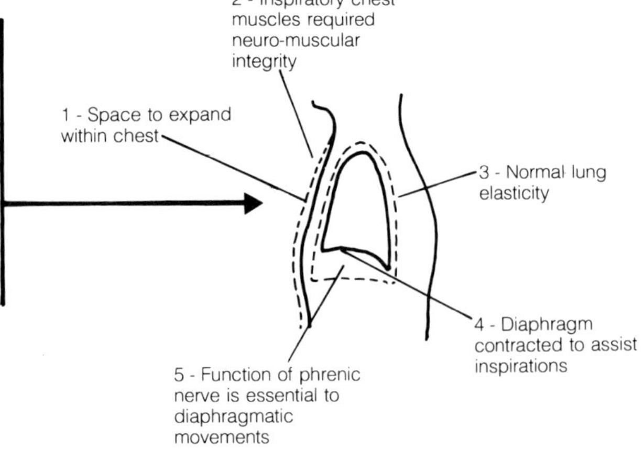

Spirometry with helium dilution methodology allows measurement of static lung volumes. The tidal volume (**TV**) is the volume of air breathed in and out during quiet respiration (approximately 500 ml) and the expiratory reserve volume (**ERV**) (approximately 1200 ml) is the extra volume of air that can be expired with effort; even then a residual volume (**RV**) of approximately 1000 – 1500 ml is left in the lungs. The total lung capacity (**TLC**) represents the volume of air in the lungs at maximal inspiration, and the volume expired between maximal inspiration and maximal expiration is the vital capacity (**VC**).

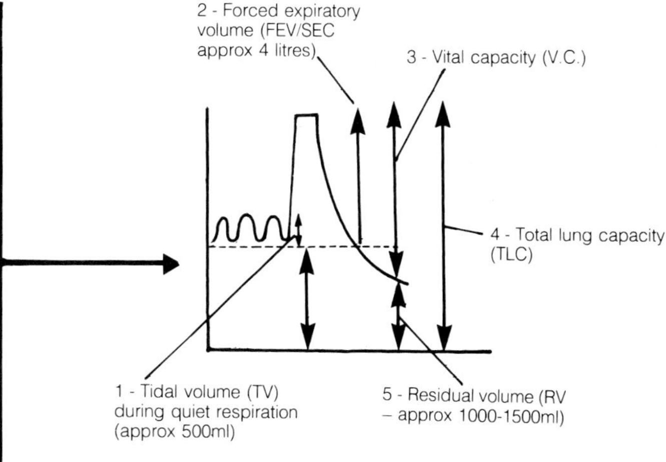

Spirometry is also used for the very important tests of dynamic ventilatory function and can be simply performed at the bedside – perhaps before and after therapy (e.g. with a bronchodilator). The two most valuable parameters measured are the forced expiratory volume in one second (**FEV1** – normal value approximately 4 litres) and the forced vital capacity (**FVC** – normal value approximately 5 litres) – requiring a maximal expiratory effort from maximum inspiration to maximum expiration.

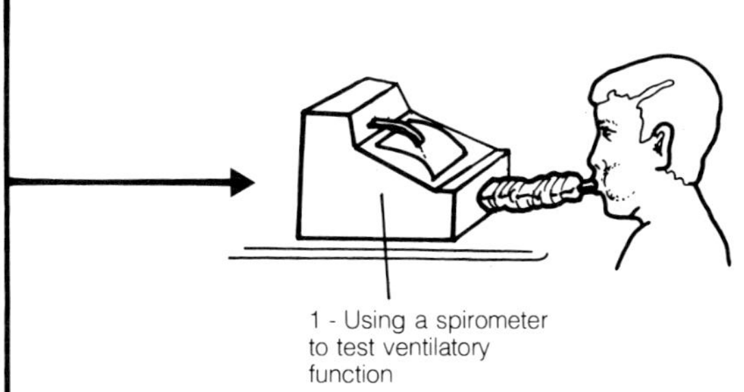

All these ventilatory parameters are subject to height, age and sex variables and the normal values for a particular individual (which will have a 15% normal variation) are obtainable from standard tables.

Patients with **obstructive ventilatory defects** have difficulty in fast expiration and the FEV1 is reduced disproportionately severely to any reduction in FVC, (low FEV1/FVC ratio). In addition, the static tests may show a high TLC, low VC and increased RV and RV/TLC ratio.

A restrictive defect (such as poorly compliant lung due to interstitial fibrosis) causes a reduction in the VC and FVC but the respiratory effort remains efficient such that the FEV1/FVC ratio remains normal. The TLC is low and the RV and RV/TLC ratio may be low or normal.

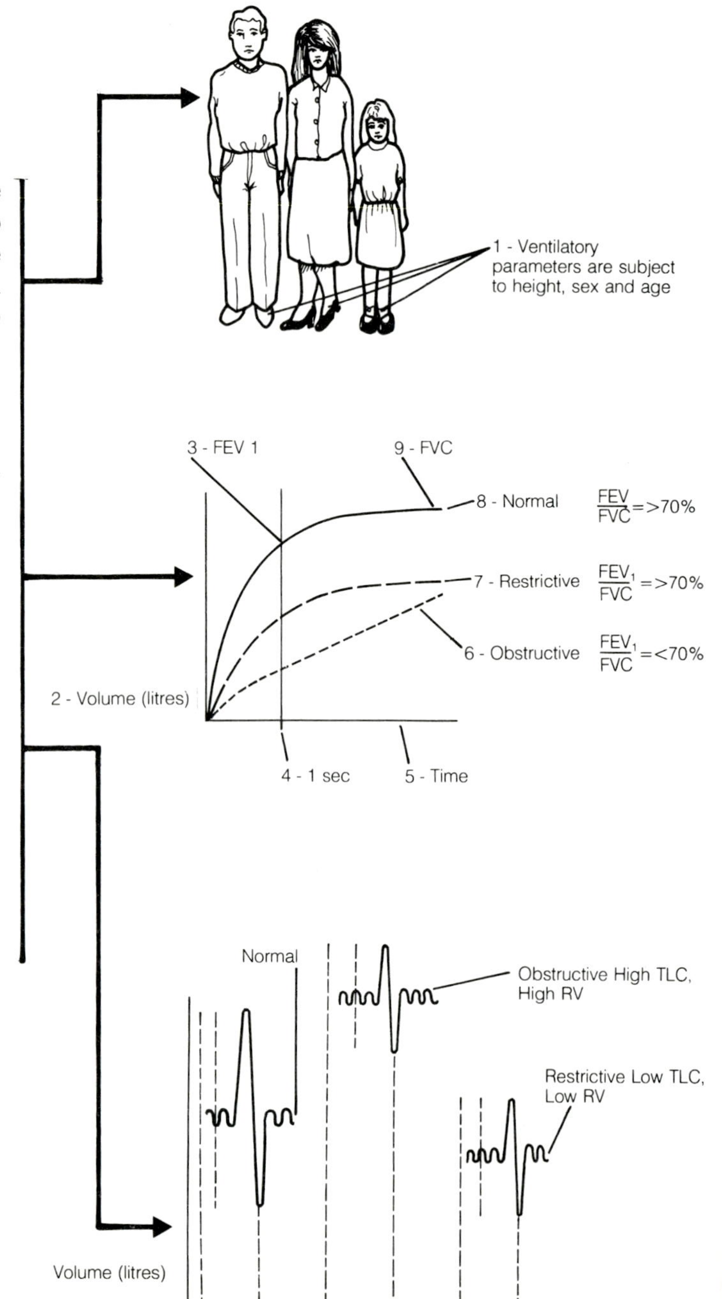

$\dfrac{FEV}{FVC} = >70\%$

$\dfrac{FEV_1}{FVC} = >70\%$

$\dfrac{FEV_1}{FVC} = <70\%$

A simple bedside test of dynamic ventilatory function is particularly useful in the serial assessment of asthma. The Wright's Peak Flow Meter measures the peak expiratory flow rate (PEFR – normal value 500 l/min), is comparable to the FEV1 measurement in some respects, and is reduced early in bronchoconstriction.

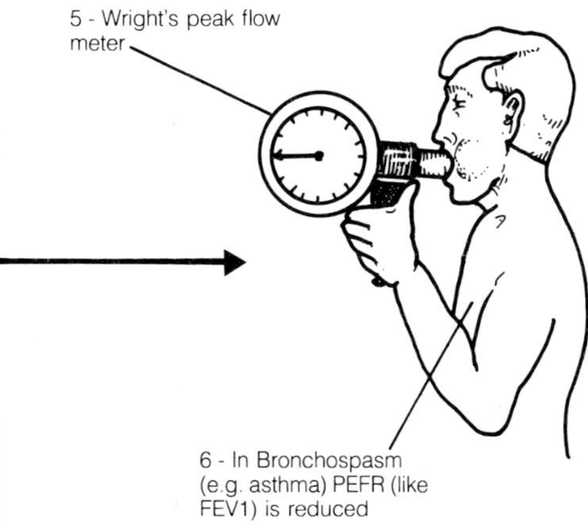

Testing Gas Exchange – The pulmonary venous blood and exhaled air composition depend on matching ventilation and blood perfusion to all the thousands of acini. Unmatched ventilation and perfusion at acinar level is the major reason for impaired gas exchange perhaps together with a reduced area of gas diffusing surface – (pneumonectomy will obviously reduce gas exchange, although the surviving lung may be normal).

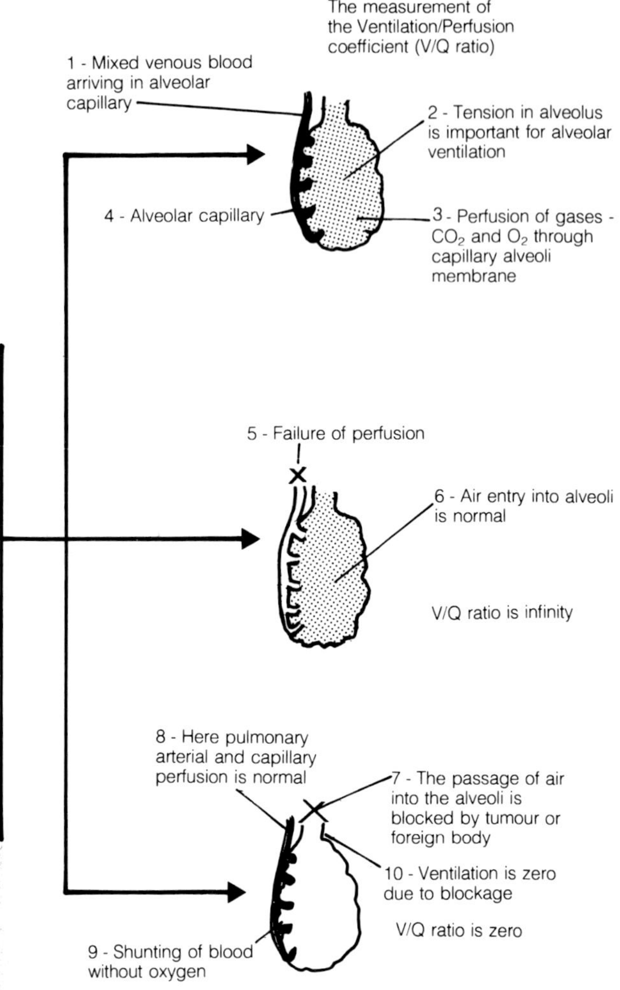

The gas tensions in blood leaving an individual alveolus depend on the tensions in the mixed venous blood that arrived in the alveolar capillary and the ratio between the alveolar ventilation (V) and perfusion (Q). The V/Q ratio may have values lying between infinity (where there is ventilation but no perfusion e.g. due to pulmonary embolism – the "dead space" situation) and zero (where there is perfusion but no ventilation – the "right to left shunt" situation). In lung disease affecting only certain lung areas, the overall result is a composite picture, but the concept of the V/Q ratio remains important.

The tendency towards hypercapnia due to perfusion of alveoli with low V/Q ratios is compensated by overventilation of alveoli with normal V/Q ratios and hypercapnia is unusual. However, due to

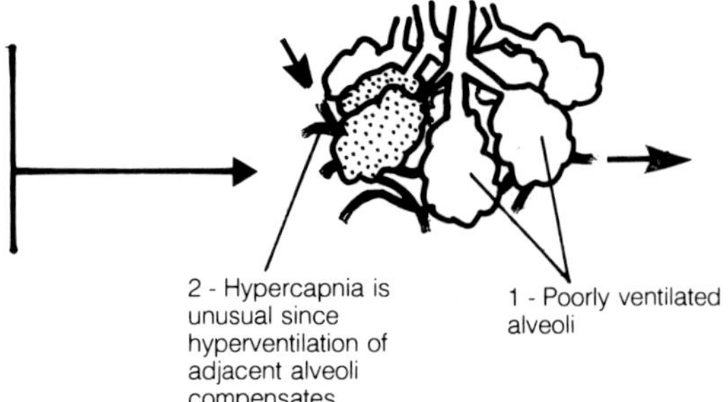

the fast saturation of haemoglobin under normal V/Q conditions, overventilation of normal alveoli will not compensate the problem of poor oxygen diffusion in low V/Q areas of lung, and hypoxaemia results.

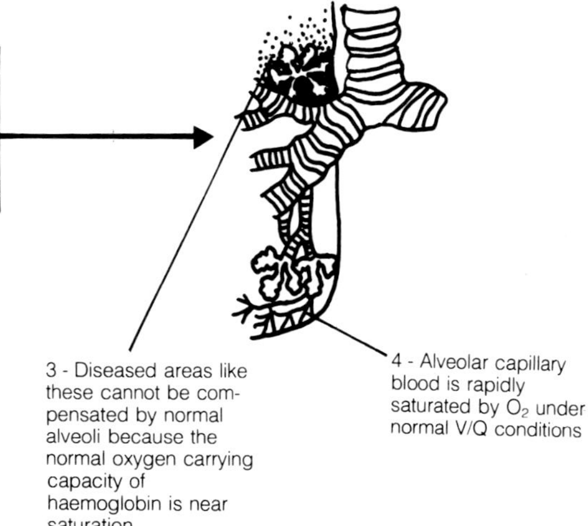

Measurement of arterial blood gas tensions is one important method of assessing adequate gas exchange – perhaps the most important as it tells us the oxygen supply to critical organs. However, the measurement of **transfer factor (DLCO)** is another measure of overall gas-exchange, which it quantifies as a measured average tension gradient from alveoli to pulmonary capillary blood. The units are mmol per minute per KPA. The method usually employs carbon monoxide (CO) at 1.5% concentration inhaled at a single inspiration, the breath being held for a fixed period (10 seconds) before the exhaled alveolar gas is collected (after washing out the dead space gas) in order to measure the quantity of CO transferred.

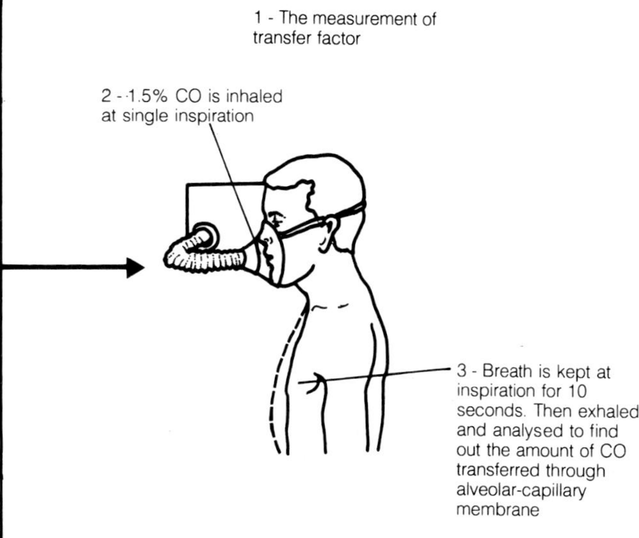

Helium is added to the inspired gas: Its dilution by dead space gas (evaluated from exhaled alveolar gas) is used to estimate the initial alveolar concentration of CO and the alveolar volume into which the inspired gases were distributed. Measurement of transfer factor is most useful in the initial and serial assessment of patients with diffuse parenchymal lung disease, but lung volumes and red cell haematology must always be studied together with any **DLCO** measurement as both may influence the result.

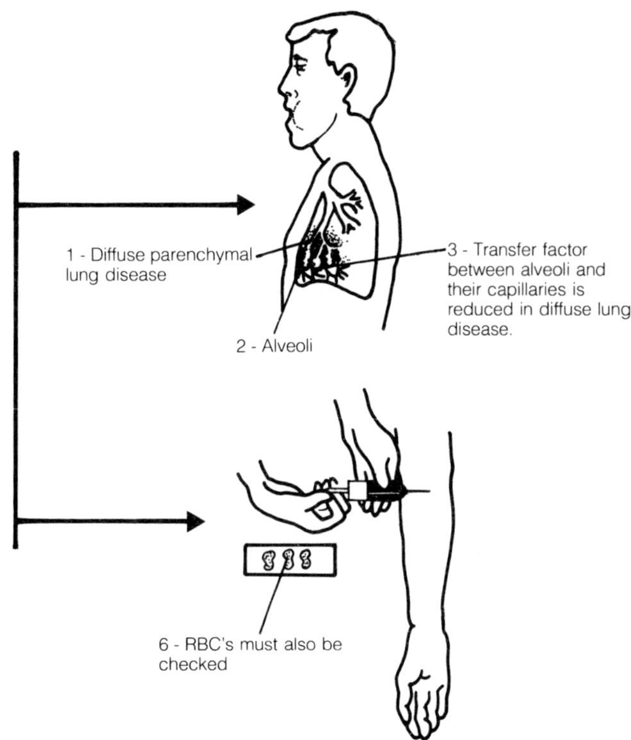

Chest X-ray Interpretation The basic preliminaries to examining the postero-anterior (PA) chest X-ray (CXR) are to check the patient's name, the date on the film, the left and right, that the film has been adequately exposed, (the posterior ribs should be discernible through the cardiac shadow and the pulmonary vessels indentifiable in the hilar regions), that the patient has taken an adequate inspiration, (such that in normal people the dome of the right hemi-diaphragm is near the anterior end of the sixth rib), and that the patient is not rotated, (that the medial ends of both clavicles are symmetrically disposed about the spinous processes). A repeat CXR may be more important than an attempted interpretation of a poor quality film.

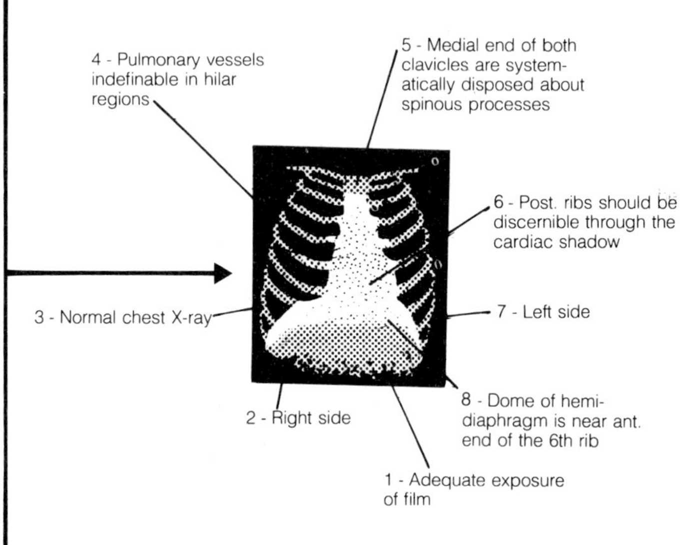

Now move on to obvious normality (or abnormality). The heart shadow is characteristic and normally lies half to two thirds to the left of the midline. The left heart border is normally that of the left ventricle and the right heart border that of the right atrium. On a standard adult film of the chest the normal maximum transverse heart diameter is 11.5 – 15.5 cm. and this should not increase by more then 1.5 cm. in serial X-rays of the same individual. The cardiothoracic ratio should be less than 50%.

The boot shaped heart of left ventricular dilatation with failure and pulmonary congestion exemplifies an abnormal situation. Above the heart, one checks the aortic arch and aortic contour as far as it is discernible. At the same time one is checking the width of the superior mediastinum and each lateral contour. Next move to the hilar regions – difficult areas for the beginner! In normal people the hilar shadows are caused by the pulmonary arteries and veins with a minor contribution from the walls of the major airways. As the left main bronchus is hyparterial (c.f. the right side), the left hilum is commonly slightly (perhaps 1 cm.) higher than the right. Both hila should be of equal radiodensity and have a concave lateral aspect due to the divergence outwards of the major upper lobe vein upwards and the basal artery downwards. The **diagnosis** of cardiac, mediastinal or hila abnormalities is made in conjunction with the lateral CXR.

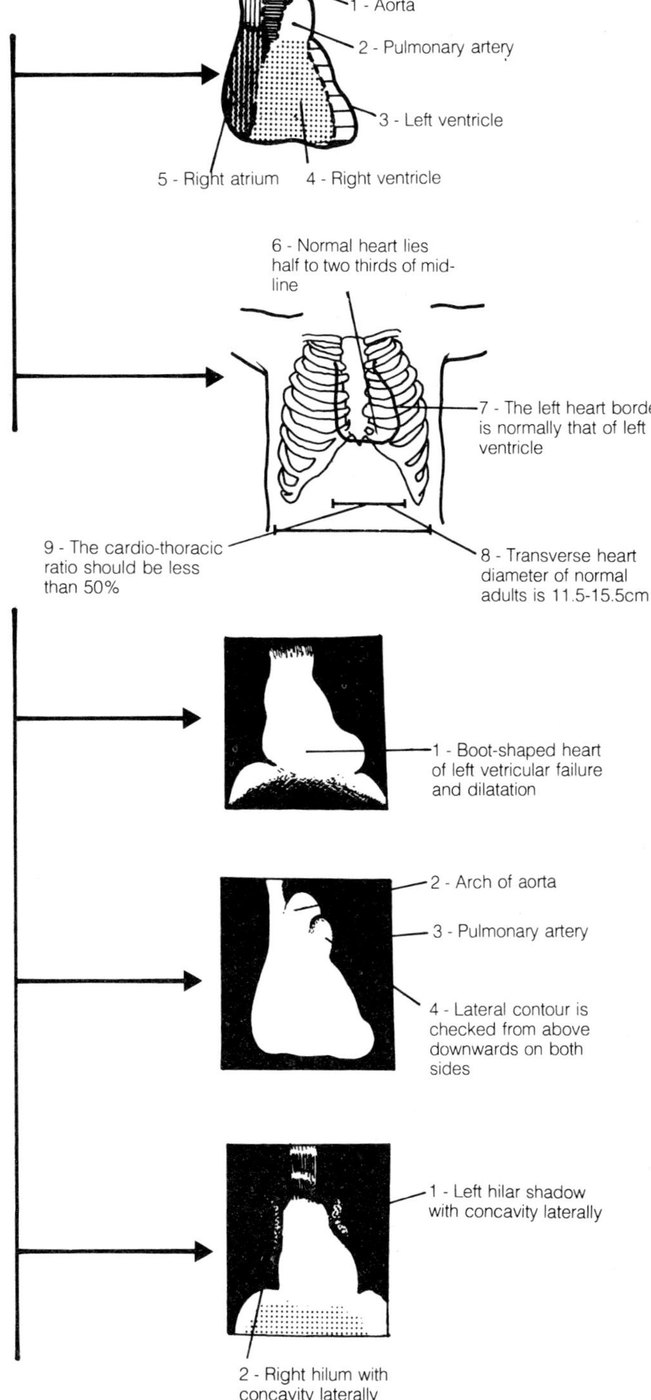

The lung vessels are rapidly screened as they radiate out from the hila. The vessels in the upper half of the lungs are of smaller calibre than those in the lower halves but they are symmetrical when comparing left and right sides. In heart failure, upper lobe vascular engorgement is an important radiological sign. When scanning the lungs, any non-vascular shadows are abnormal. The lungs are normally symmetrically transradient (but may appear different if the patient is rotated).

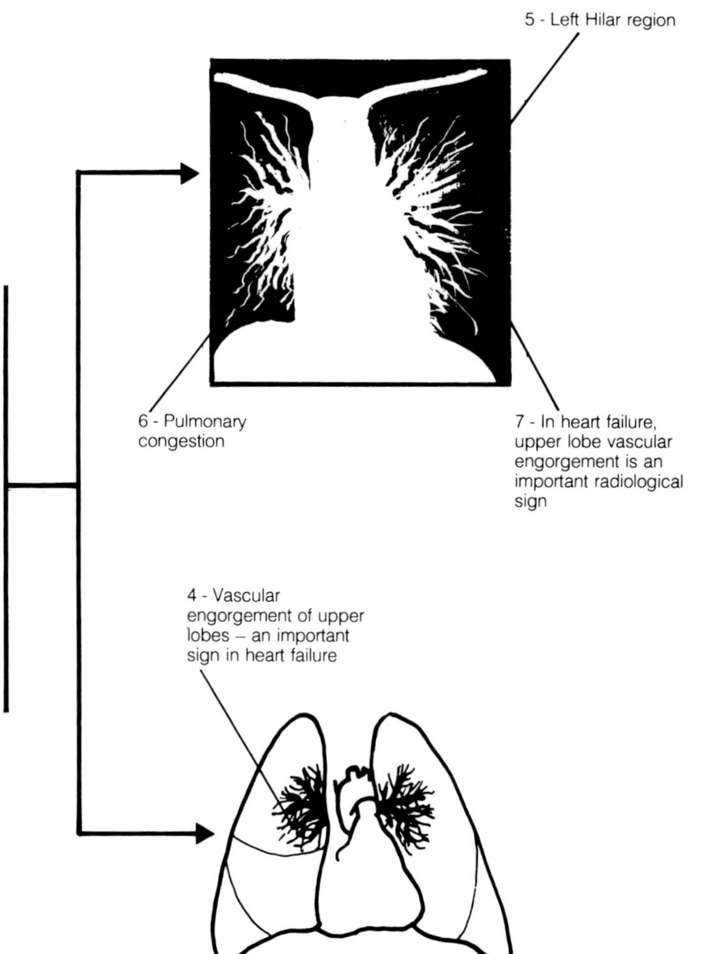

Areas of opacification can be due to many pathologies and the radiologist can only describe **"consolidation"**, (although he may well be able to distinguish lobar consolidation, patchy consolidation throughout a lobe or lung, probable pleural effusion, pleural thickening, discrete intrapulmonary mass or masses, or atelectasis').

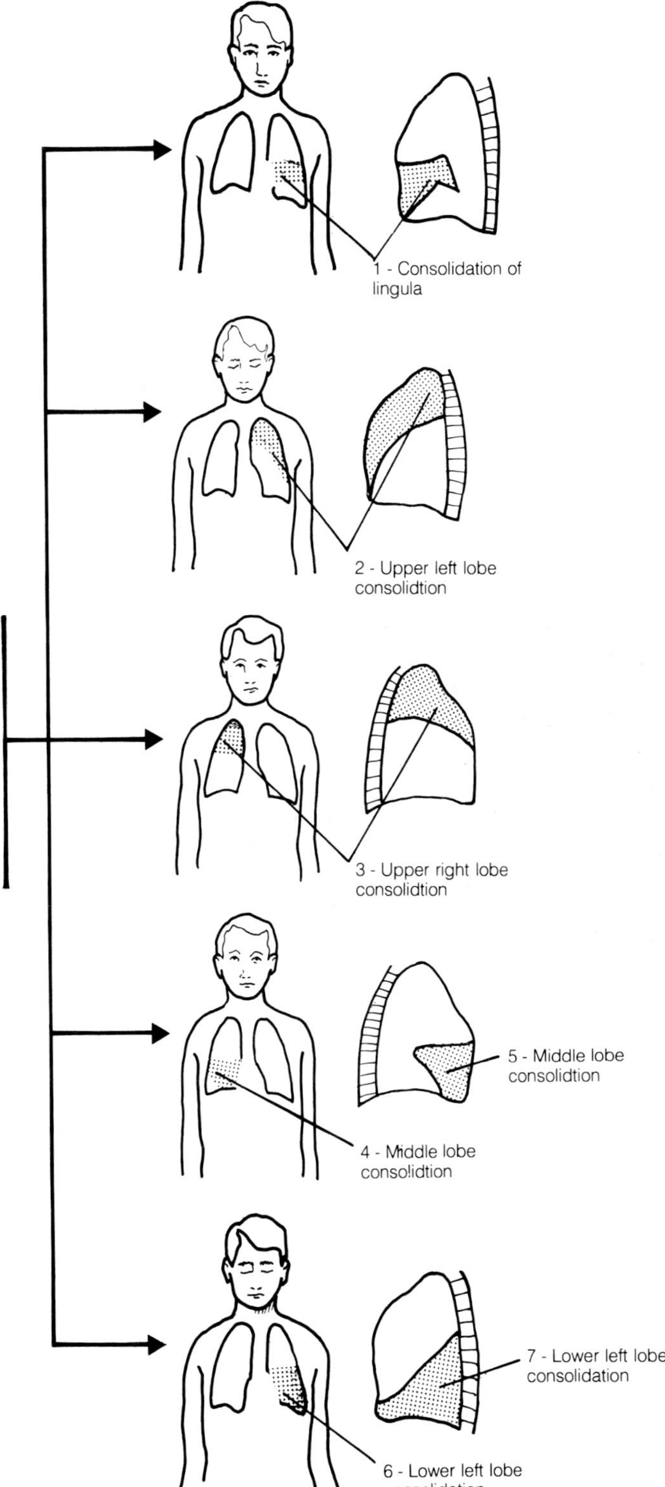

Collapse (atelectasis) should be radiologically distinguishable from consolidation. An upper lobe collapse produces a triangular opacity with its base on the lung apex and its apex at the hilum. A lower lobe collapse produces a triangular opacity with its base on the diaphragm and its apex at the hilum. A middle lobe collapse again produces a triangular opacity with its base on the right side of the heart and apex projecting into the lung field.

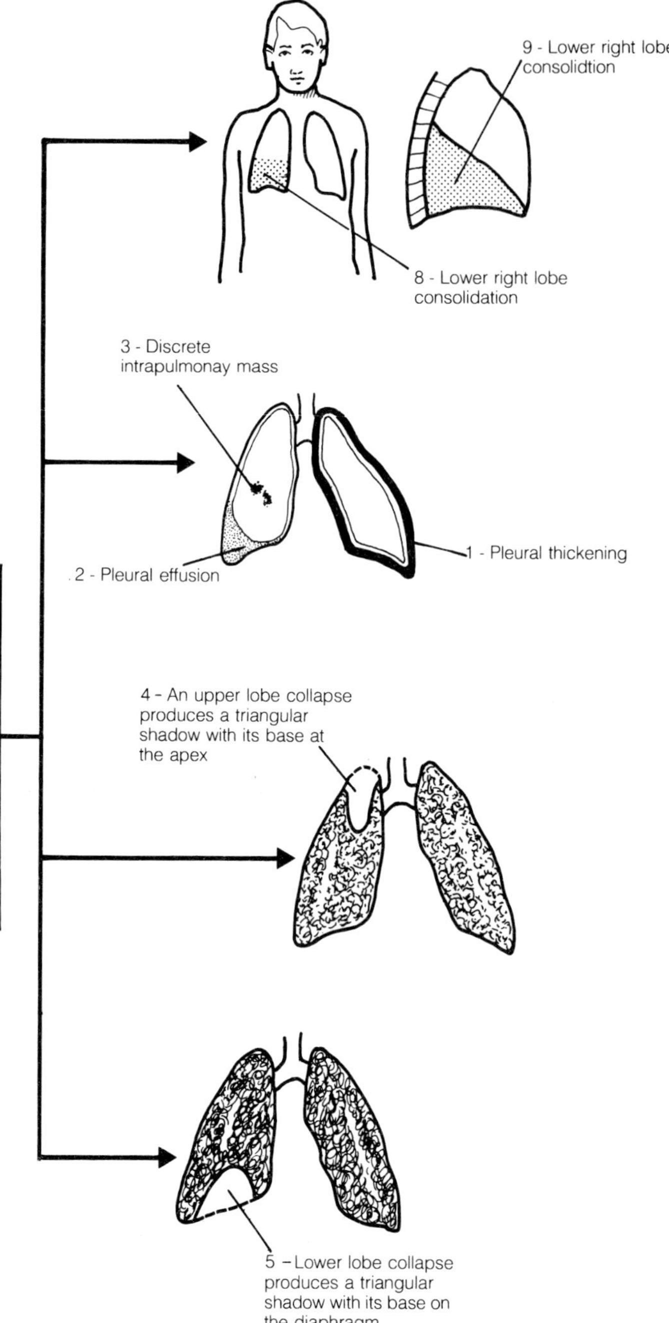

Variable degrees of mediastinal shift occur toward the lost lung volume together with compensatory overinflation of the functioning lobe. Atelectasis of a whole lung produces more marked mediastinal shift towards that side, diaphragmatic elevation on that side and a radiological "white-out" of the lung field on the CXR.

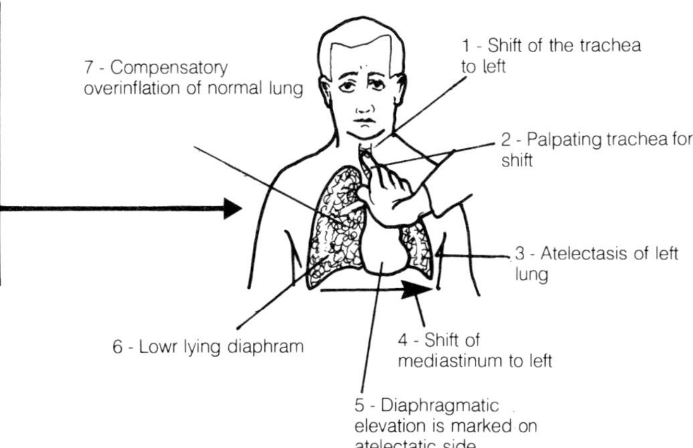

The causes of major atelectasis include aspirated foreign body, endobronchial tumour, bronchial stenosis or compression – the latter being more common in children whose bronchi are extremely soft and malleable.

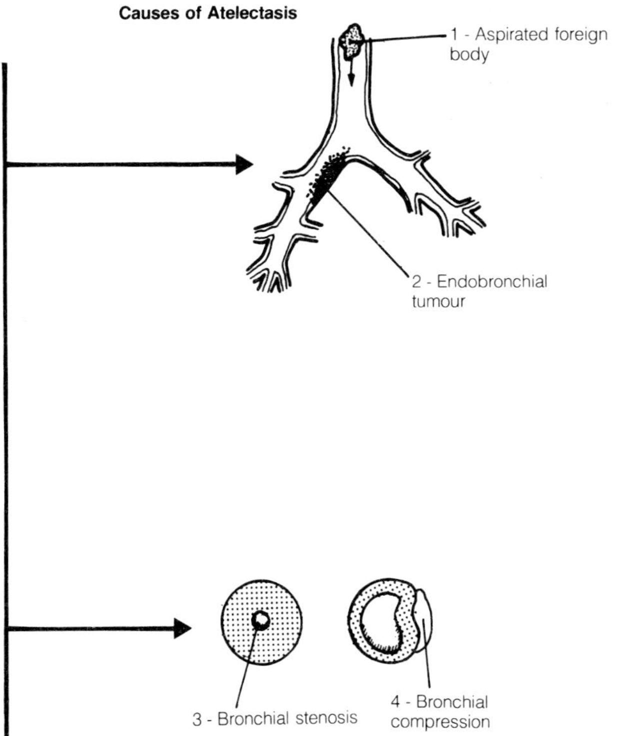

An increase in pulmonary transradiancy may occur with the compensatory overinflation of a lobe (after adjacent lobar collapse), or in pulmonary emphysema when the lungs are overexpanded with a low-lying diaphragm and often, loss of pulmonary vessels.

The dome of the right hemidiaphragm should lie near the 5th – 6th ribs anteriorly and is normally 1 – 2 cm. higher than the left dome. The **costophrenic angles** are normally clearly visible as acute angles although the cardiophrenic angles are often obscured by the cardiac fat pads (particularly on the left). In emphysema, the diaphragm is flatter and often up to two interspaces lower and the costophrenic angles are not clear. Blunting of the costophrenic angles is the earliest radiological sign of a pleural effusion.

The horizontal fissure is usually visible as a white hair-line shadow running from the right hilum to meet the 5th – 6th rib in the axilla.

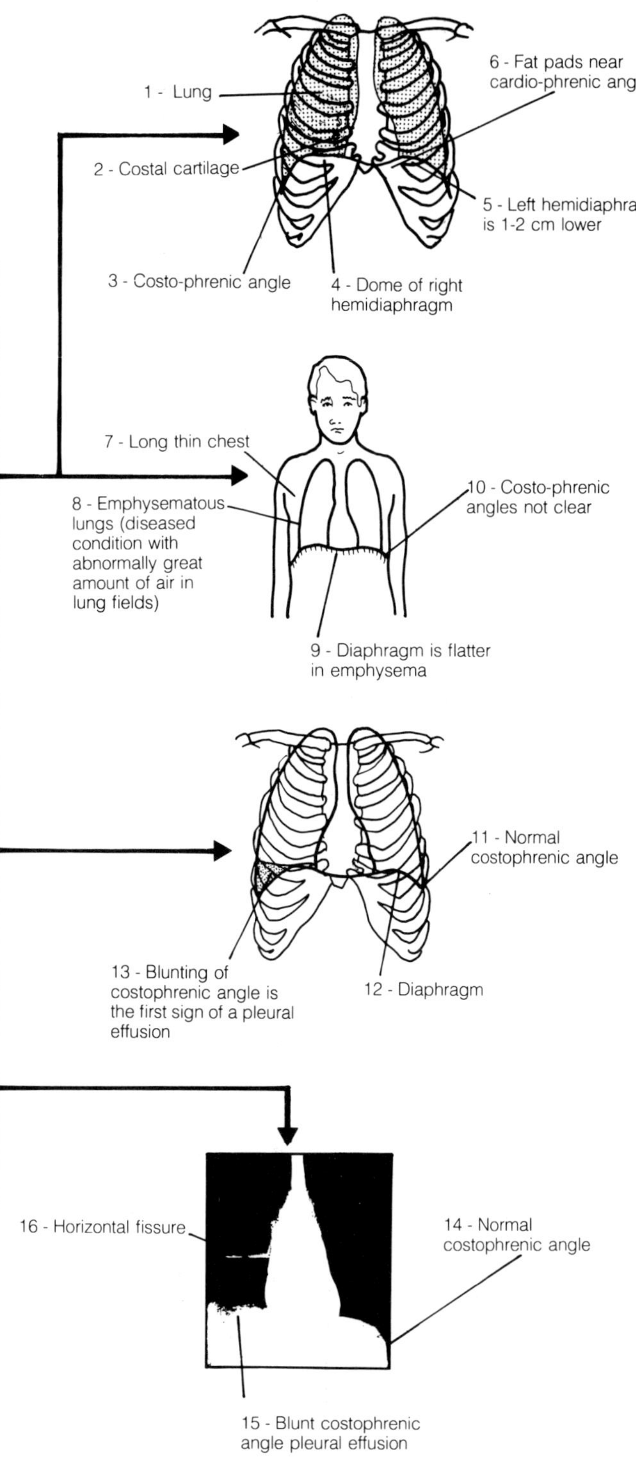

Lastly, **checks** are made of areas difficult to see – particularly the region behind the heart (is there some extra contour here?) and then the apices (is there a small pneumothorax or apical TB focus?) and the regions underlying the clavicles. Now move on to examine the bony skeleton examining carefully and methodically for holes, fractures or abnormal ossification.

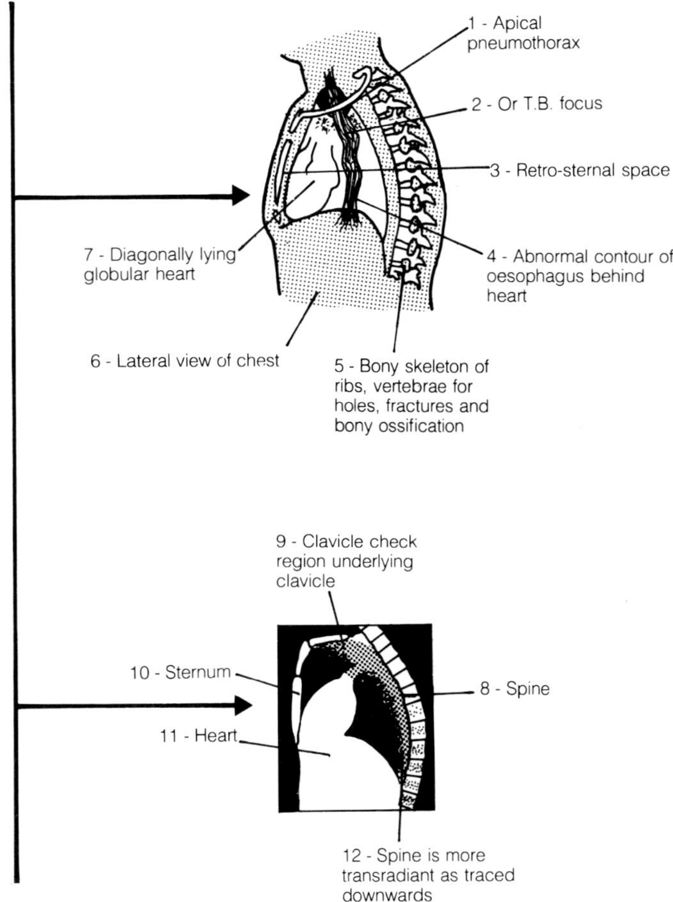

The lateral CXR is an essential complement to the PA film. Although initially difficult to interpret, a logical approach always helps:– Identify the diagonally-lying globular heart shadow; the retrosternal space (anterosuperior to the heart) should be as transradiant as the retrocardiac space. Another rule is that the vertebral bodies normally appear more transradiant as the spine is traced downwards.

Obviously, a posteriorly placed pleural effusion could cause both these normal rules to be broken.

Both leaves of the diaphragm are normally identified as smooth, well-differentiated humps, with the gastric air bubble just below the left. In a left lateral film (that is

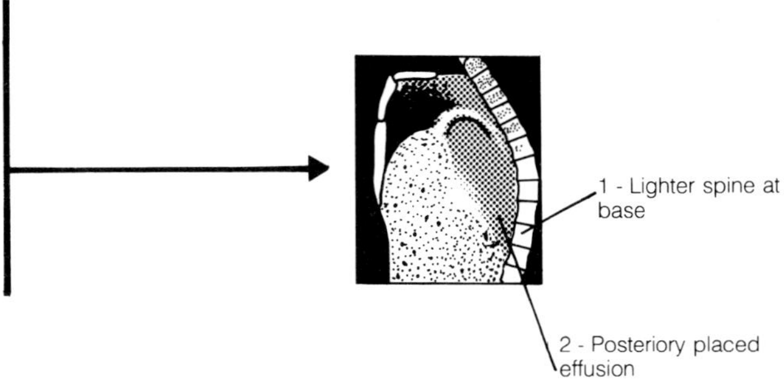

with the patient's left side against the X-ray plate and away from the X-ray source), the right hemidiaphragm is the one arising from the most magnified ribs. The oblique fissure should be defined in its normal position and then if possible the horizontal fissure found. The assessment of hila and mediastinal pathology is performed together with the PA film.

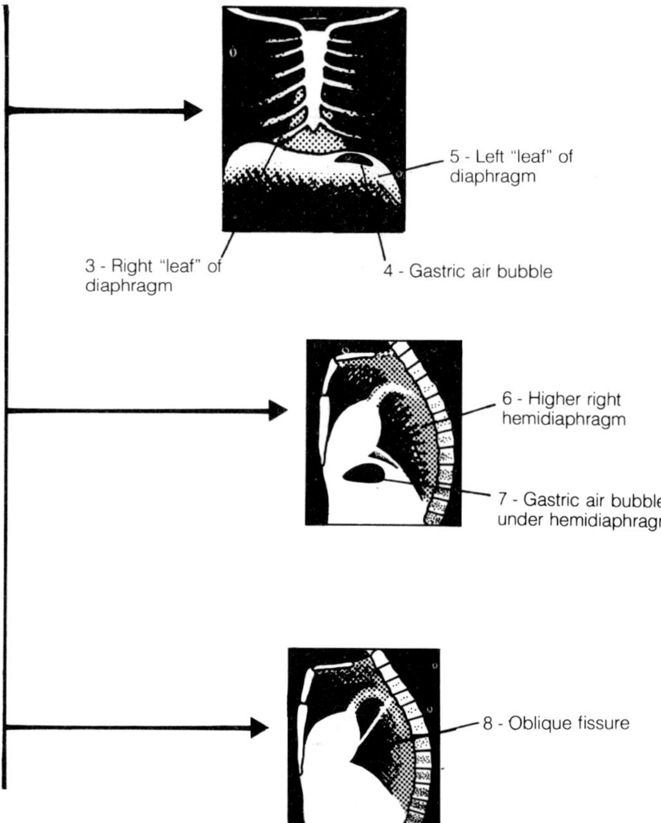

Although various imaging procedures, notably CT scanning, have refined the interpretation of chest radiological signs, every clinician must be capable of the initial, careful, CXR review.

THE SYMPTOMS AND SIGNS OF CHEST DISEASE

Symptoms – There are certain symptoms of chest disease:–

(1) **Cough** – Cough results from contraction of the expiratory muscles, initially against a closed glottis and then following the sudden opening of the glottis, the rapid expulsion of air and debris from the major airways. The cough reflex is stimulated from irritant receptors in major airways, chemoreceptors and stretch receptors in the more distal airways; although it is a protective reflex, coughing may become counter-productive and exhausting in both laryngeal and tracheobronchial diseases. Where a vocal cord

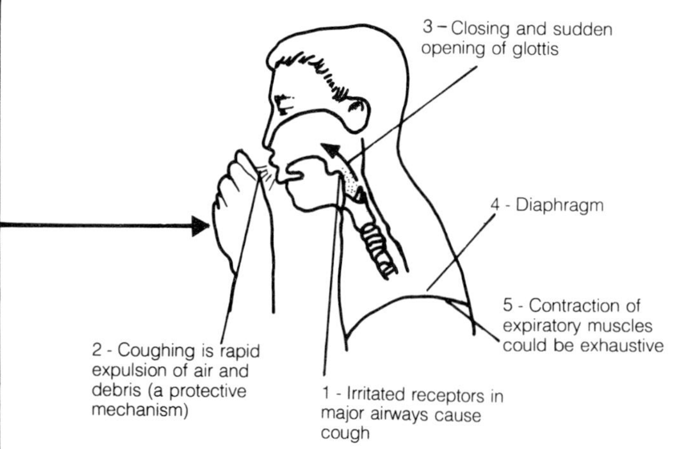

is paralysed, coughing loses its explosive force and ceases to clear the respiratory tract of secretions.

(2) **Sputum** – A cough is described as dry or productive; the latter refers to the production of sputum, whose daily expectorated volume, colour, texture and odour are all relevant to the enquiring physician. Sputum may be described as serous (e.g. the clear frothy sputum expectorated in acute pulmonary oedema), mucoid (e.g. the tenacious, grey or white sputum of chronic bronchitis), purulent or mucopurulent (e.g. the thick yellow or green sputum expectorated by a chronic bronchitic in an infected spell, or in large quantities in bronchiectasis). Purulent sputum may also be due to an excess of eosinophils (e.g. in asthma, and bronchopulmonary aspergillosis).

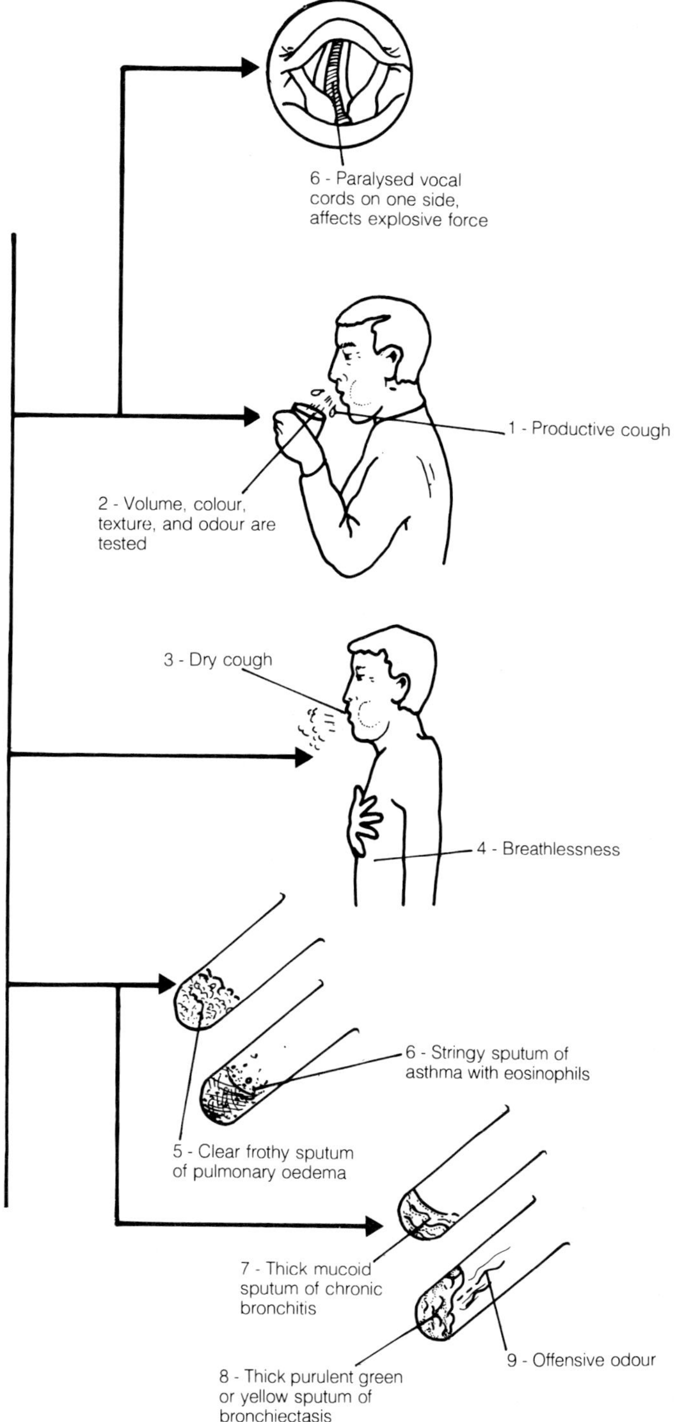

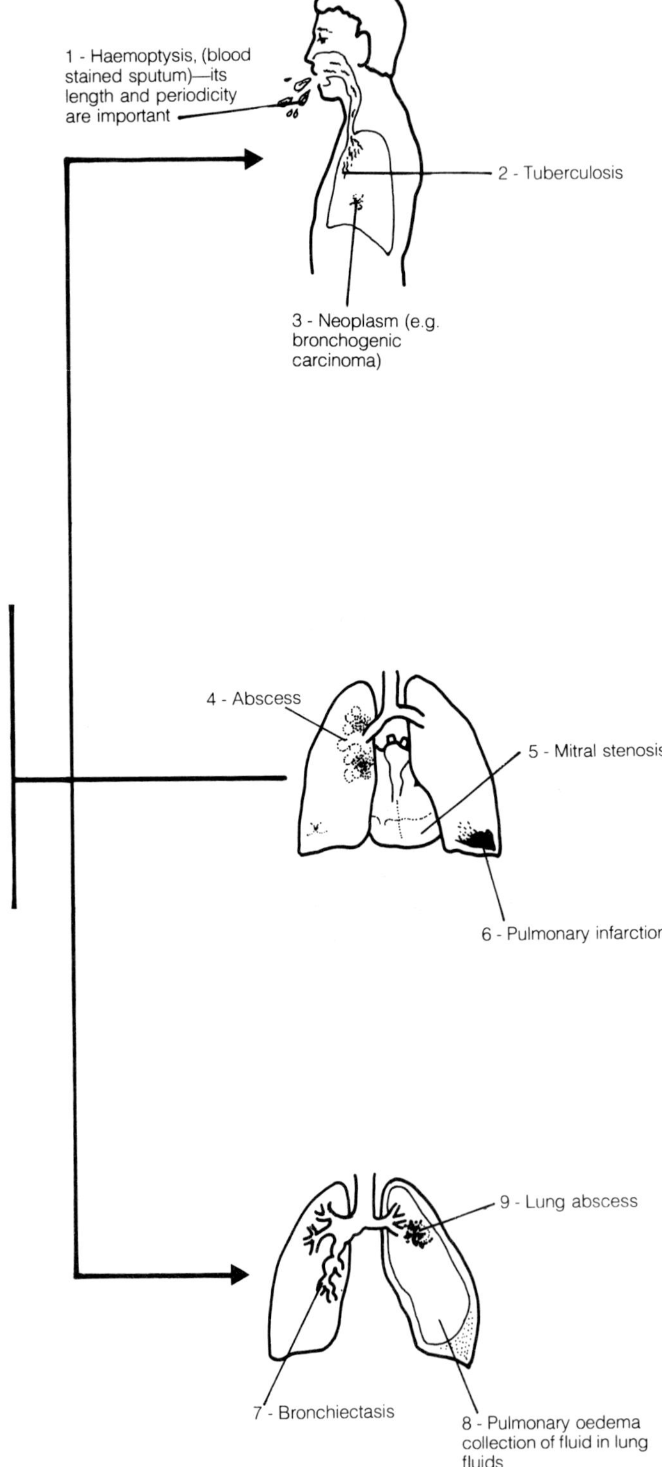

(3) **Haemoptysis** – Haemoptysis is always a symptom to be taken seriously; it may denote pulmonary pathology (e.g. neoplasm, tuberculosis, infarction, bronchiectasis or lung abscess) or cardiovascular pathology (e.g. mitral stenosis or acute pulmonary oedema) although occasionally no cause is found. The length of history of haemoptysis, periodicity and severity are all sought.

(4) Breathlessness (Dyspnoea) – Breathlessness is a complex symptom. Whilst chemical causes such as changes in PaO_2, PaCO and blood pH can be reasonably understood as causes of reflex changes in breathing patterns to re-establish homeostasis, there are situations of obstructive ventilatory defects (e.g. chronic obstructive airways disease, COAD, and asthma) and of restrictive ventilatory defects (e.g. widespread fibrosing alveolitis or oedema) where lung receptors stimulate breathing mechanisms and create the sensation of breathlessness. Further, higher centres can stimulate both breathlessness and hyperventilation (e.g. hysteria).

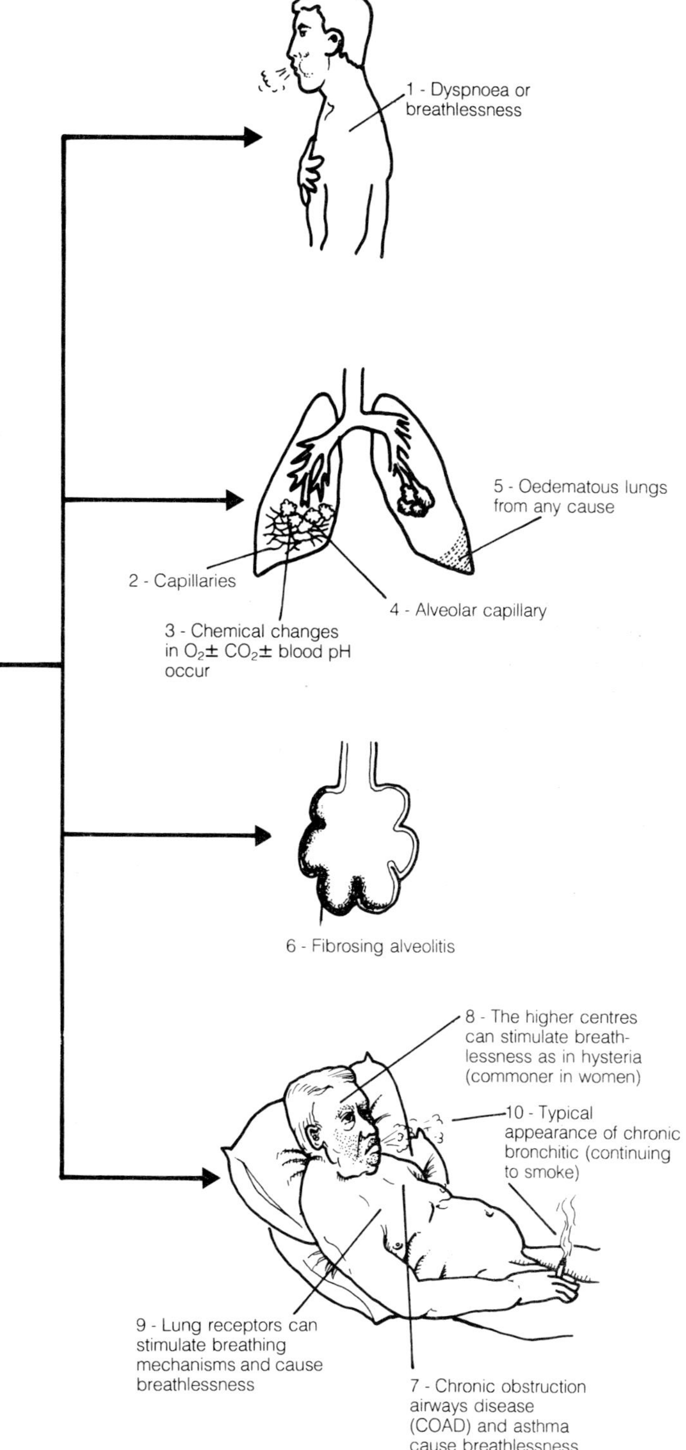

The pattern of breathlessness helps in diagnosis – a sudden onset (e.g. pneumothorax, pulmonary embolism), nocturnal episode (e.g. acute left ventricular failure), nocturnal episodes or episodic with wheeze (e.g. asthma), worsening breathlessness over weeks (e.g. pleural effusion) or over a year or more (e.g. fibrosing alveolitis). The severity of breathlessness can be graded from the patient's history:

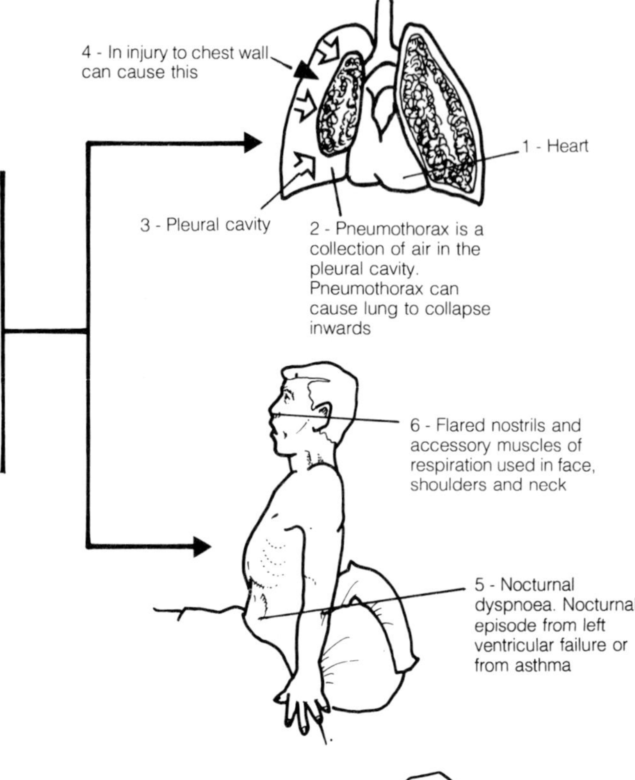

The exercise tolerance can be quantified as the distance along the flat that the patient can walk or the number of flights of stairs he can climb before requiring a stop "for breath". Also record whether the patient feels breathless at rest and whether he feels breathless when lying flat; (how many pillows does he sleep with at night?). **Orthopnoea** refers to breathlessness on lying flat.

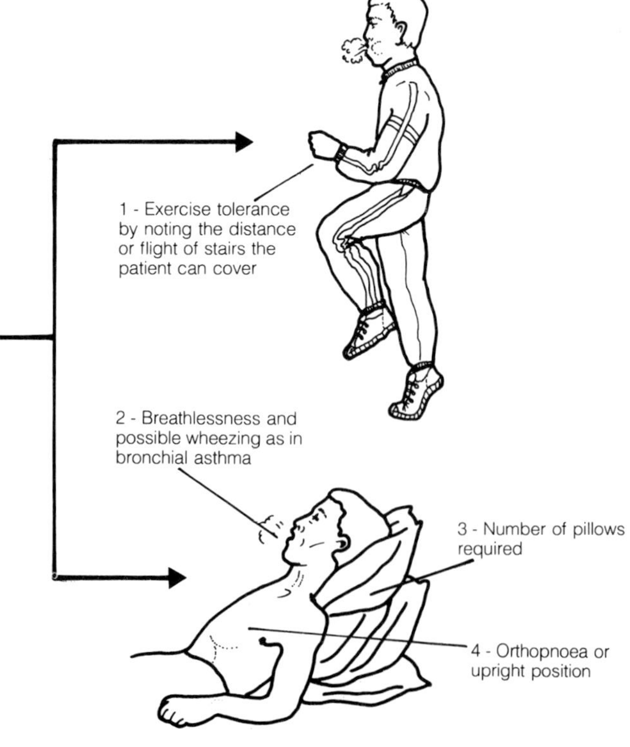

(5) **Wheezes (Rhonchi)** – Wheezes are musical sounds originating from the lower respiratory tract. They are generated by airways oscillating near the point of closure – like the reed of a wind instrument. Wheeze with breathlessness is a characteristic complaint in asthma and also in COAD – auscultation of the chest detects these predominantly expiratory rhonchi in both lung fields. Partial obstruction of the larynx or trachea may cause the inspiratory wheeze termed **stridor**.

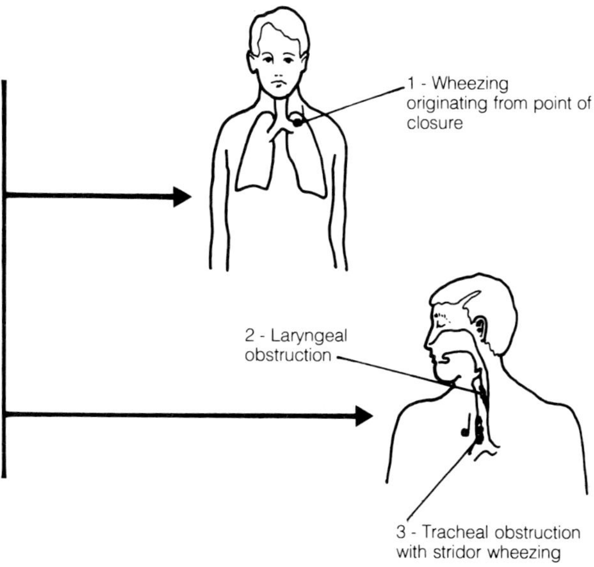

(6) **Chest Pain** – Chest pain tends to be central (tracheal pain – a central rawness) or lateral (pleuritic pain – a stabbing peripheral pain). Both are brought on by deep inspiration and coughing. Pleuritic pain implies pleural inflammation often due to adjacent pneumonia or pulmonary infarction, and the pain may be well localised over the diseased region.

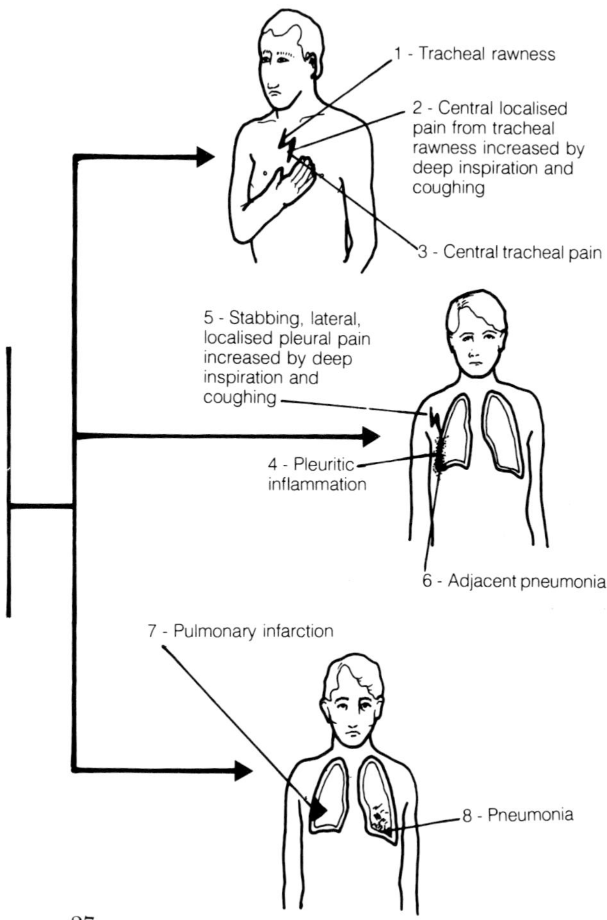

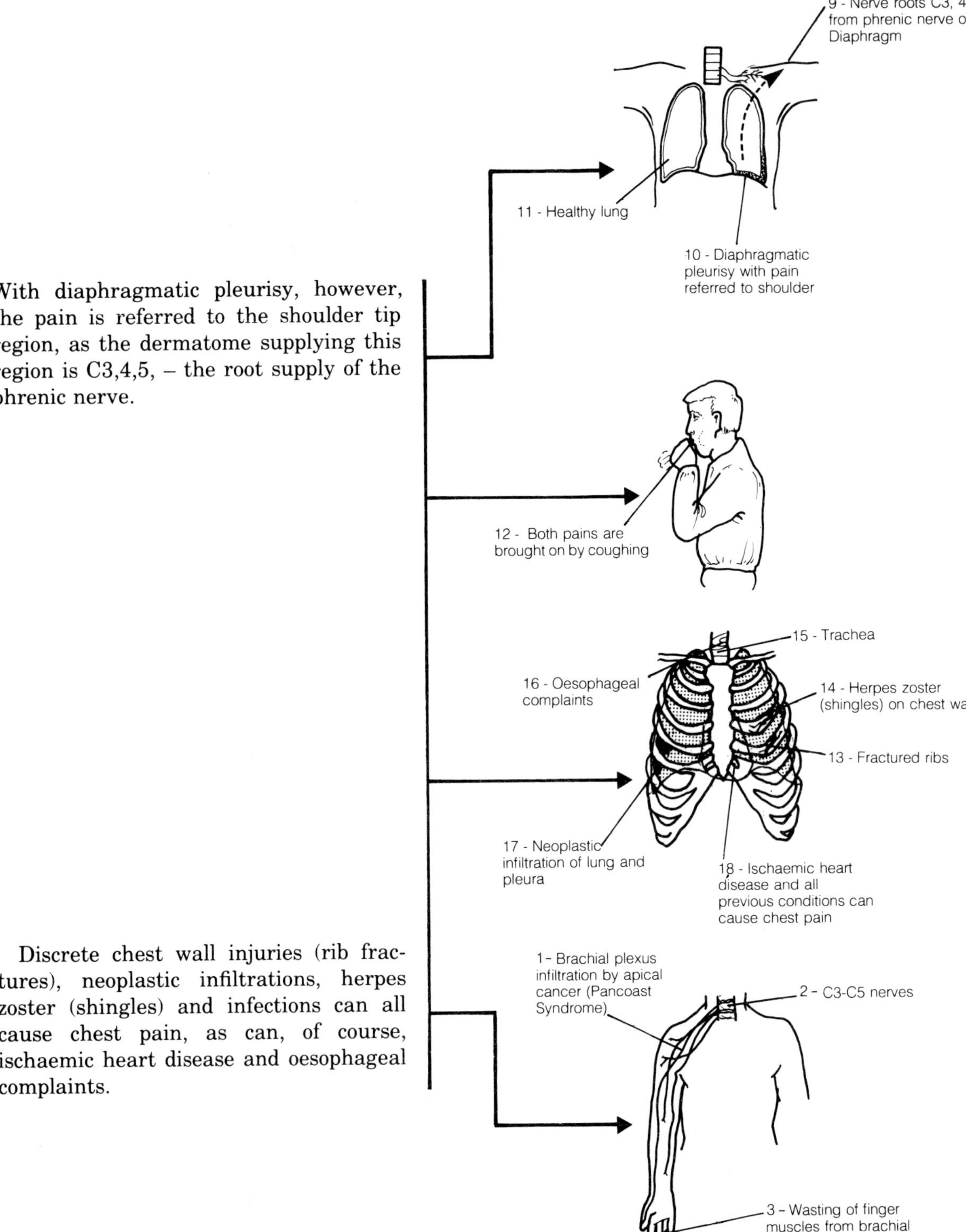

With diaphragmatic pleurisy, however, the pain is referred to the shoulder tip region, as the dermatome supplying this region is C3,4,5, – the root supply of the phrenic nerve.

Discrete chest wall injuries (rib fractures), neoplastic infiltrations, herpes zoster (shingles) and infections can all cause chest pain, as can, of course, ischaemic heart disease and oesophageal complaints.

Signs – The general examination of the patient precedes all specific examinations and may detect generalised wasting or signs of metastatic disease, or more specific pointers to respiratory disease such as cyanosis or finger clubbing.

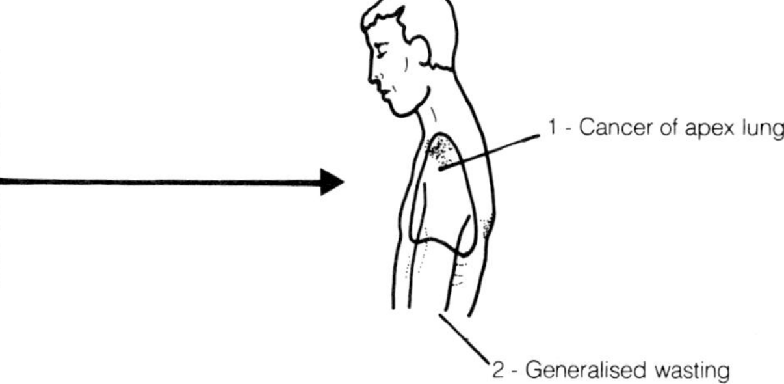

Central Cyanosis – The blue hue of the tongue, the inner aspect of the lips and conjunctivae is due to a circulating arterial deoxyhaemoglobin concentration of at least 1.5 g/dl and denotes severe respiratory disease (or a right to left shunt within the cardiovascular system – cyanotic heart disease).

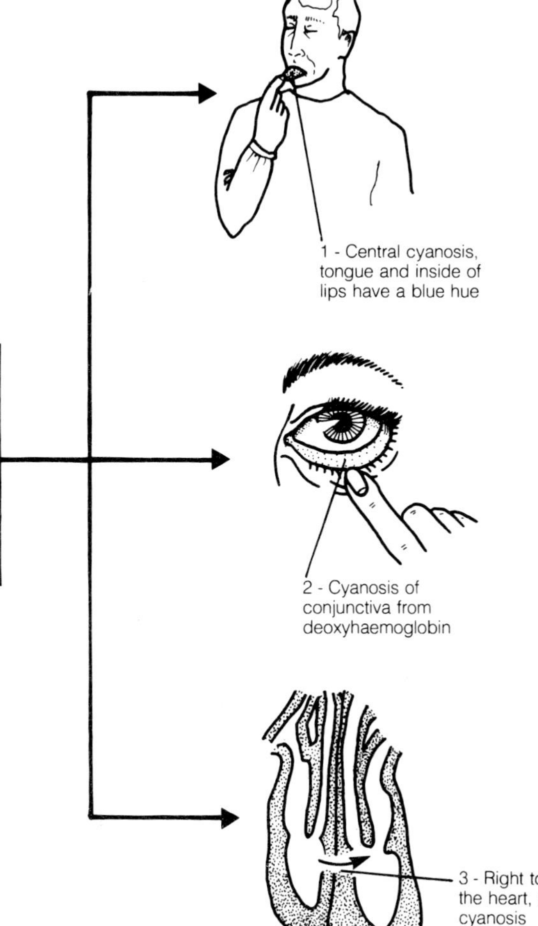

Hand Signs – Finger clubbing is the phenomenon where there is a progressive loss of the angle between the nail and the oedema of the nail bed. (There is rarely pain and swelling of wrists and ankles with gynaecomastia in a dramatic syndrome termed hypertrophic pulmonary osteoarthropathy HPOA). Clubbing is an important feature in chronic suppurative chest disease, squamous bronchial carcinoma, fibrosing alveolitis, cyanotic heart disease and bacterial endocarditis; rarely it can be familial and without significance. Finger clubbing is an unusual accompaniment of cirrhosis and some intestinal inflammations.

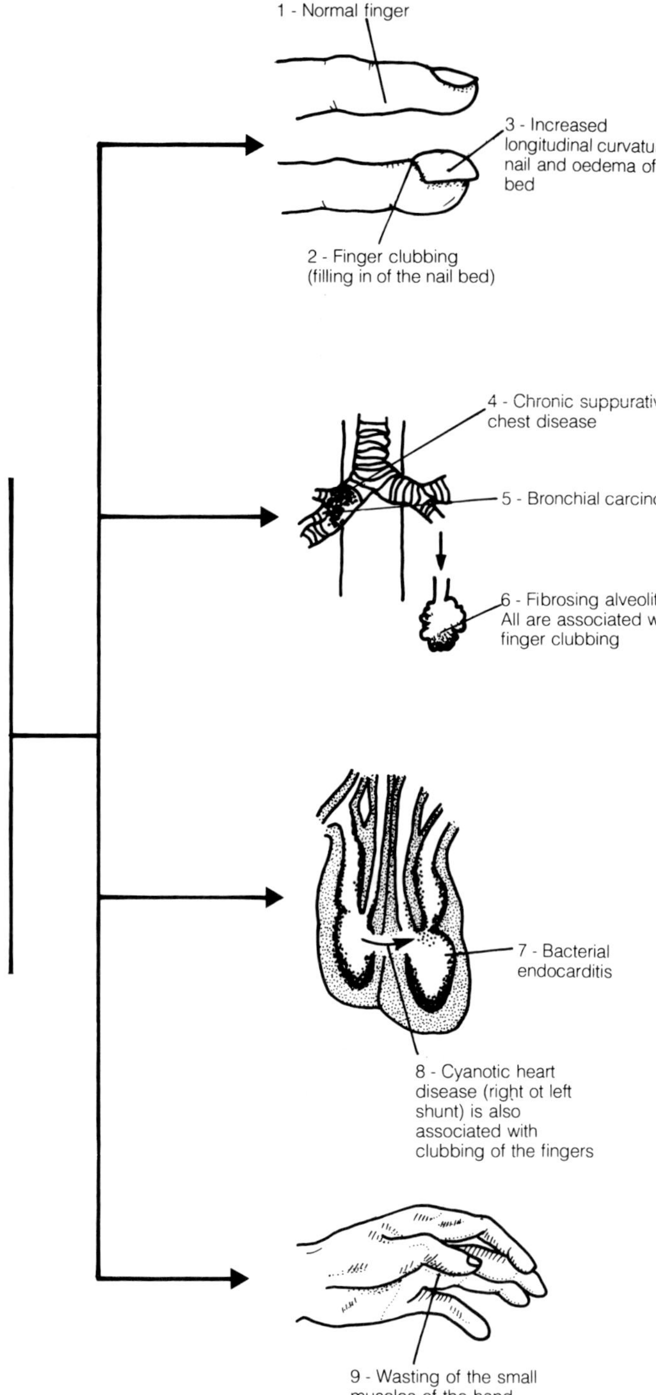

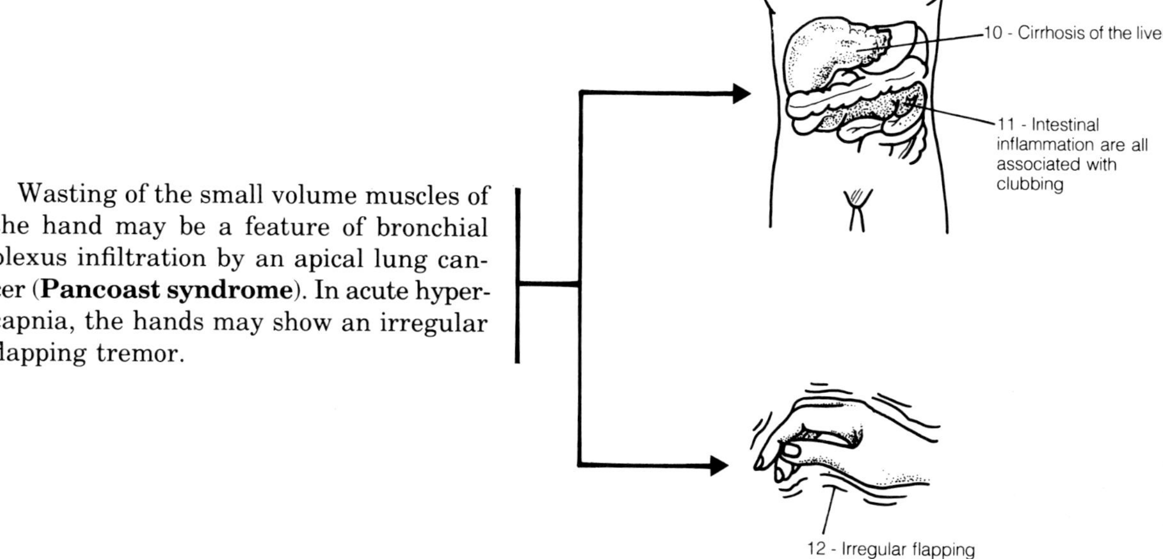

Wasting of the small volume muscles of the hand may be a feature of bronchial plexus infiltration by an apical lung cancer (**Pancoast syndrome**). In acute hypercapnia, the hands may show an irregular flapping tremor.

Chest Inspection The chest of a child is cylindrical. As age advances it broadens, although tending towards cylindrical again in old age, (particularly with emphysema). The strong, active subject has a broad chest with a wide costal

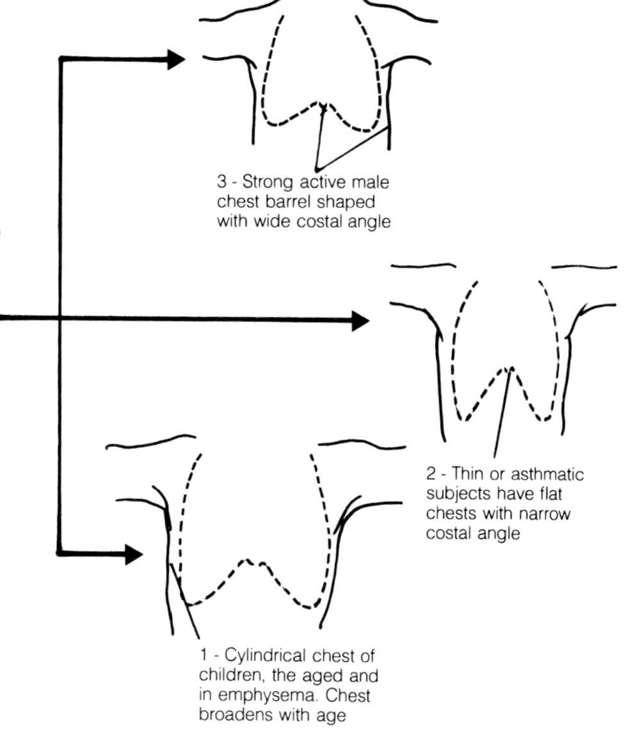

angle. Spinal curvature is of importance, as this may severely impair ventilatory function: **kyphosis** increases the antero-posterior (A–P) diameter of the chest whilst reducing the VC. **Scoliosis** produces chest asymmetry. Severe obstructive respiratory disease in childhood leads to a localised prominence of the sternum (**pectus carinatum**) often with a gutter-like deformity of the 3rd–6th ribs on each side (**Harrison's sulcus**). The "rosary" of the prominent costochondral junctions in rickets is now rare. A simple developmental malformation comprises a deep depression at the lower end of the sternum (**pectus excavatum**).

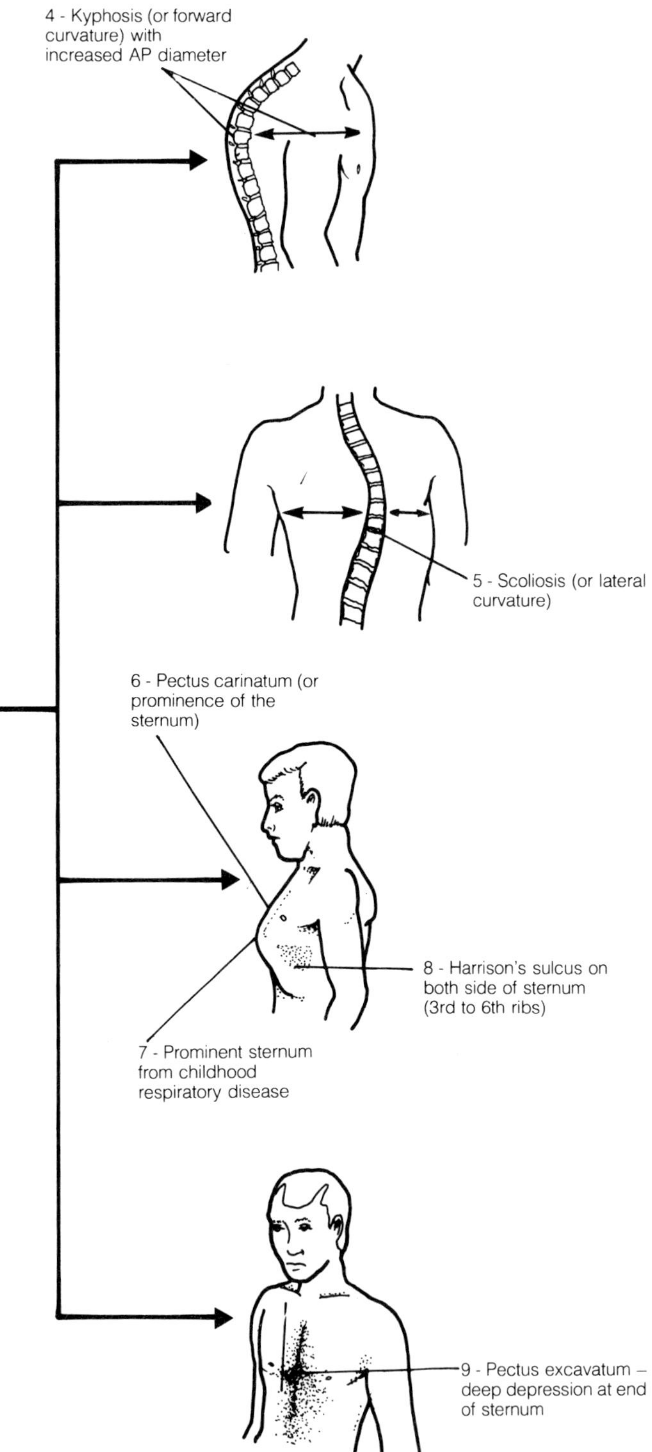

Over-inflation of the lungs (e.g, asthma, emphysema) leads to an increased A–P diameter and a "barrel chest".

Contraction of the accessory muscles of inspiration (e.g. alae nasi, sternomastoid) during respiration is also pathological.

Bilateral indrawing of the intercostal spaces on inspiration also indicates hyperinflation.

Localised flattening of an area of the chest may indicate underlying fibrosis (especially towards the apices).

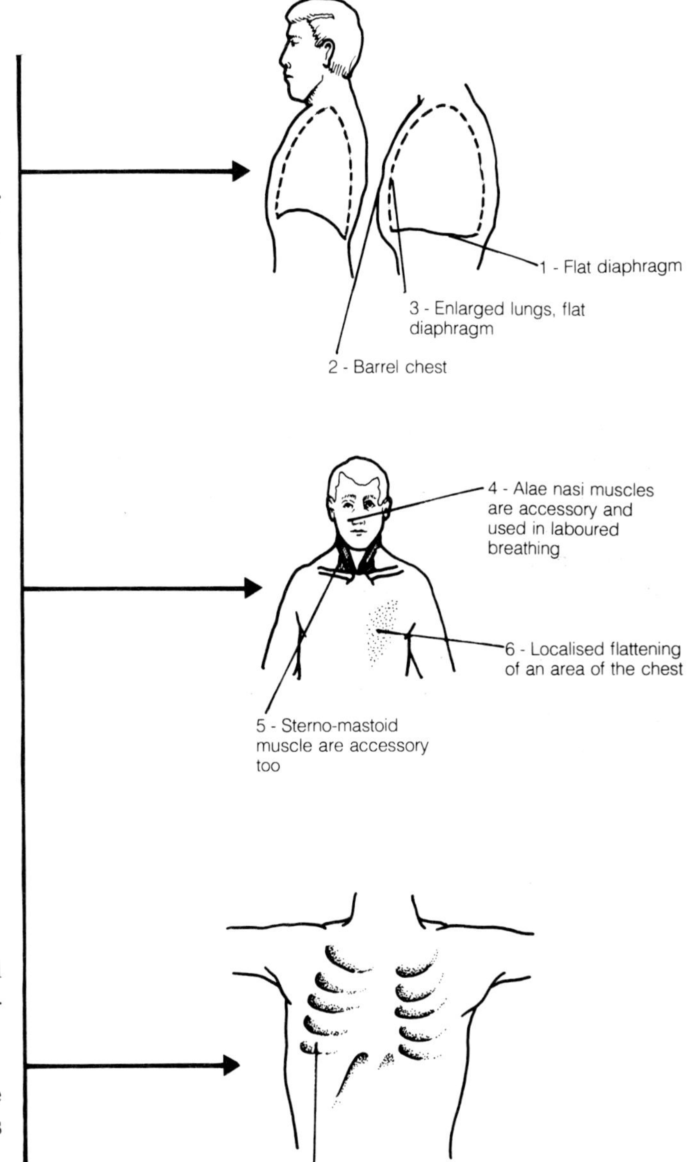

Observation of Respiratory Movements First note the position and comfort of the patient (e.g. the upright, laboured, "pursed-lip" breathing of an emphysema cripple, e.g. the metabolic "air-hunger" of the comatose diabetic, e.g. the terminal waxing and waning, periodic or Cheyne-Stokes breathing of the dying victim of heart failure). Observe the respiratory frequency (normally 18-20/minute), the depth of respirations (e.g. the

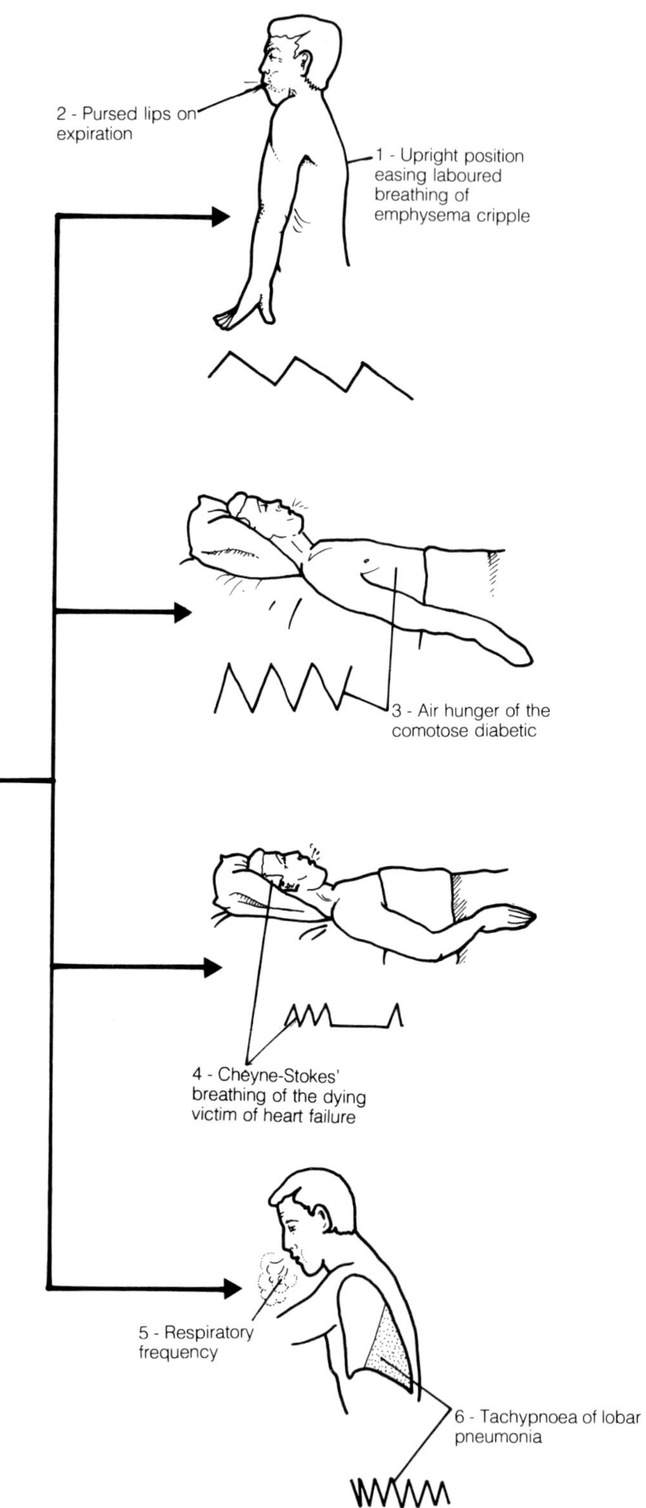

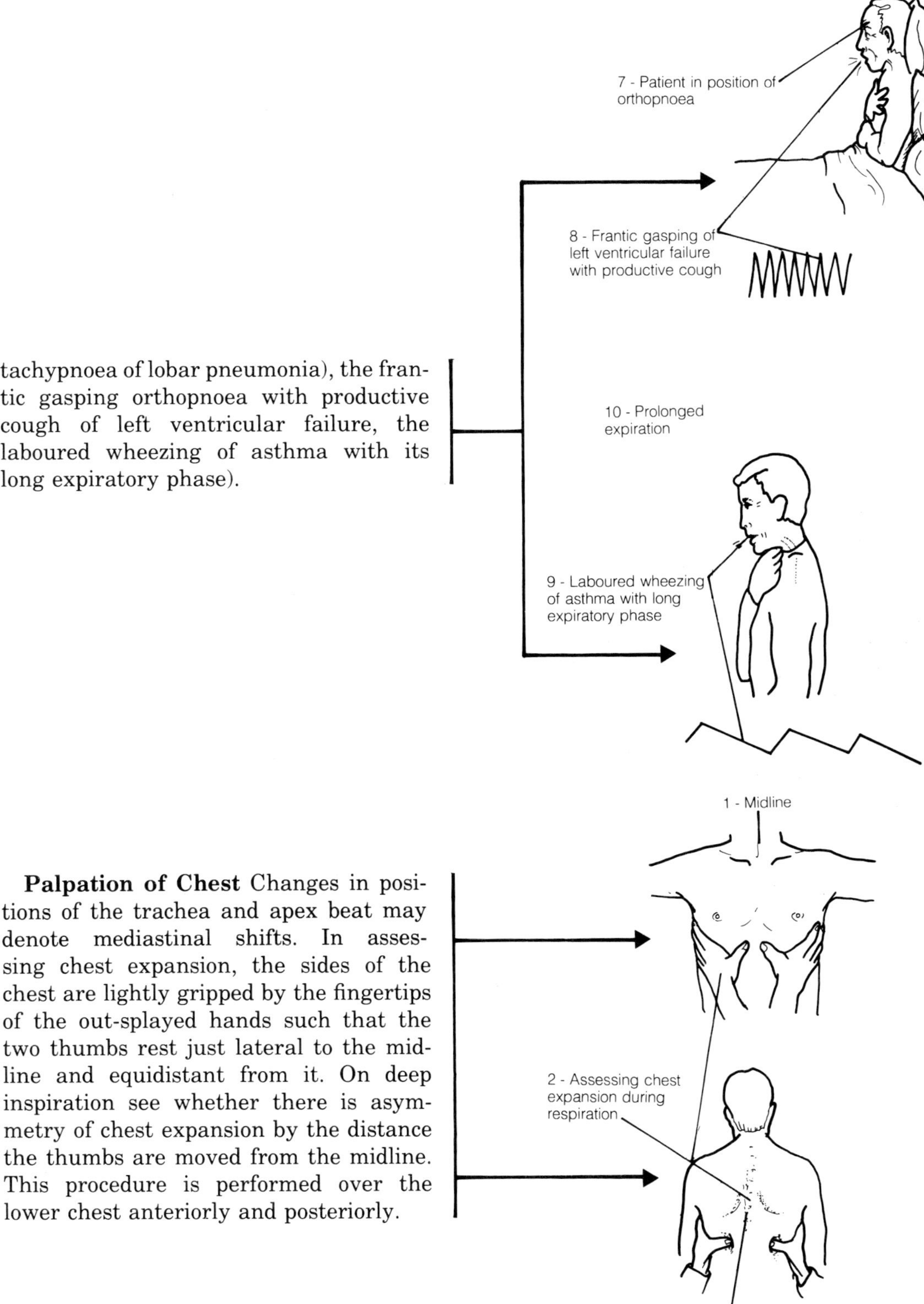

tachypnoea of lobar pneumonia), the frantic gasping orthopnoea with productive cough of left ventricular failure, the laboured wheezing of asthma with its long expiratory phase).

Palpation of Chest Changes in positions of the trachea and apex beat may denote mediastinal shifts. In assessing chest expansion, the sides of the chest are lightly gripped by the fingertips of the out-splayed hands such that the two thumbs rest just lateral to the midline and equidistant from it. On deep inspiration see whether there is asymmetry of chest expansion by the distance the thumbs are moved from the midline. This procedure is performed over the lower chest anteriorly and posteriorly.

Percussion The finger to be struck (left middle finger) must be held flat and firmly against the chest wall and the striking finger (right middle finger) brought lightly but suddenly against it. The percussion note is felt and heard. The note is compared on the two sides. The percussion note loses its normal resonance when normal air-filled lung is separated from the chest wall by pleural thickening or fluid or when the underlying lung itself is consolidated, fibrotic or collapsed. Hyperresonance is found over a pneumothorax. It should be noted that there is a physiological area of dullness to percussion overlying the heart and that liver dullness may start as high as the right fifth intercostal space in the supine subject.

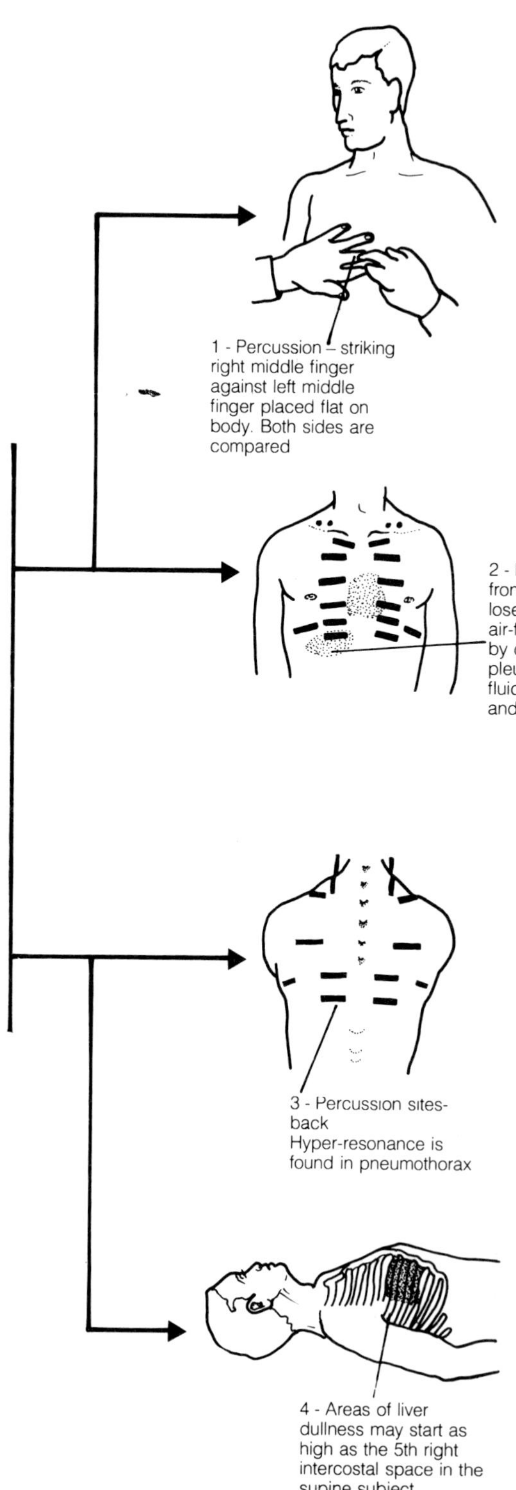

1 - Percussion — striking right middle finger against left middle finger placed flat on body. Both sides are compared

2 - Percussion sites on front. Percussion note loses its resonance over air-filled lungs replaced by consolidation or pleural thickening or fluid or over the heart and liver

3 - Percussion sites- back Hyper-resonance is found in pneumothorax

4 - Areas of liver dullness may start as high as the 5th right intercostal space in the supine subject

Although tactile vocal fremitus (TVF) is really part of palpation, the author recommends that this test only be performed after the clinician has detected dullness over the lung field. The ulnar border of the examiner's hand is placed firmly against the chest wall over the dull area whilst the patient says "99". The resonance or fremitus transmitted is compared to that over normal lung. A dull area with increased fremitus denotes consolidation or fibrosis whilst decreased fremitus denotes pleural thickening or effusion or pulmonary collapse. The mechanism is the same as for bronchial breathing and bronchophony.

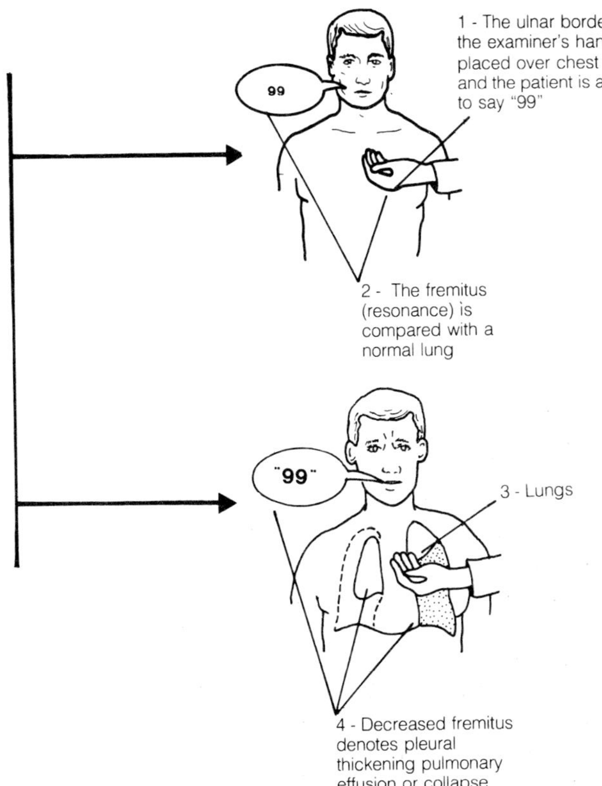

Auscultation The majority of sounds heard from the chest are in the low frequency range and so the stethoscope bell is chosen for chest auscultation and multiple areas on both sides listened to and compared as the patient mouth breathes. The auscultation comprises listening to the breath sounds (and voice sounds) and added sounds.

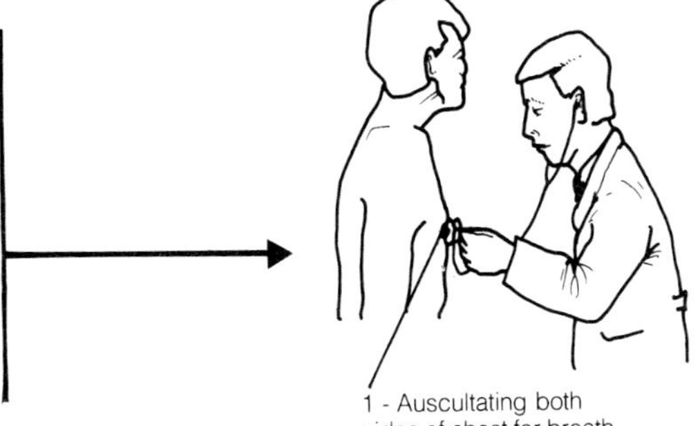

The Breath Sounds (and voice sounds) – The breath sounds are due to air turbulence and eddying in the trachea and larger bronchi. Vesicular breathing is heard over the majority of normal lungs. The inspiratory phase is long and distinct and is followed immediately by a short, rustling and indistinct expiratory phase. Louder, bronchial breathing is normally heard over the trachea and main bronchi: the breath sounds are harsh, there is a pause between inspiration and expiration and the expiratory phase is prolonged.

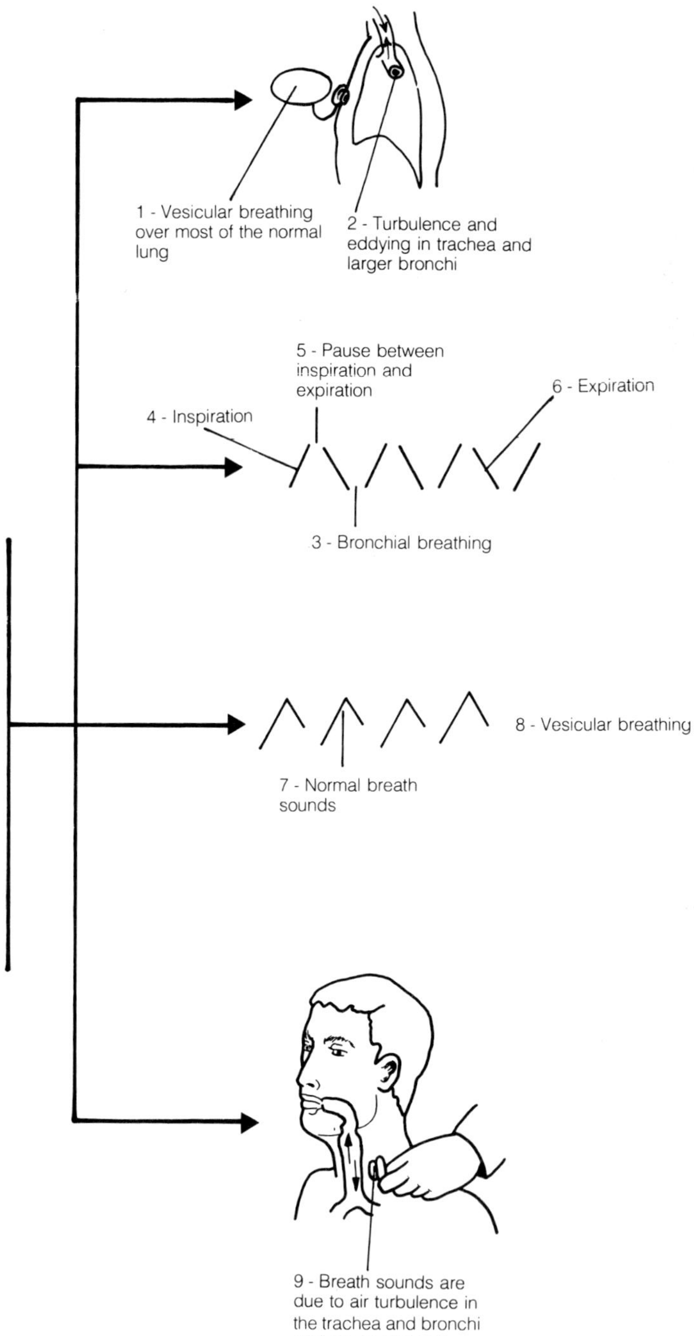

Bronchial breathing occurs pathologically when there is consolidated lung, a displaced bronchus or in compressed airless lung with patent bronchi (e.g. fibrosis). Voice sounds conducted through consolidated lung tissue are louder and more distinct than over normal lung (**bronchophony**); sometimes, the whispered voice is transmitted very clearly (**whispering pectoriloquy**) whereas at other times high pitched voice sounds have a bleating quality (**aegophony**) often over the compressed lung above a pleural effusion.

The breath and voice sounds are diminished over a pleural effusion, thickened pleura, a pneumothorax, emphysematous lung or a collapsed lung or lobe due to an obstructed bronchus.

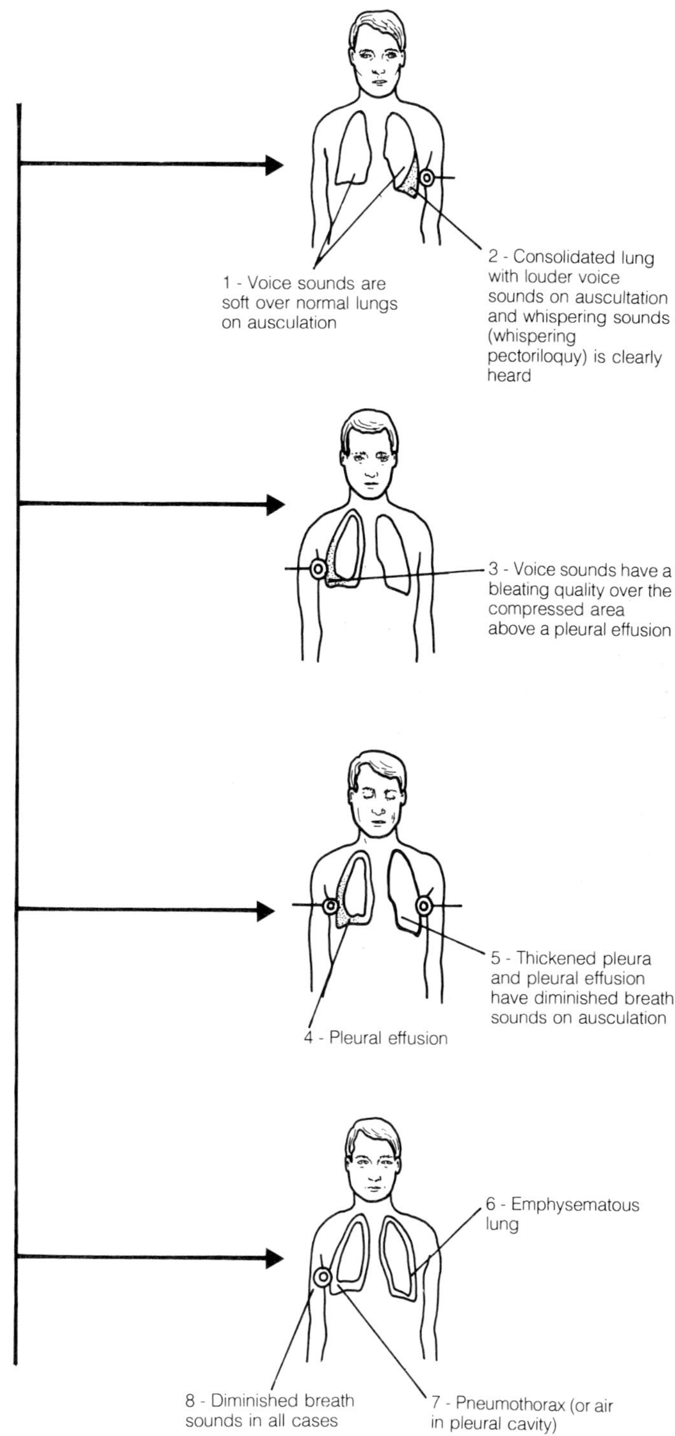

Added sounds – Wheezes or rhonchi are produced by air flowing through bronchi narrowed due to external compression (e.g. from hilar lymphadenopathy), due to spasm of the bronchial musculature (e.g. asthma) or intraluminal contents (bronchial secretions or neoplasm). Rhonchi are best heard in expiration; coughing may shift or eliminate the rhonchi due to pooled endobronchial secretions.

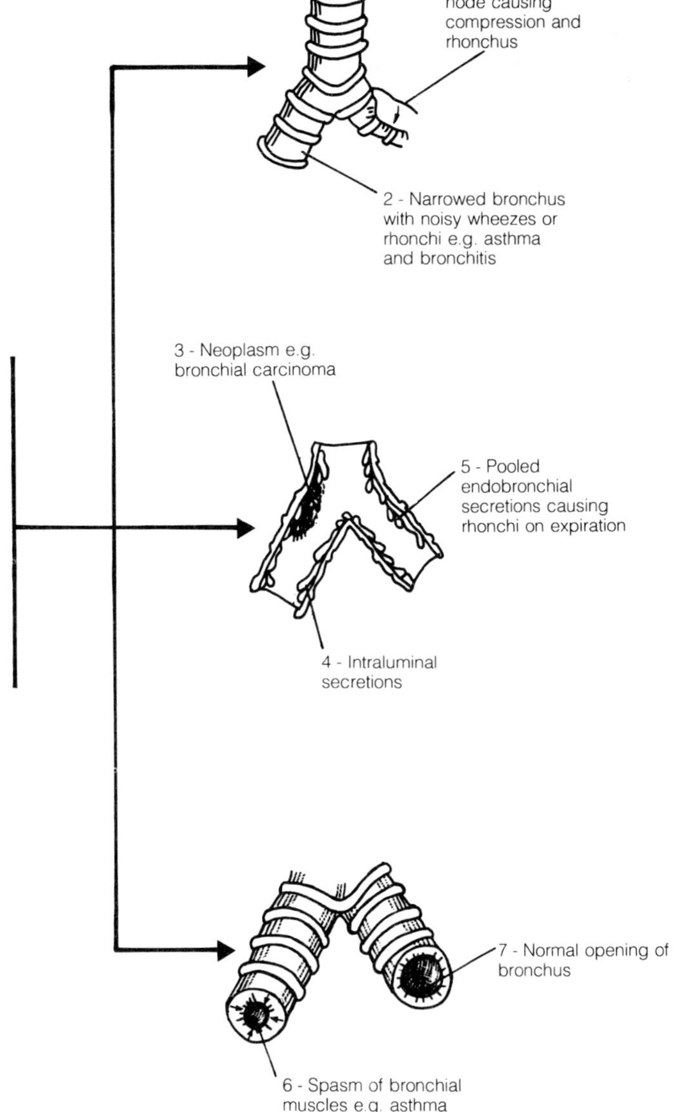

Crepitations are crackling sounds probably caused by the explosive reinflation of collapsed alveoli; they occur where there is parenchymal lung fluid as in acute left ventricular failure (LVF) or bronchopneumonia. Crepitations are an early and remarkable sign in fibrosing alveolitis and said to be due to delayed opening of distal airways. The crepitations of acute LVF and fibrosing alveolits are typically end-inspiratory and tend to be basal in situation.

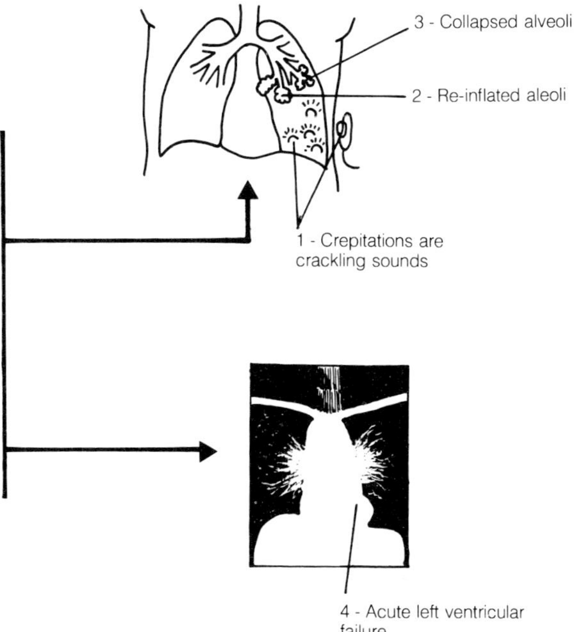

Inflamed or roughened pleura gives rise to a coarse "creaking" or "to-and-fro" rubbing sound during inspiration and expiration. This is the **pleural rub** and is often very well localised and seems to originate from very close to the stethoscope.

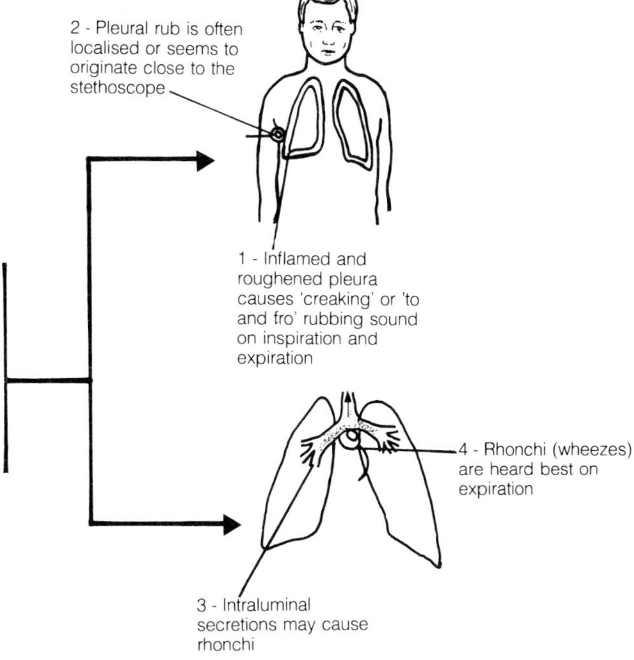

Diseases of the Upper Respiratory Tract

ACUTE CORYZA (THE COMMON "COLD")

This is a viral infection of the mucous membrane of the nasal passages and caused most commonly by rhinoviruses, spread from other sufferers by droplet infection. The disease is particularly common in the cold, damp weather.

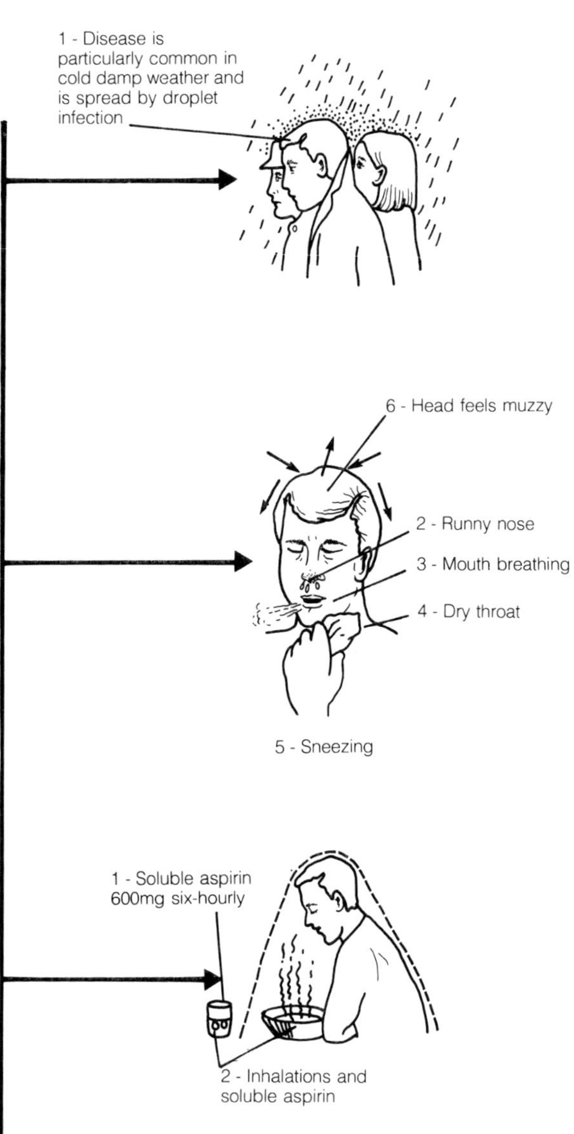

Reactive and excessive watery nasal discharge occurs for several days accompanied by sneezing, whilst the throat feels dry (exacerbated by mouth breathing) and the head feels "muzzy". Any fever is slight and transient.

The disease is mild and usually self limiting. A warm environment with soluble aspirin (600 mg) six-hourly for the minor discomforts and inhalations for nasal congestion may all help the symptoms, but there is no specific therapy.

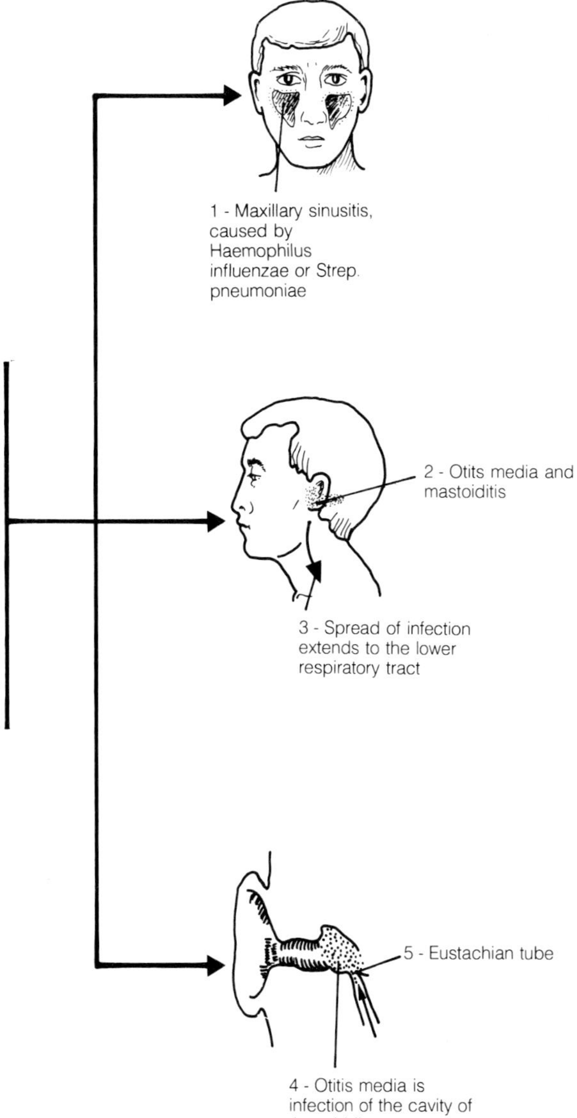

1 - Maxillary sinusitis, caused by Haemophilus influenzae or Strep. pneumoniae

2 - Otits media and mastoiditis

3 - Spread of infection extends to the lower respiratory tract

5 - Eustachian tube

4 - Otitis media is infection of the cavity of the middle ear

Complications include spread of the virus infection or secondary bacterial infection (particularly with Haemophilus influenzae or Streptococcus pneumoniae) to cause sinusitis (particularly maxillary sinusitis), "eustachian catarrh" with complicating **otitis media** or spread of infection to the lower respiratory tract. In all these secondary conditions, the systemic symptoms are worse, the fever more marked and there are localising signs according to the site of infection,

HAY FEVER (SEASONAL ALLERGIC RHINITIS)

This condition occurs in sensitive individuals at the local pollination season – the commonest pollens involved are those from trees and grasses. Skin allergen testing will usually confirm an individual's specific hypersensitivity to a particular pollen. The symptoms, due to sensitisation of the nasal mucosa to the inhaled allergen, are blocked and then runny nose (watery discharge) with sneezing, and red, itchy and watery eyes.

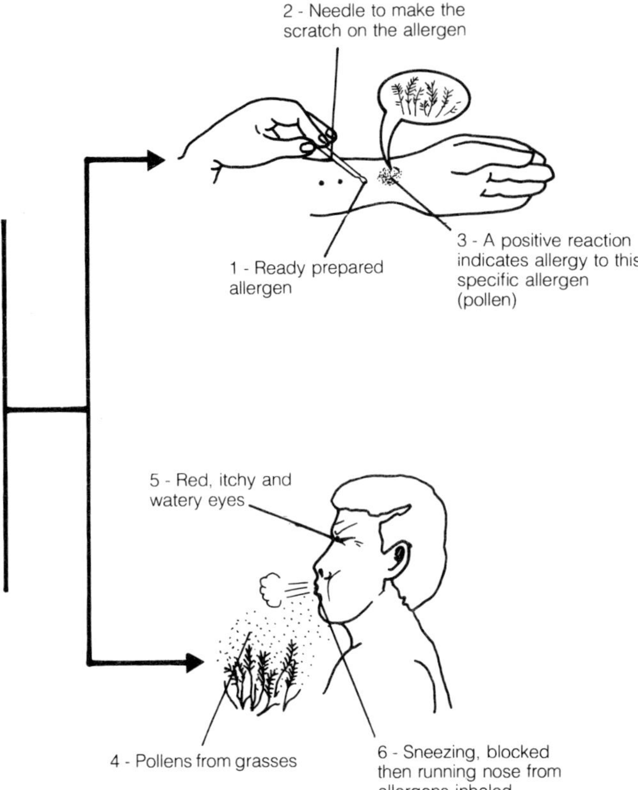

Treatment may be prophylactic in the form of a course of hyposensitising injections. This is most successful for those allergic to grass pollens and comprises 9-10 subcutaneous injections of a standard pollen vaccine, performed a couple of months before the pollination season.

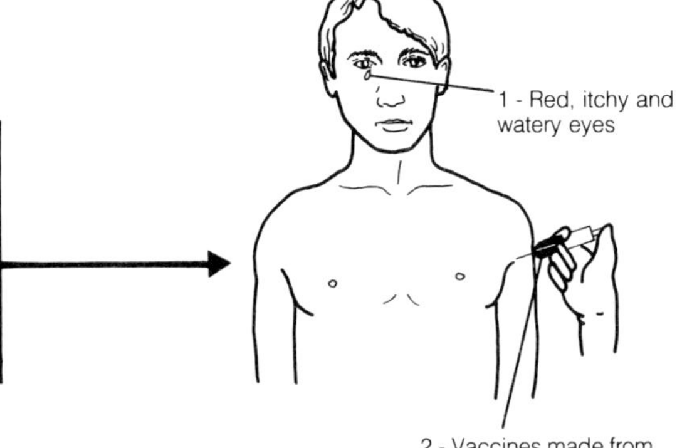

Disodium chromoglycate inhibits the release of mediators from mast cells but is only effective if taken before exposure to the allergen; it is best administered as a nasal spray. Antihistamines (e.g. promethazine 25 mg b.d., or chlorpheniramine 4 mg b.d.) are of great value in the attack, but they produce, (like most antihistamines), drowsiness that is exacerbated by alcohol. A steroid nasal spray (e.g. beclomethasone diproprionate 50 μg metered nasal dose delivered by inhalation up each nostril q.d.s.) is also very useful but not immediately acting. Systemic steroids are effective but rarely indicated. Tachyphylaxis tends to render the usefulness of ephedrine based nasal decongestants to short-lasting relief, but this can be welcome.

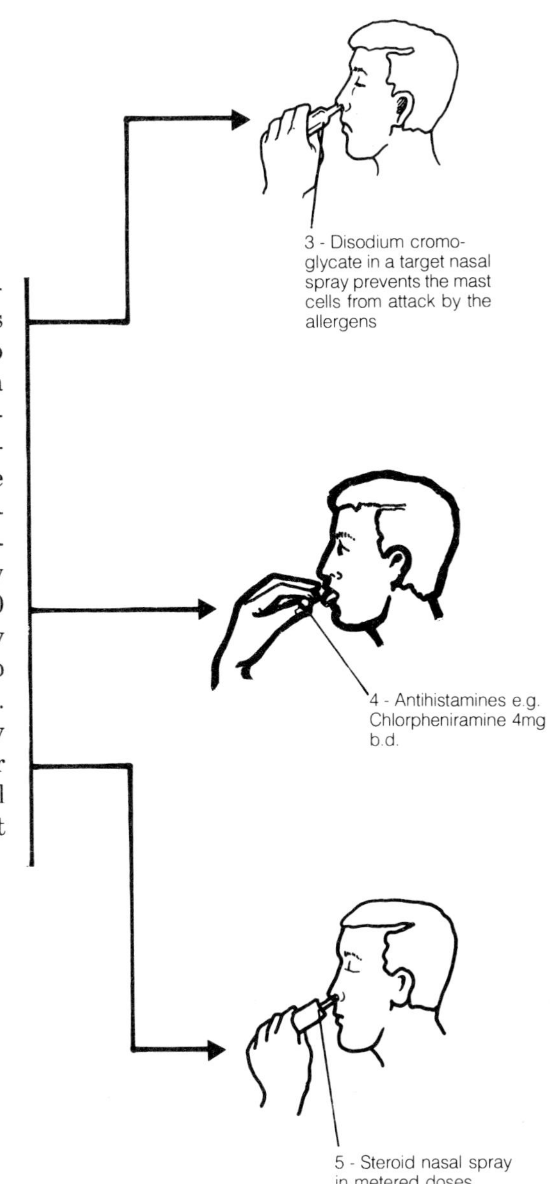

3 - Disodium cromoglycate in a target nasal spray prevents the mast cells from attack by the allergens

4 - Antihistamines e.g. Chlorpheniramine 4mg b.d.

5 - Steroid nasal spray in metered doses

LARYNGITIS

Acute laryngitis: Often the complication of a viral "cold" but influenza and parainfluenza viruses are common pathogens as well as rhino-, entero- and adenoviruses. The symptoms are hoarse voice, laryngeal discomfort of varying intensity but usually accompanied by frequent coughing bouts. This cough is usually dry and "hacking". Mild fever and malaise is common. Indirect laryngoscopy reveals an erythematous larynx.

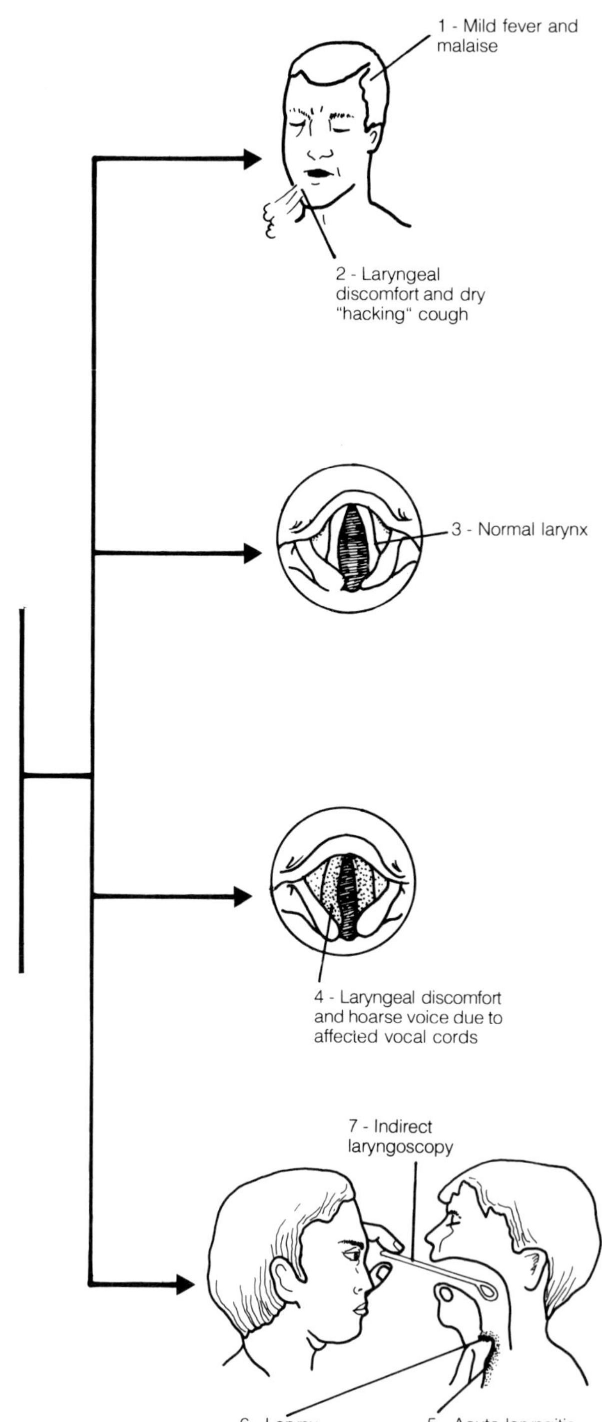

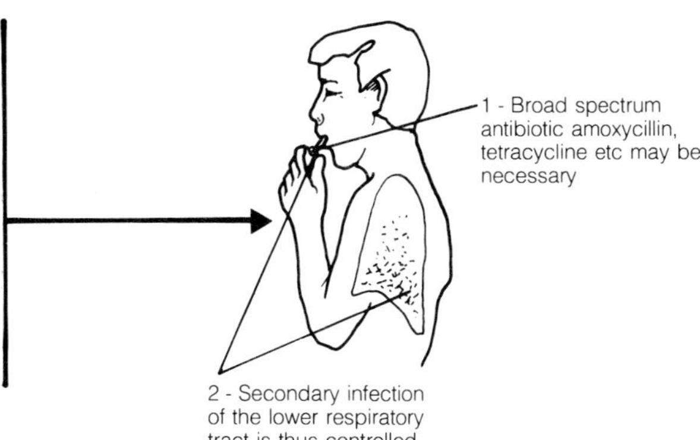

The disease is self-limiting and curtailed if the patient is nursed in warm, well ventilated surroundings and supplied with a cough suppressant such as codeine linctus. He must rest his voice. Steam inhalations may be soothing.

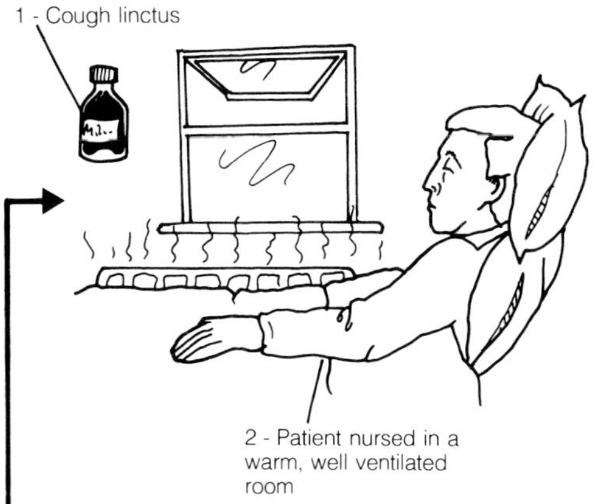

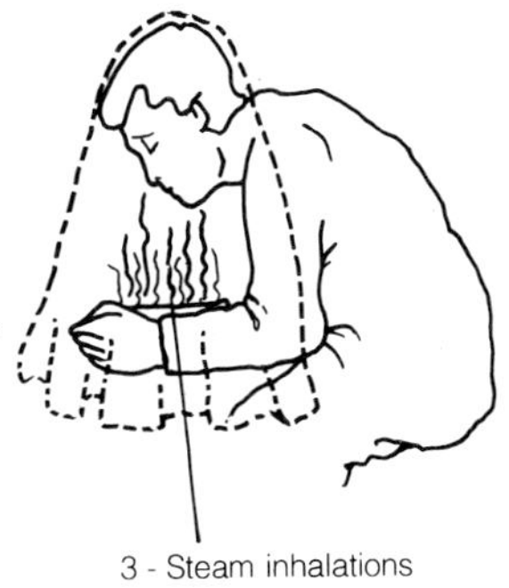

As with other viral upper respiratory infections, should the condition persist for longer than a few days or should the systemic symptoms worsen or the patient expectorate purulent sputum, then a broad spectrum antibiotic (e.g. amoxycillin or co-trimoxazole or tetracycline) is indicated as secondary infection or complicating lower respiratory tract infection may have occurred.

Chronic laryngitis and we must not forget tuberculous laryngitis, is an altogether more indolent process. The student must remember that hoarse voice is always an important complaint: it may signify cord paralysis, laryngitis or laryngeal cancer. It should never be ignored and requires indirect laryngoscopy to investigate it.

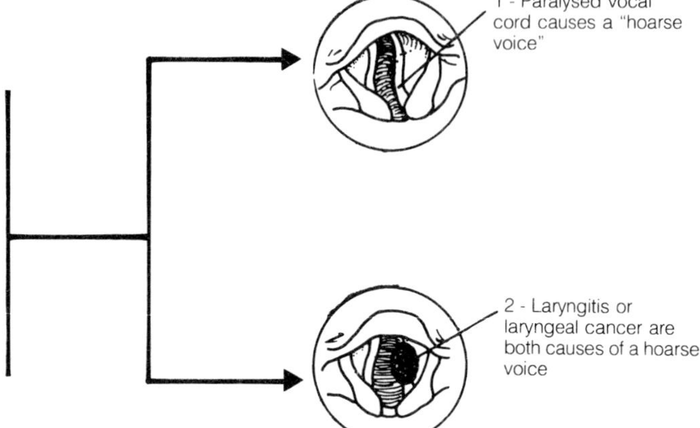

INFLUENZA

This short but sometimes severe viral illness is usually caused by influenza viruses A or B, (RNA myxo-viruses). The illness is spread by droplet infection and the viruses infect the respiratory epithelial cells, initially of the upper respiratory

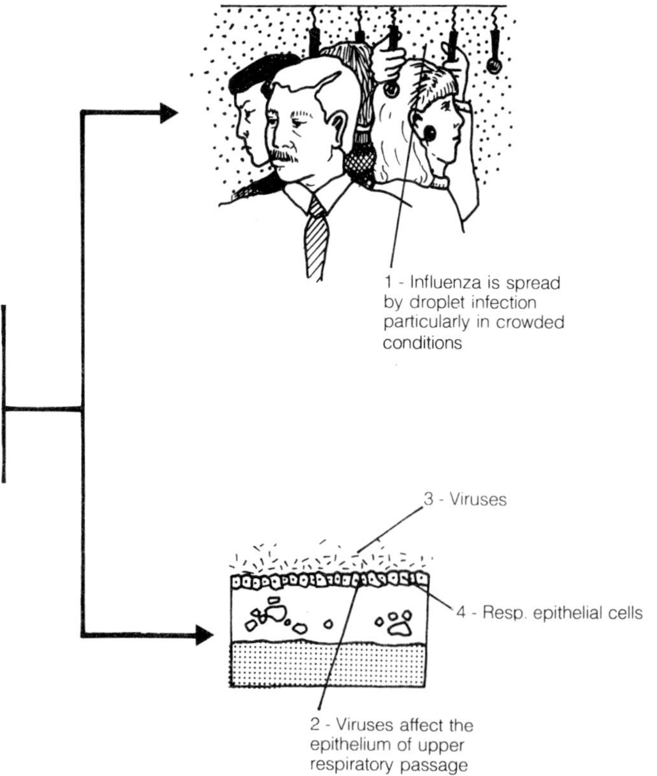

passages. After approximately 2 days' incubation, fever with shivering, malaise, diffuse aches and pains and often headache are followed by nasal congestion, a sore throat and a dry persistent cough. The disease is self-limiting within approximately 3 days but the languor and cough may persist for longer.

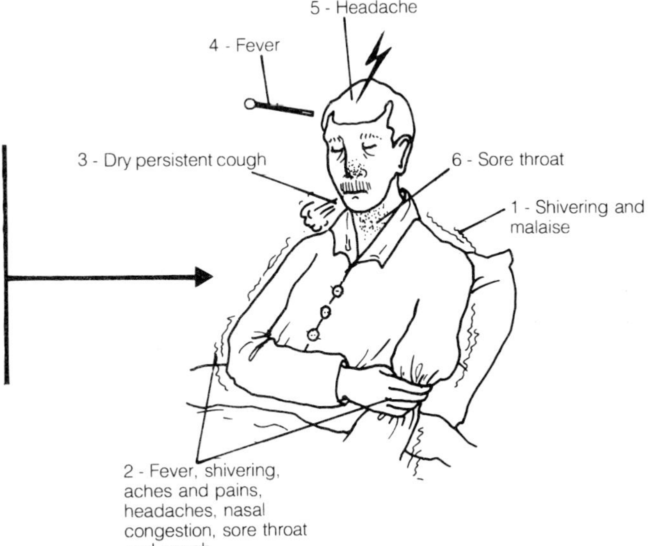

Prophylactic treatment with influenza vaccine gives enhanced immunity against influenza infection and is to be recommended in the autumn season for immunosuppressed patients and chronic respiratory cripples. Treatment of the

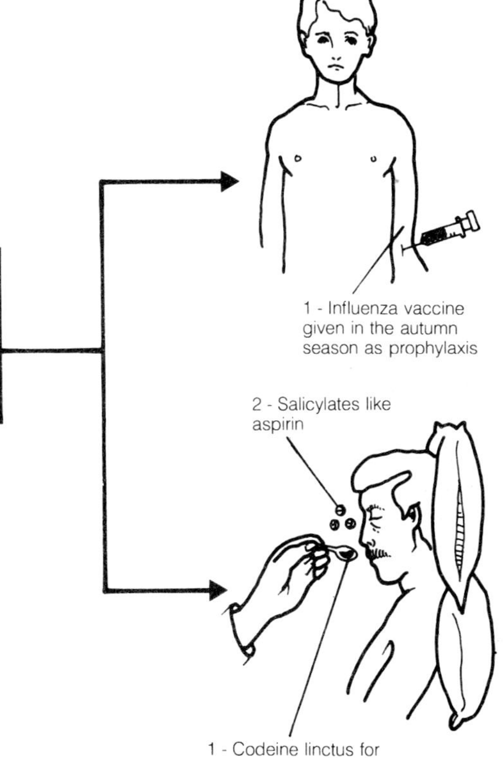

established case is symptomatic with salicylates for discomfort, codeine linctus for cough and a warm, well ventilated and not too dry environment for rest; steam inhalers as required for catarrhal or laryngeal symptoms or for the not uncommon tracheobronchitis of influenza.

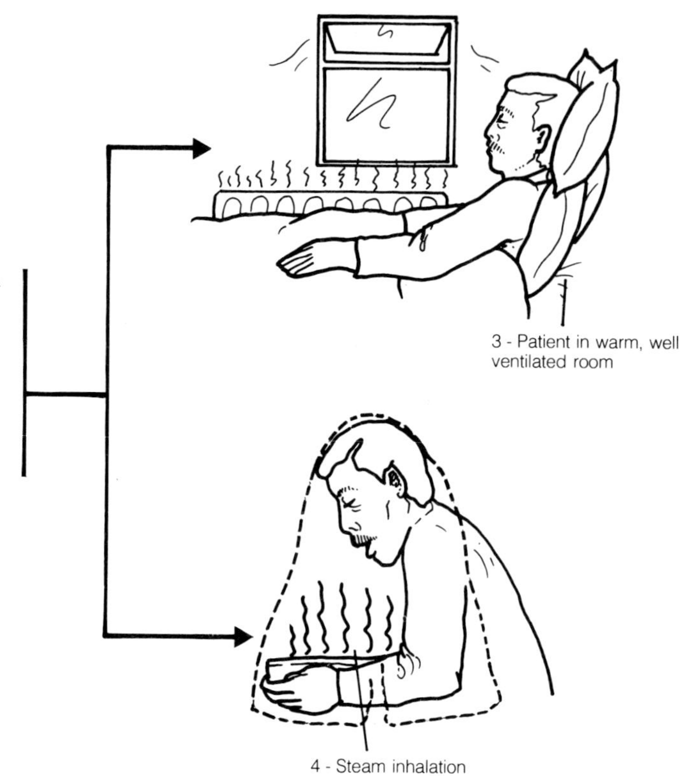

Spread of the influenza infection to the lower respiratory tract may be more serious particularly when it predisposes to secondary bacterial infection; the production of purulent sputum is an indication for prompt introduction of broad spectrum antibiotics.

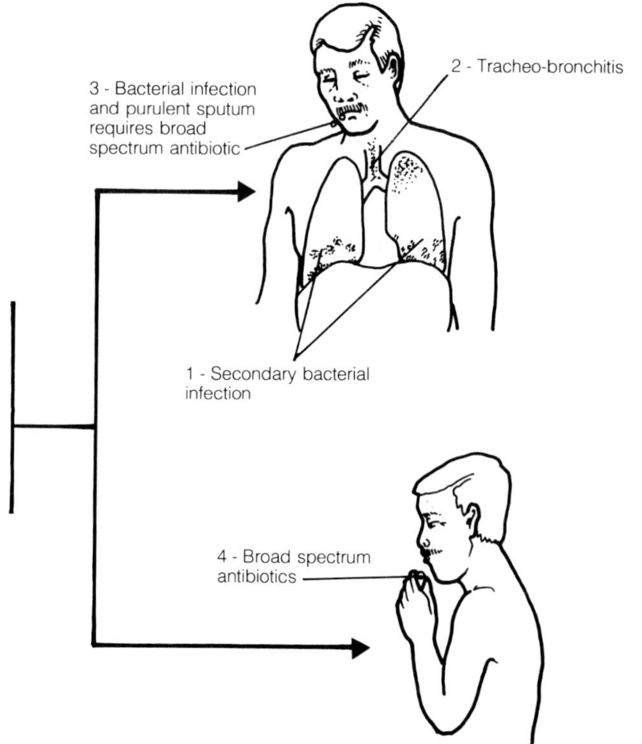

Pneumonia with respiratory death and heart failure are both recognised complications of influenza in the debilitated. A viral encephalomyelitis is an unusual, potentially serious but usually self-limiting complication of influenza.

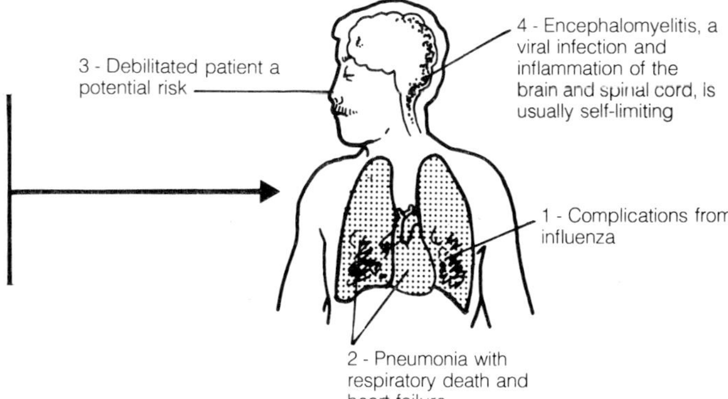

Diseases of the Lower Respiratory Tract

INFECTIONS

THE BACTERIAL PNEUMONIAS

Pneumonia is a general term for inflammation of the lung parenchyma and although many opportunistic infectious agents (and indeed some chemical and physical agents) may be the cause, nevertheless the most common forms of pneumonia are caused by a finite list of

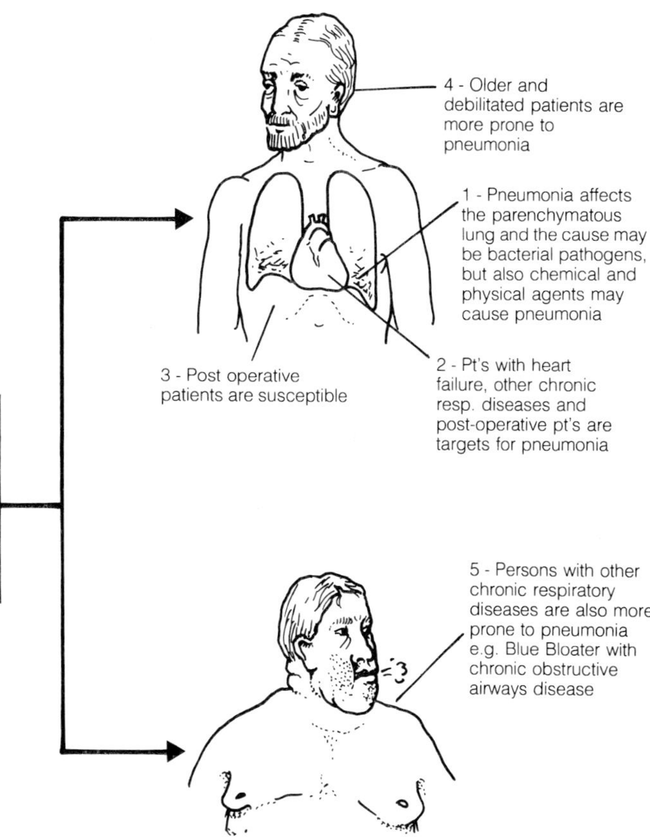

infective pathogens. Although no one is exempt, certain adults are more prone to pneumonia:– the ageing, those with chronic respiratory disease or heart failure and the post-operative or debilitated patients who are prone to aspiration. Pneumonia is more common in the winter and in areas of polluted urban air.

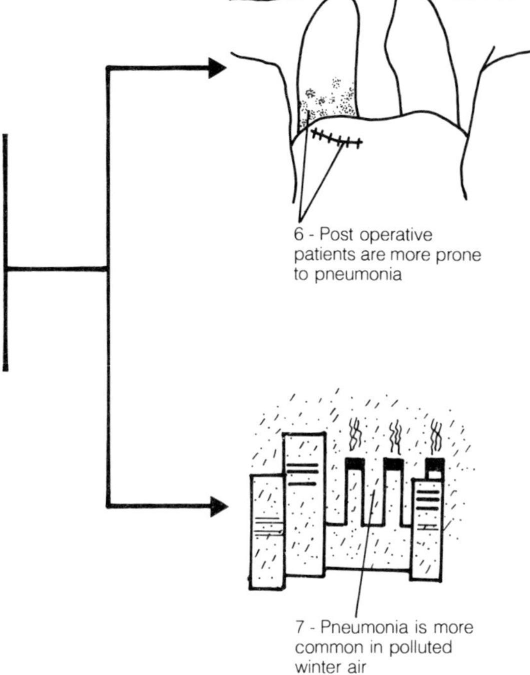

6 - Post operative patients are more prone to pneumonia

7 - Pneumonia is more common in polluted winter air

Pneumonia primarily impairs gas exchange, so the arterial PO_2 tends to fall whilst increased ventilation tends to keep the PCO_2 steady, (except those respiratory failure patients already hypercapnic).

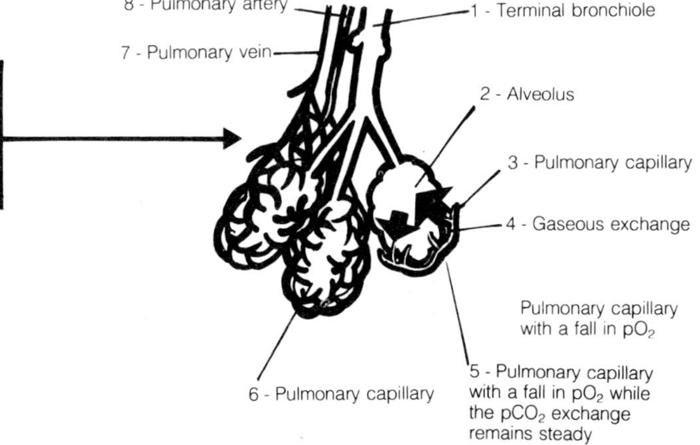

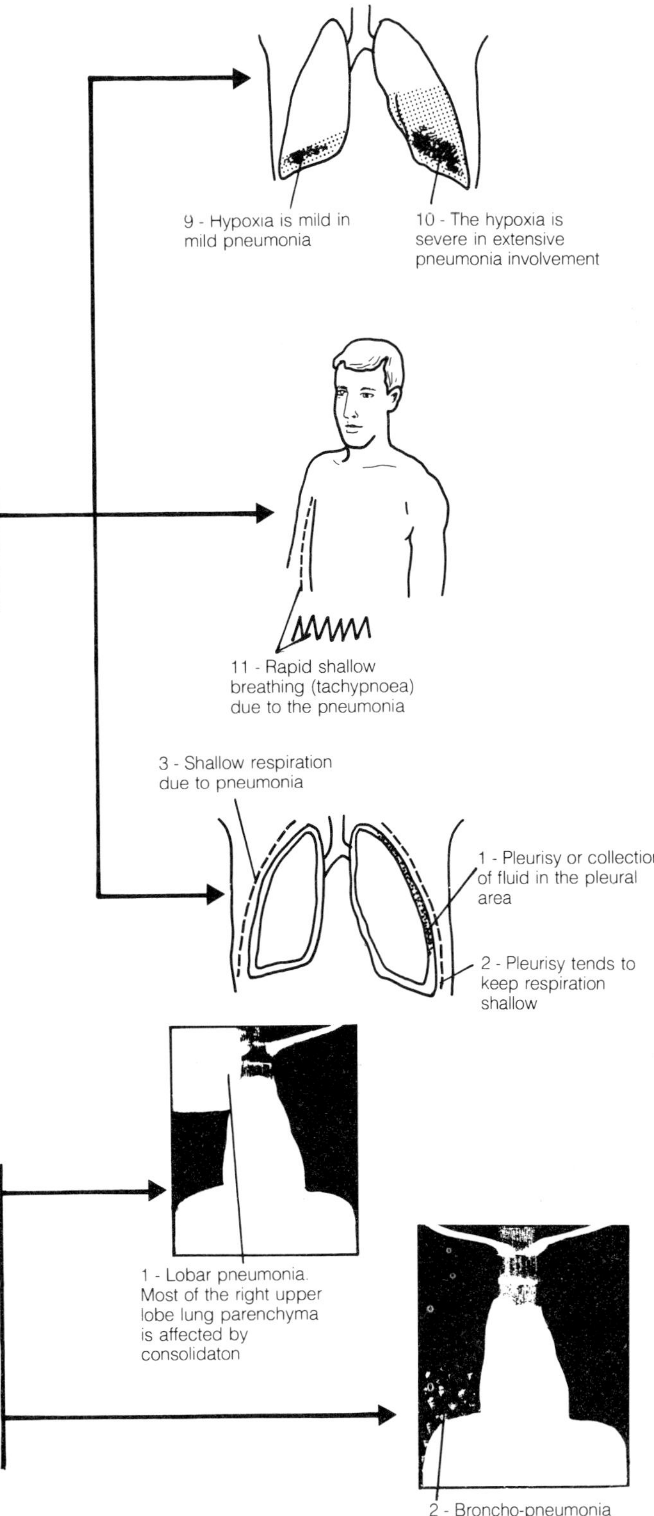

The severity of the hypoxia depends upon the extent of the pneumonia. The energy expended in ventilating the less compliant lung is kept to a minimum by rapid breathing (tachypnoea) and a small tidal volume. If pleurisy is present, this also tends to keep the respiration shallow.

Radiologically, it is useful to distinguish lobar pneumonia from bronchopneumonia. In lobar pneumonia, most or all of the parenchyma of one lobe is affected by consolidation, although the patent bronchi leading to the lobe are visible on X-ray as an air-bronchogram. Bronchopneumonia tends to be basal and often bilateral and produces patchy areas of consolidation on X-ray.

(We might here note that one clinical consequence of this patchiness is that the physical signs of consolidation are less clear but crepitations common).

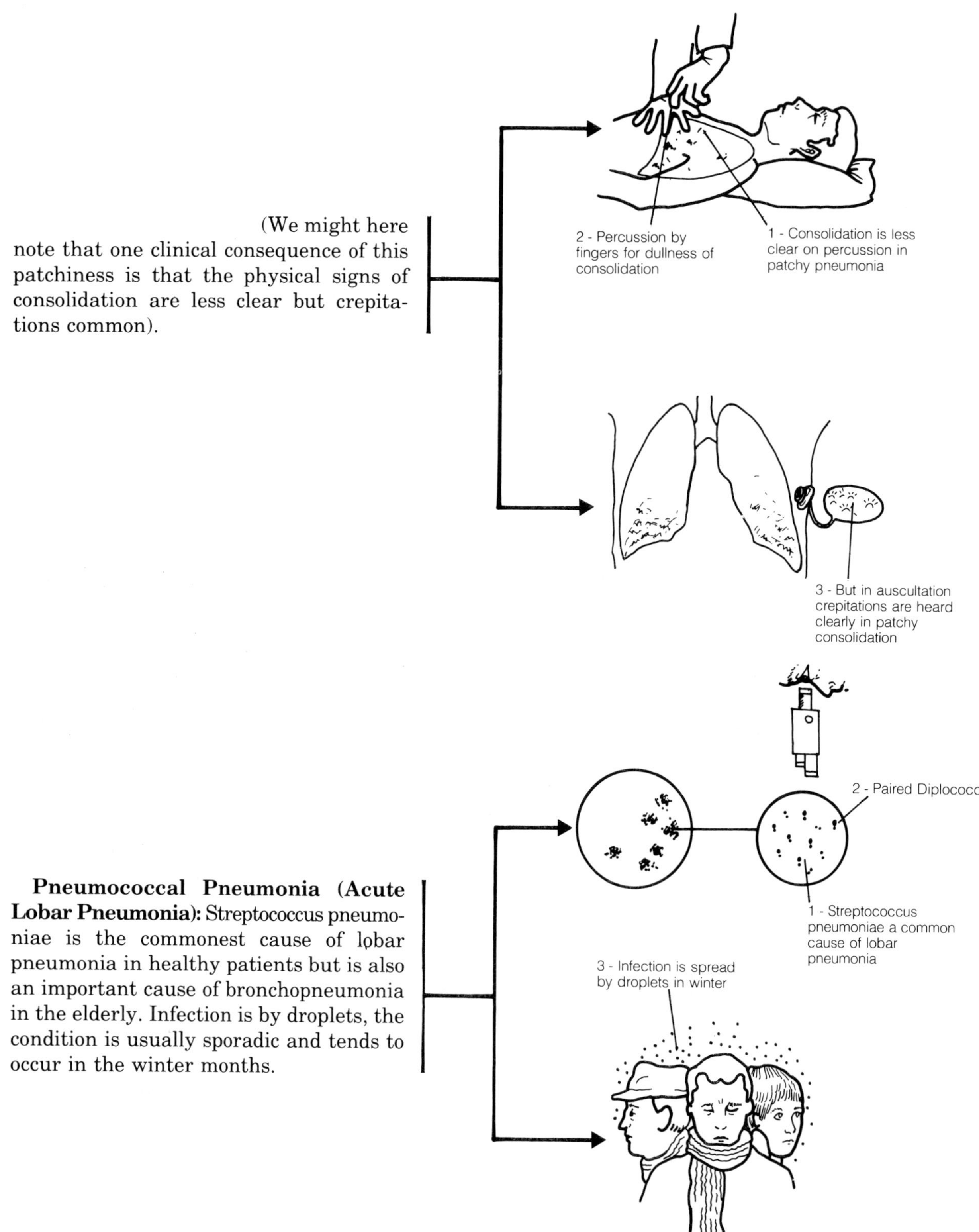

Pneumococcal Pneumonia (Acute Lobar Pneumonia): Streptococcus pneumoniae is the commonest cause of lobar pneumonia in healthy patients but is also an important cause of bronchopneumonia in the elderly. Infection is by droplets, the condition is usually sporadic and tends to occur in the winter months.

The affected lobe (segments) undergoes consolidation due to a profuse exudation of fibrin, erythrocytes and some polymorphs (red hepatization). The polymorphs then predominate in the consolidated area and macrophages become more numerous and the process slowly resolves (grey hepatization – so-called because the lung has a colour and texture resembling liver at this time). A very severe inflammatory reaction may lead to necrosis within the lung parenchyma and abscess formation.

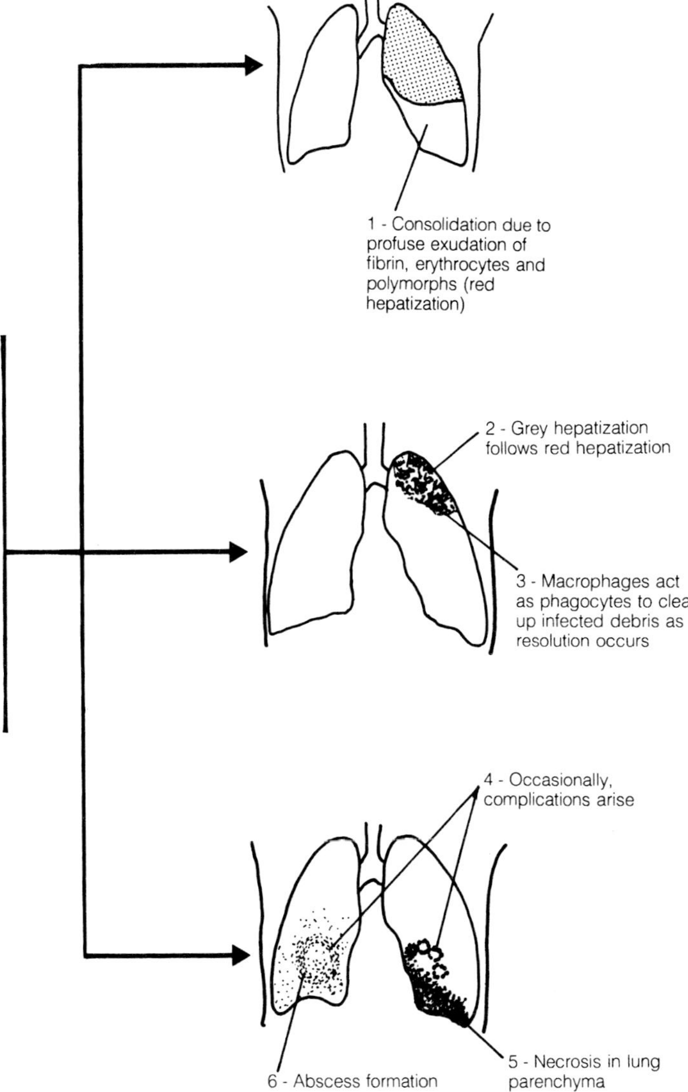

The clinical onset is sudden with shivering or rigor as a fever develops abruptly. The patient becomes tachypnoeic with languor, generalised aches and often pleuritic chest pain over the affected lobe. Interestingly, reactivation of herpes labialis is a common accompaniment. A painful dry cough may soon become productive of blood containing sputum. Respiration is rapid, shallow and painful with, on examination, diminished chest movements and the signs of consolidation develop over the affected region: a pleural rub and crepitations may precede the development of classic consolidation signs.

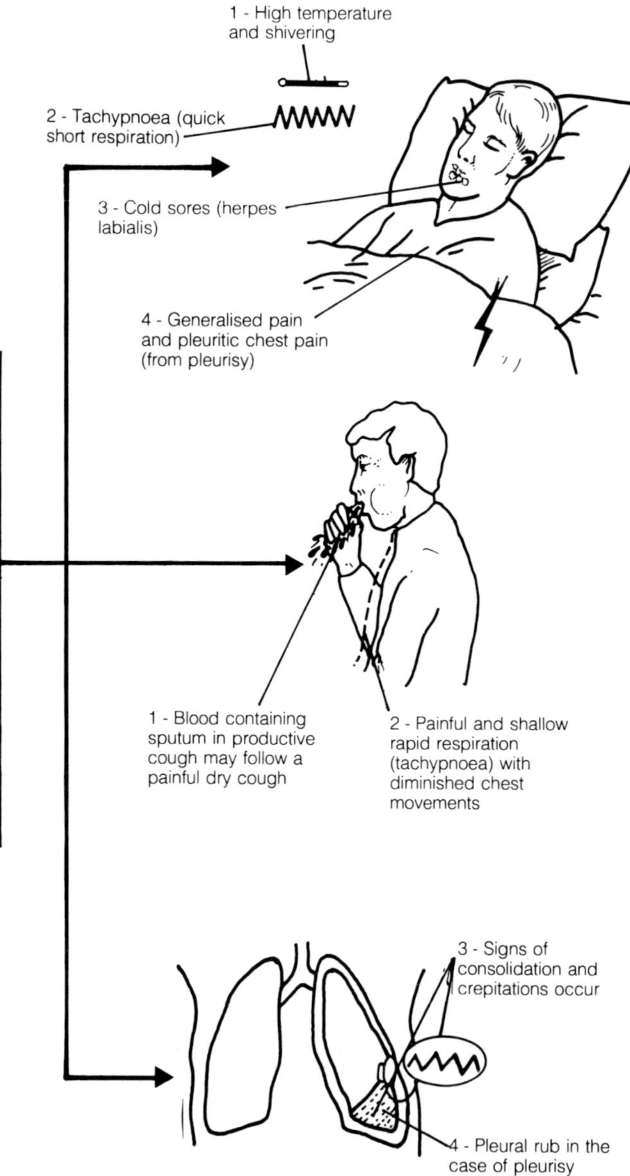

The peripheral blood film shows a polymorphonuclear leucocytosis and the pneumococcus may be grown from a blood culture, although sputum culture (or Gram staining showing the characteristic diplococci) is the usual method of diagnosis.

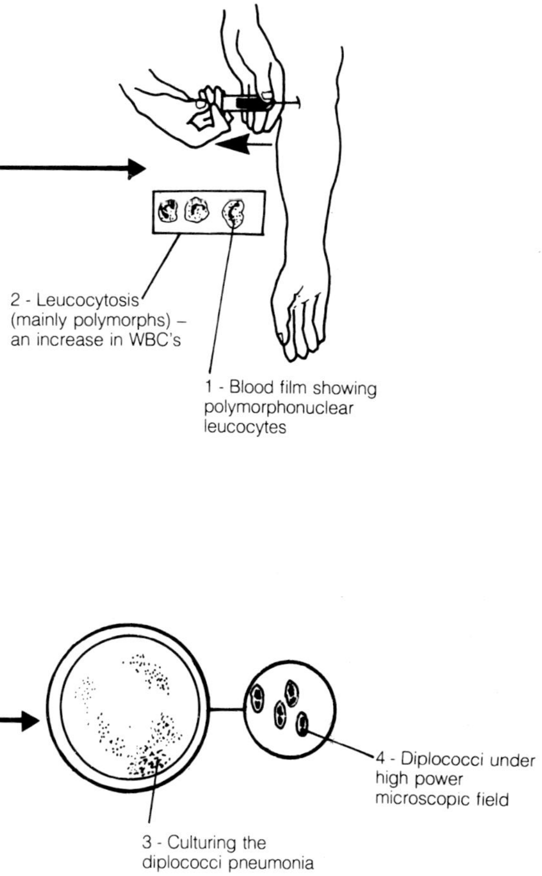

Treatment is with benzyl penicillin 600 mg i.m. b.d. (or q.d.s. intravenously in the severely ill). Amoxycillin 250 mg p.o. q.d.s. is equally effective from the outset

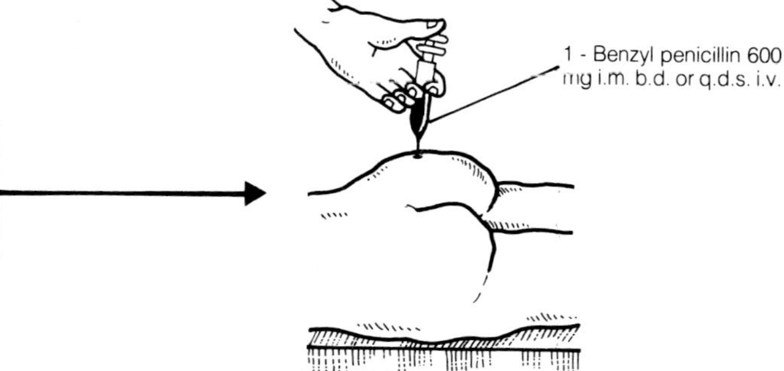

but it is usual to commence with parenteral therapy and change to oral therapy in responding patients, maintaining them on treatment for 7-10 days. Erythromycin substitutes in penicillin-sensitive patients. The disease usually responds well to treatment but radiological resolution may take 2 weeks.

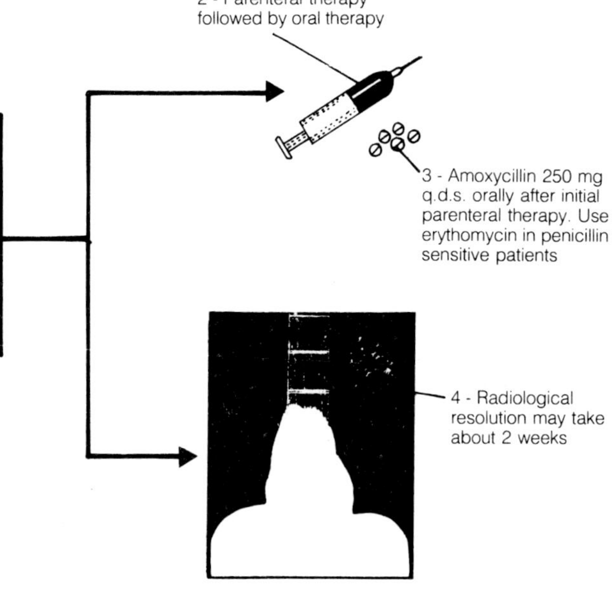

Delayed resolution of the pneumonia is not uncommon in the debilitated but raises the possiblity of some other predisposing lung condition (e.g. bronchial carcinoma), which may require further investigation (e.g. bronchoscopy) to diagnose.

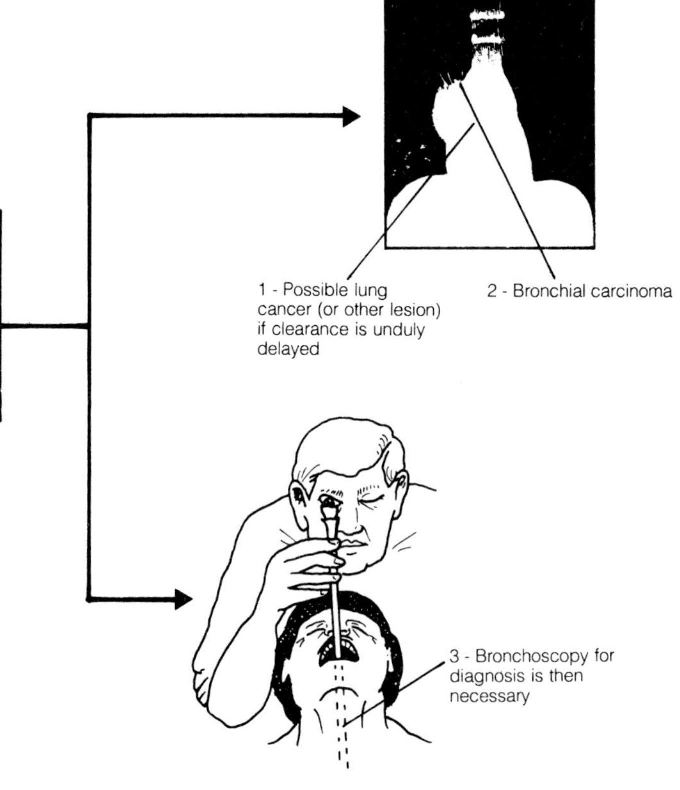

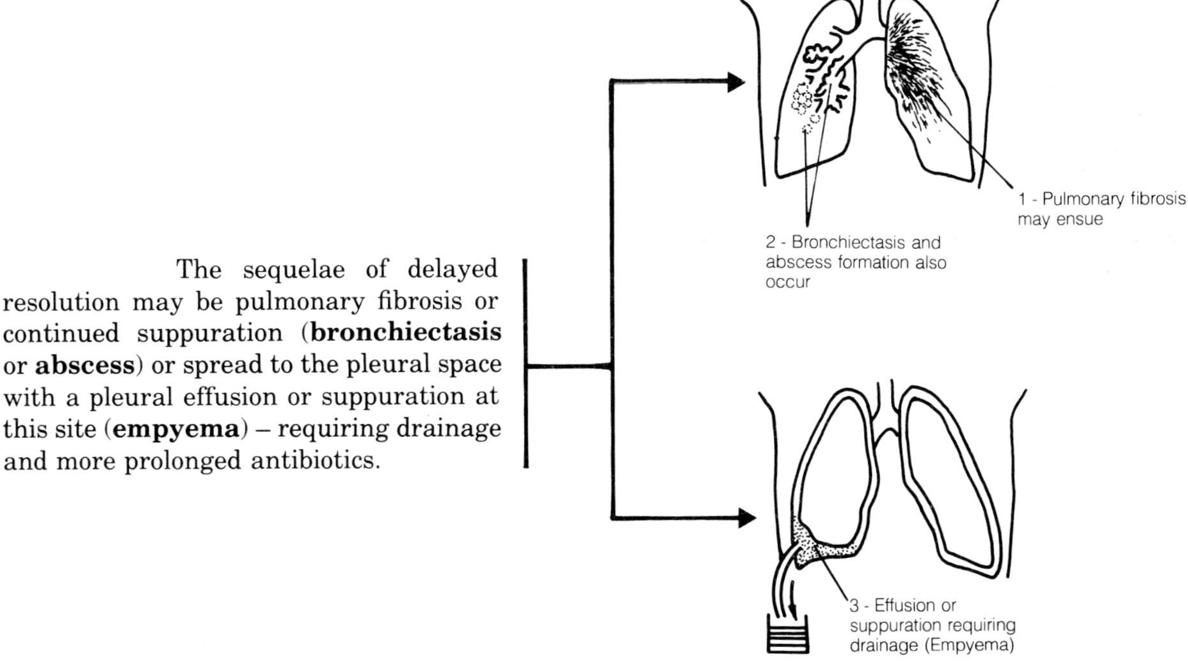

The sequelae of delayed resolution may be pulmonary fibrosis or continued suppuration (**bronchiectasis** or **abscess**) or spread to the pleural space with a pleural effusion or suppuration at this site (**empyema**) – requiring drainage and more prolonged antibiotics.

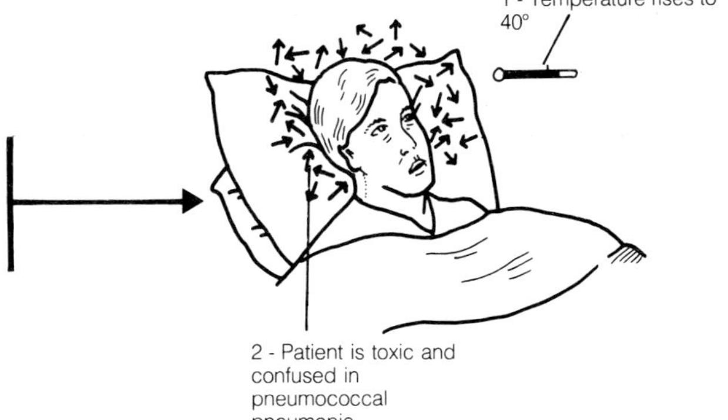

In the **acute illness** of pneumococcal pneumonia the patient may become toxic and confused as the temperature rises to 40 degrees centigrade.

Meningism is not uncommon in children at this time but a specific pneumococcal meningitis may occur and a lumbar puncture may need to be performed to exclude this: it is rare, however. Also in the acute phase of the illness, a toxic circulatory collapse is recognised – particularly in the elderly and infirm. A specific pneumococcal pericarditis or endocarditis is rare.

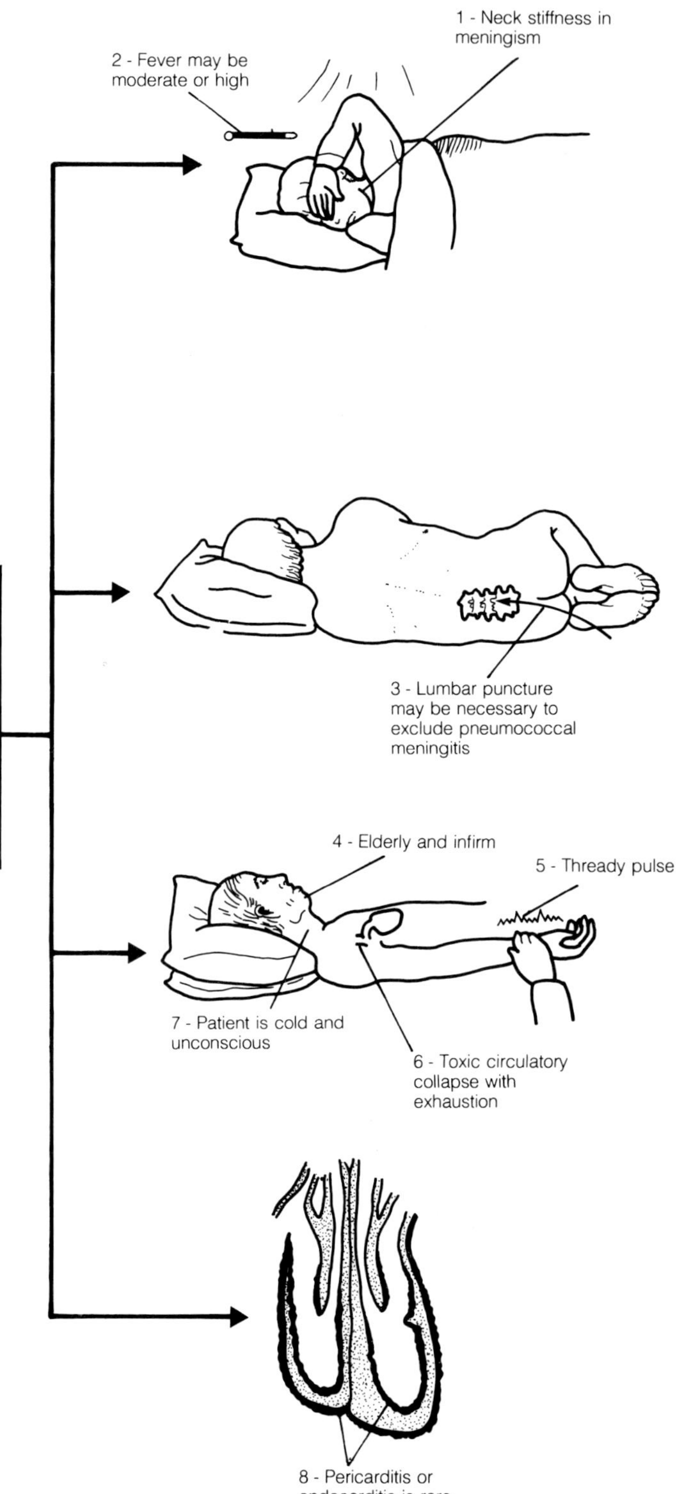

The acute onset of lobar pneumonia could be confused with pulmonary infarction and haemoptysis and pleuritic pain but cough and pyrexia are only minor features here and there is often a perceptible site of embolus. Pulmonary tuberculosis should not normally be confused with pneumococcal pneumonia but, in some situations, all pulmonary pathogens can mimic others.

Staphylococcal Pneumonia: This serious pneumonia may occur sporadically at any age (often spreading via the blood stream from an established pre-existing site of staphylococcal infection (e.g. boil, osteomyelitis etc), or secondarily complicating pre-existing respiratory disease (e.g. influenza, pulmonary infarction).

The clinical onset is severe malaise, remittent fever, cough productive of purulent sputum and often pleurisy. The physical signs vary but crepitations are more often a feature than classic consolidation signs. Chest radiography shows areas of patchy consolidation more often than lobar consolidation; ring shadows or cyst-like abscesses are typical of staphylococcal pneumonia.

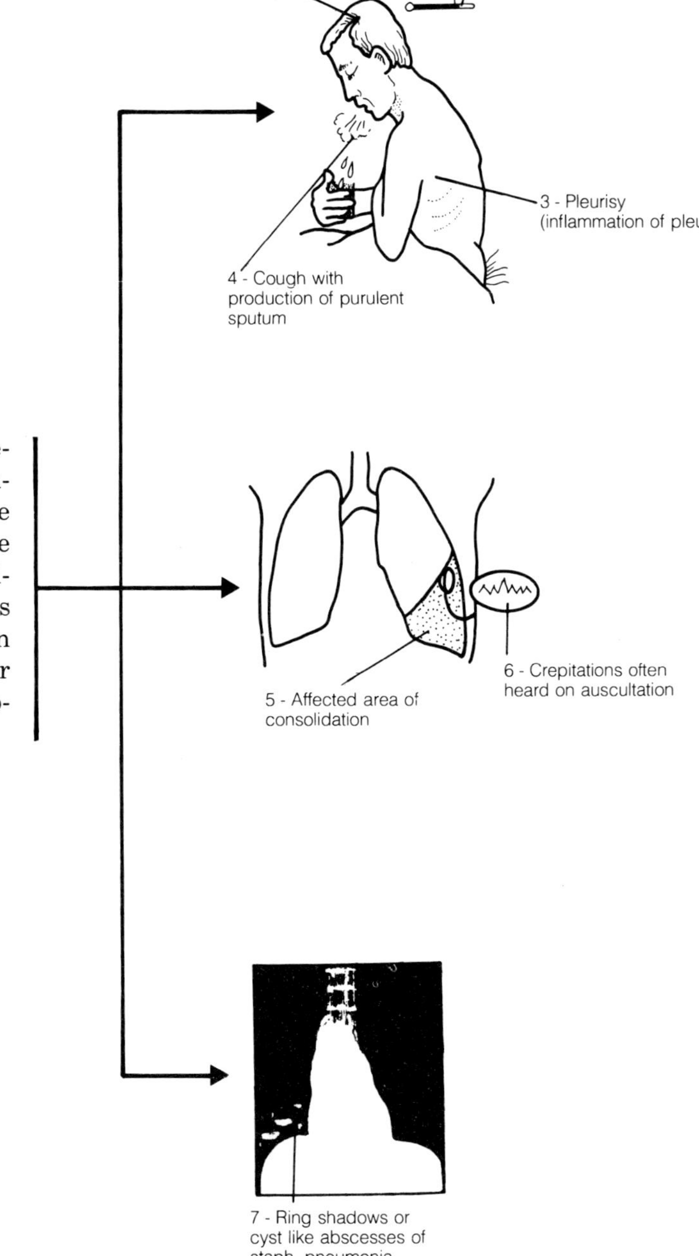

Staphylococcal pneumonia is a potentially fulminating infection with areas of lung necrosis and multiple abscesses, with attendant septicaemia. The diagnosis must be confirmed from sputum culture (and Gram stain) or blood cultures and parenteral cloxacillin (500 mg q.d.s.) initiated, together with chest physiotherapy. After the patient has responded and the pneumonia is resolving then oral flucloxacillin (250-500 mg q.d.s.) is continued.

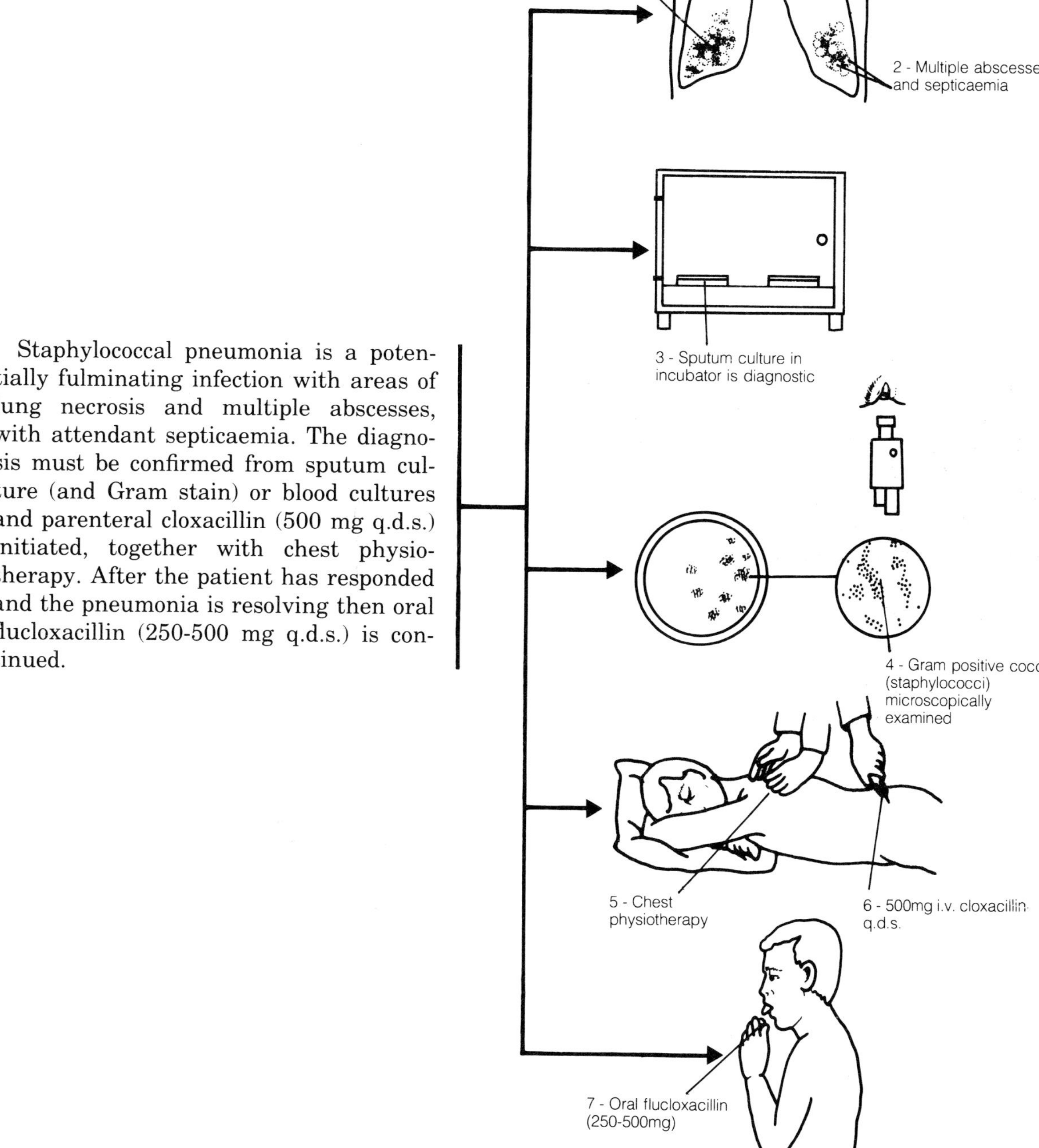

"Gram Negative" Pneumonia: Pneumonia caused by Klebsiella pneumoniae (Friedlander's bacillus) or Pseudomonas aeruginosa or other coliforms (e.g. E. coli) tends to affect patients with previous lung disease. The pneumonia is accompanied by a high fever, severe systemic symptoms and chest symptoms with a productive cough with purulent sputum, culture of which gives the diagnosis.

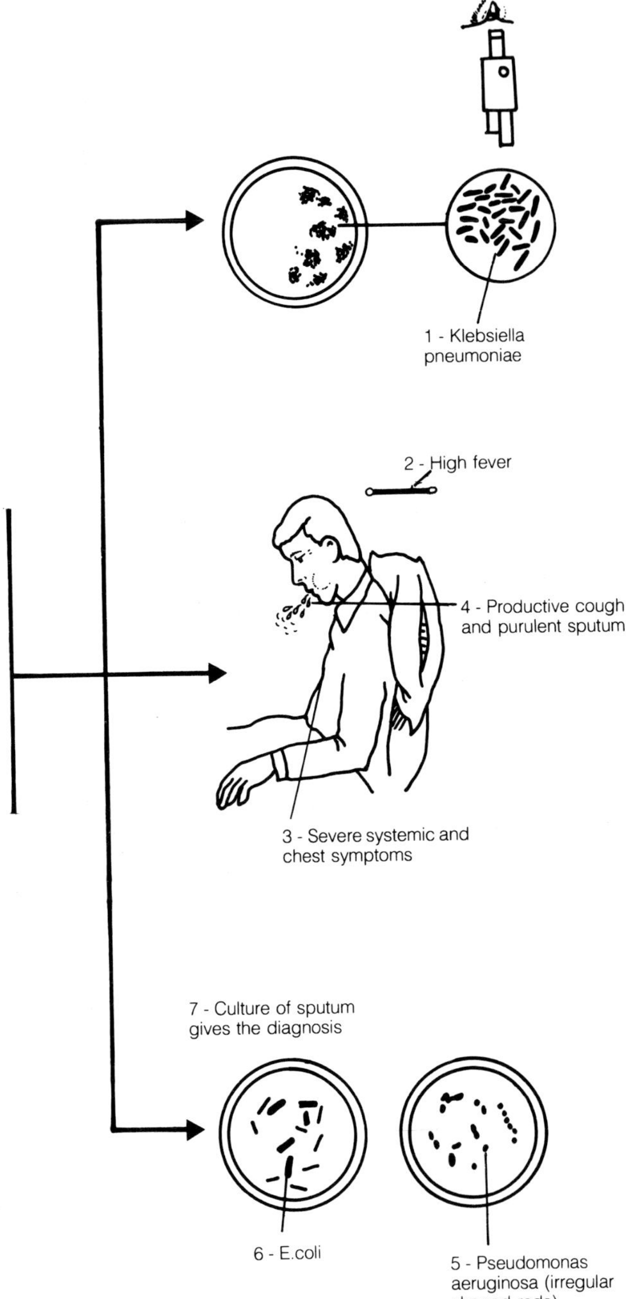

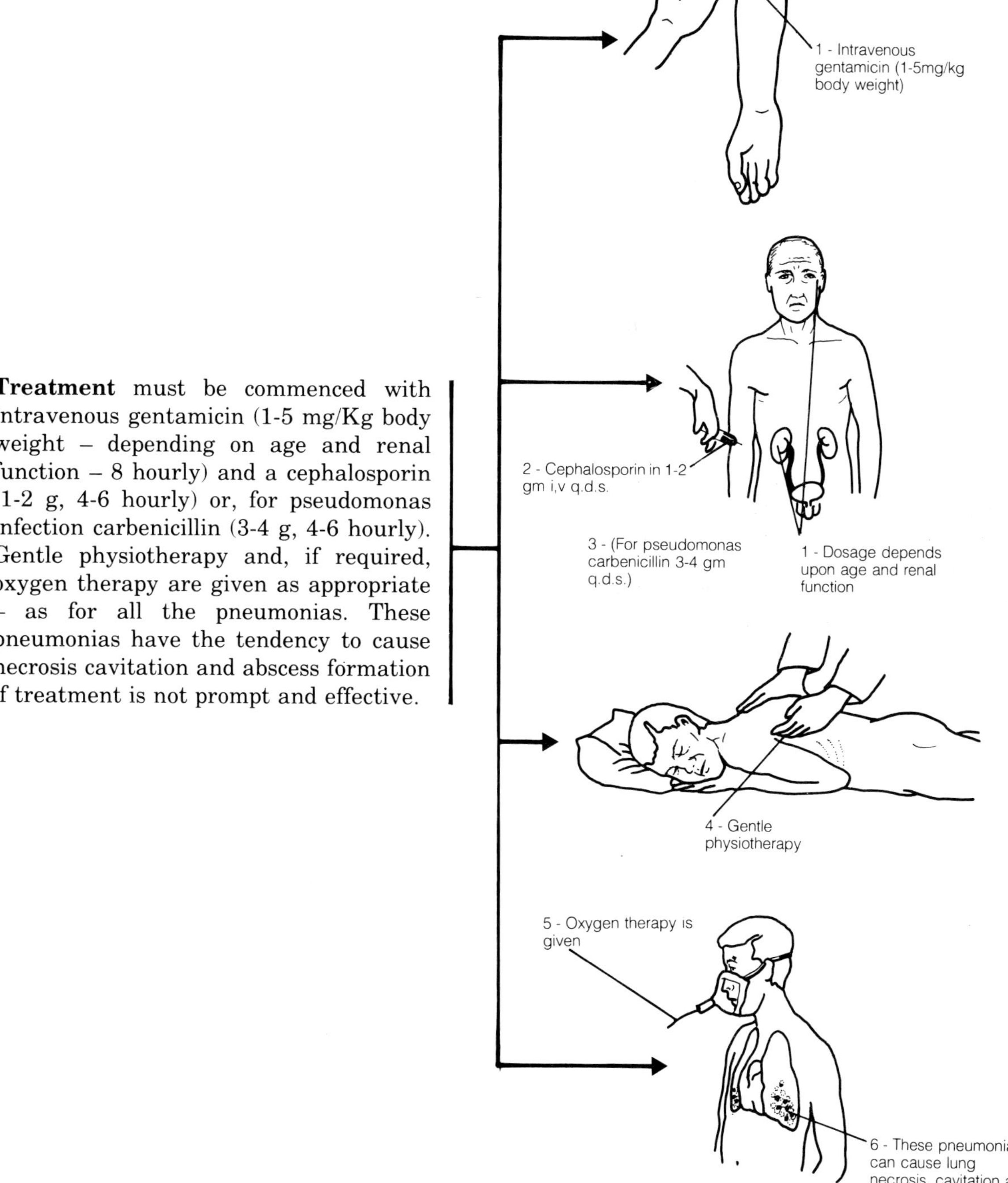

Treatment must be commenced with intravenous gentamicin (1-5 mg/Kg body weight – depending on age and renal function – 8 hourly) and a cephalosporin (1-2 g, 4-6 hourly) or, for pseudomonas infection carbenicillin (3-4 g, 4-6 hourly). Gentle physiotherapy and, if required, oxygen therapy are given as appropriate – as for all the pneumonias. These pneumonias have the tendency to cause necrosis cavitation and abscess formation if treatment is not prompt and effective.

Legionnaires's Disease: Legionella pneumophila causes a severe pneumonia with marked systemic features, particularly mental confusion and gastrointestinal upset. Culture of the organism remains difficult and the diagnosis is usually made by a rising antibody titre to the organism. Erythromycin (500 mg q.d.s. for 3 weeks) is the optimal management, and it is for this reason that erythromycin is popular as initial treatment in undiagnosed pneumonia.

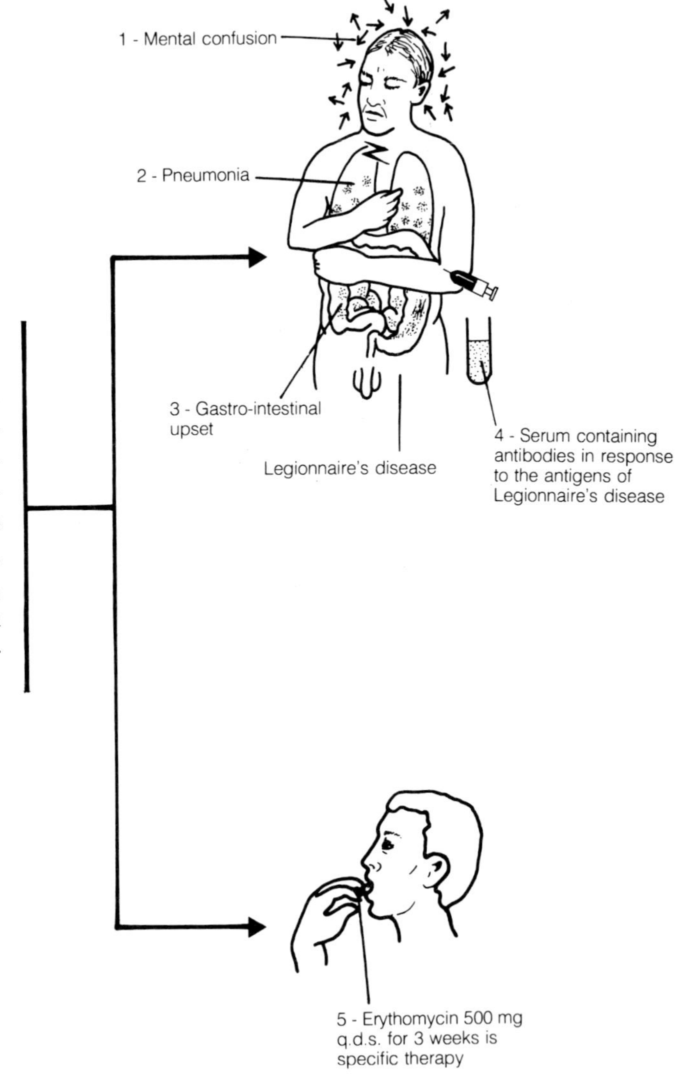

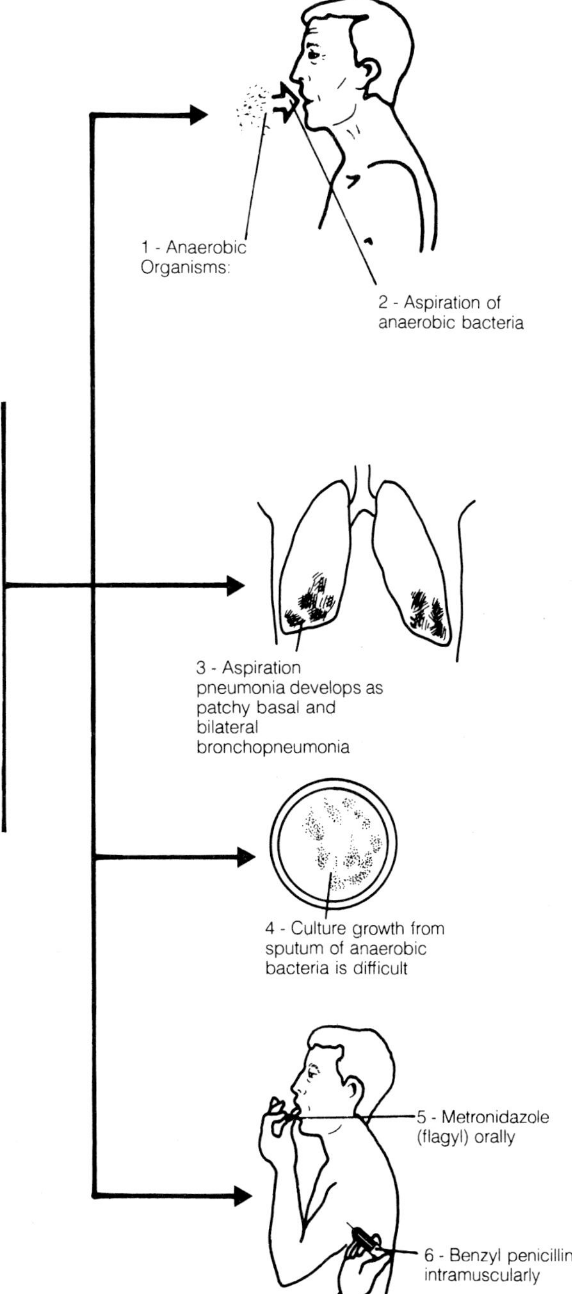

Anaerobic Organisms: Anaerobic bacteria will cause an aspiration bronchopneumonia in the debilitated. Basal, patchy bilateral bronchopneumonia (the classic aspiration pneumonia – whatever the organism) would be a common presentation and unless the pneumonia is cleared quickly, fatal suppuration may follow. Most anaerobes are difficult to grow but can be cultured from sputum with special care, and chromatograpy of sputum can also be diagnostic. Penicillin and metronidazole are optimal therapy in most cases.

NON-BACTERIAL PNEUMONIAS

Several general comments may be made concerning this group of pneumonias. Systemic clinical symptoms are often pronounced including languor, generalised aches and headache. The fever is often mild. The respiratory symptoms are often less dramatic than in bacterial infections, the sputum more mucoid and the chest signs less marked: crepitations over the diseased area of lung are often the only detectable sign apart from mild tachypnoea. However, radiological signs (which may be lobar, or lobular and patchy consolidation) are often greater, and often unexpectedly marked when compared with the paucity of physical signs. There is less commonly a peripheral blood leucocytosis than in bacterial pneumonia.

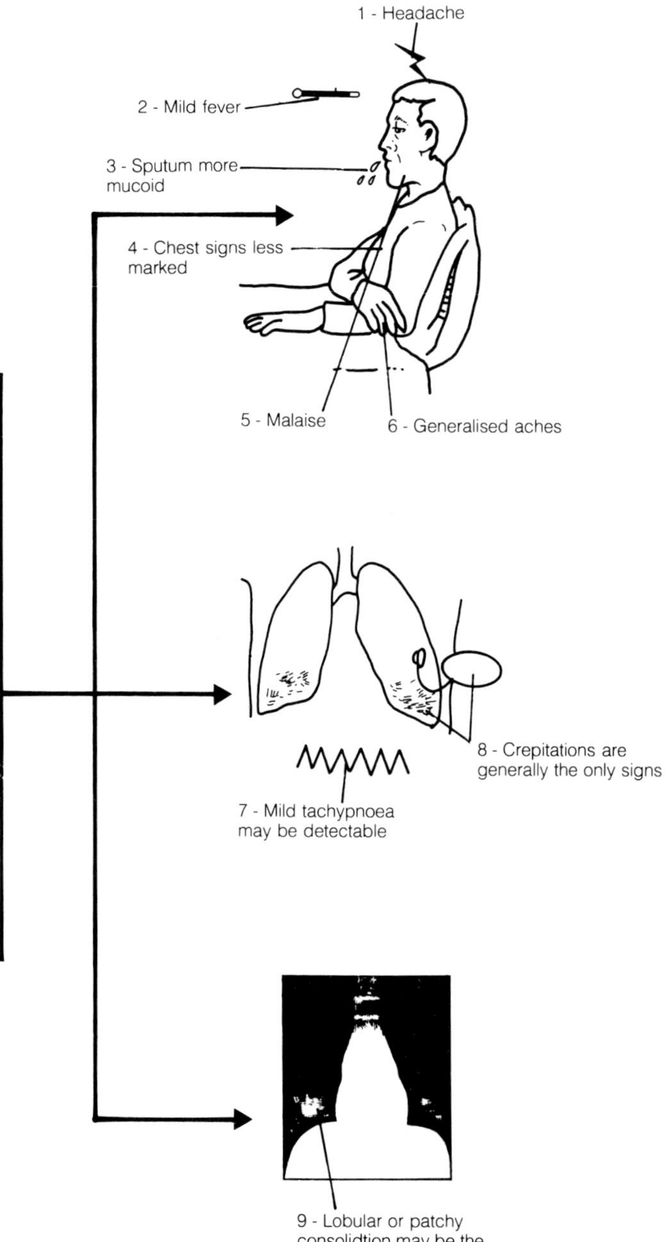

Mycoplasma Pneumonia: Mycoplasma pneumoniae is a relatively common cause of pneumonia in young and previously healthy adults. The illness obeys all the general remarks made above. Although the organism can be cultured from the sputum, it is slow to grow (up to 2 weeks) and diagnosis is made on a rising antibody titre. Cold agglutinns appear in the

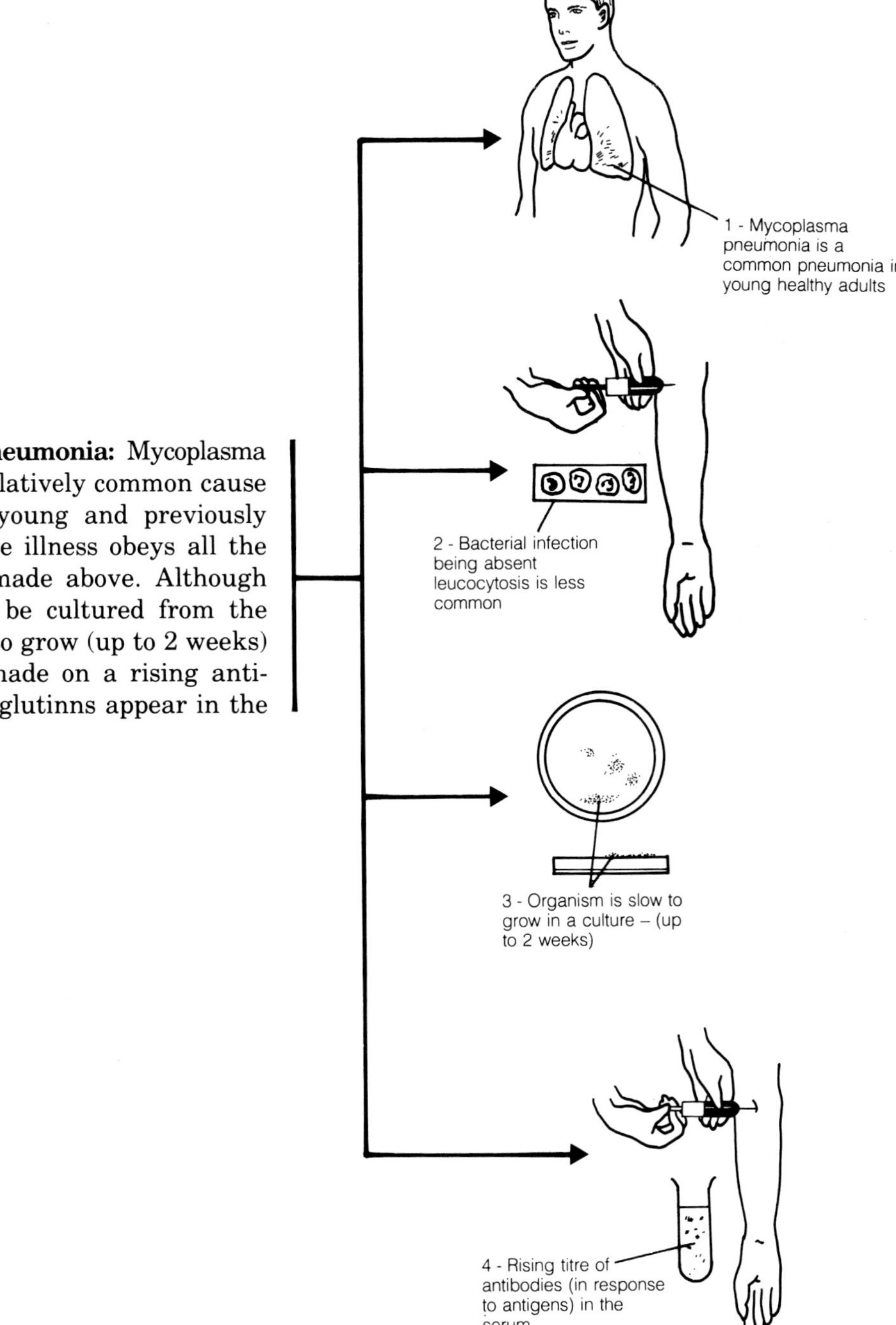

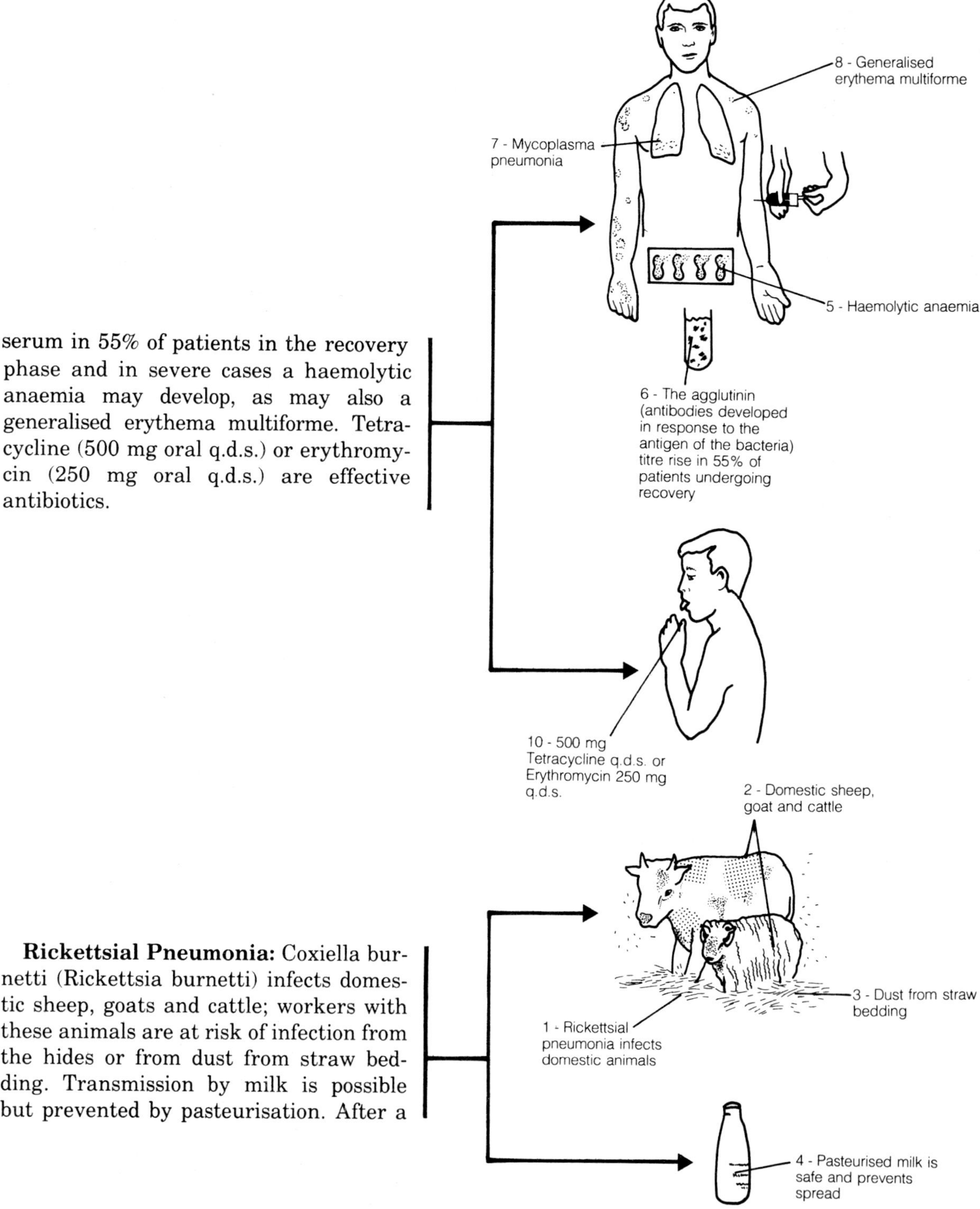

serum in 55% of patients in the recovery phase and in severe cases a haemolytic anaemia may develop, as may also a generalised erythema multiforme. Tetracycline (500 mg oral q.d.s.) or erythromycin (250 mg oral q.d.s.) are effective antibiotics.

Rickettsial Pneumonia: Coxiella burnetti (Rickettsia burnetti) infects domestic sheep, goats and cattle; workers with these animals are at risk of infection from the hides or from dust from straw bedding. Transmission by milk is possible but prevented by pasteurisation. After a

2-3 weeks incubation period a pneumonia develops that is usually self-limiting although it may be long lasting; (it is rarely accompanied by an endocarditis – much more serious). Diagnosis is by the demonstration of a rising titre of antibody in paired sera and treatment is by tetracycline or erythromycin.

Chlamydial Pneumonia: Chlamydia psittaci causes psittacosis in members of the parrot family including pigeons and poultry. The rare human pneumonia caused by this organism can often be traced to contact with birds and may be a severe pneumonia that is slow to clear. It is diagnosed by serological testing and treated best by tetracycline (500 mg oral t.d.s. for 2 weeks).

It is noteworthy that the causative organism of trachoma and conjunctivitis is also a chlamydia (Chlamydia trachomatis) and is a rare cause of pneumonia in infants.

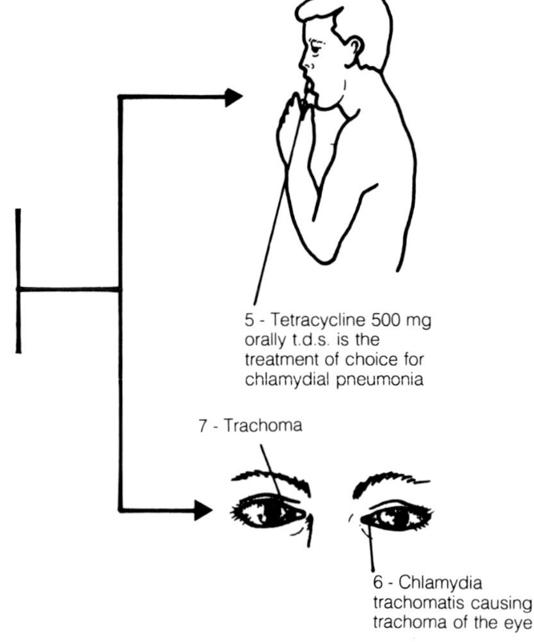

Virus Pneumonia: Influenza has already been described as an important pathogen capable of spread to the lungs themselves or predisposing to secondary pneumonic pathogens. Several viruses may cause pneumonia in children and include the respiratory syncytial virus which produces yearly winter epidemics of bronchiolitis and/or bronchopneumonia in children under 5 years, and severe pneumonia in infants.

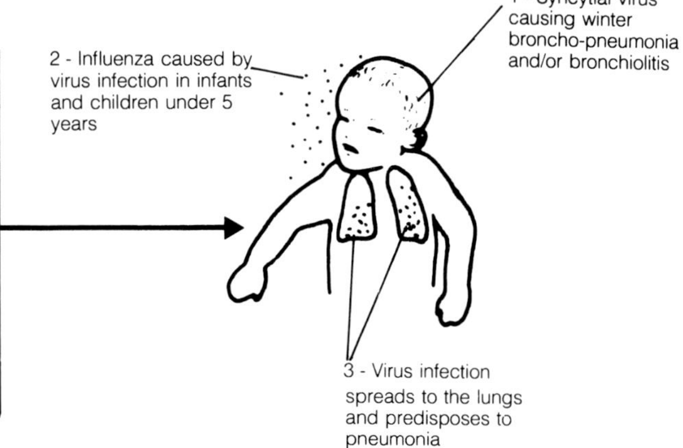

Measles virus often causes a mild tracheo-bronchitis or pneumonitis and rarely severe pneumonitis or "giant cell" pneumonia. **Severe chickenpox** (varicella) particularly in adults may be complicated by a characteristic and severe pneumonia which develops several days after the rash: its development is accompanied by a cough with haemoptysis, chest pain and usually dyspnoea. The chest X-ray shows typically diffuse, bilateral shadowing of a small nodular nature, and interestingly, this often heals with nodular calcification.

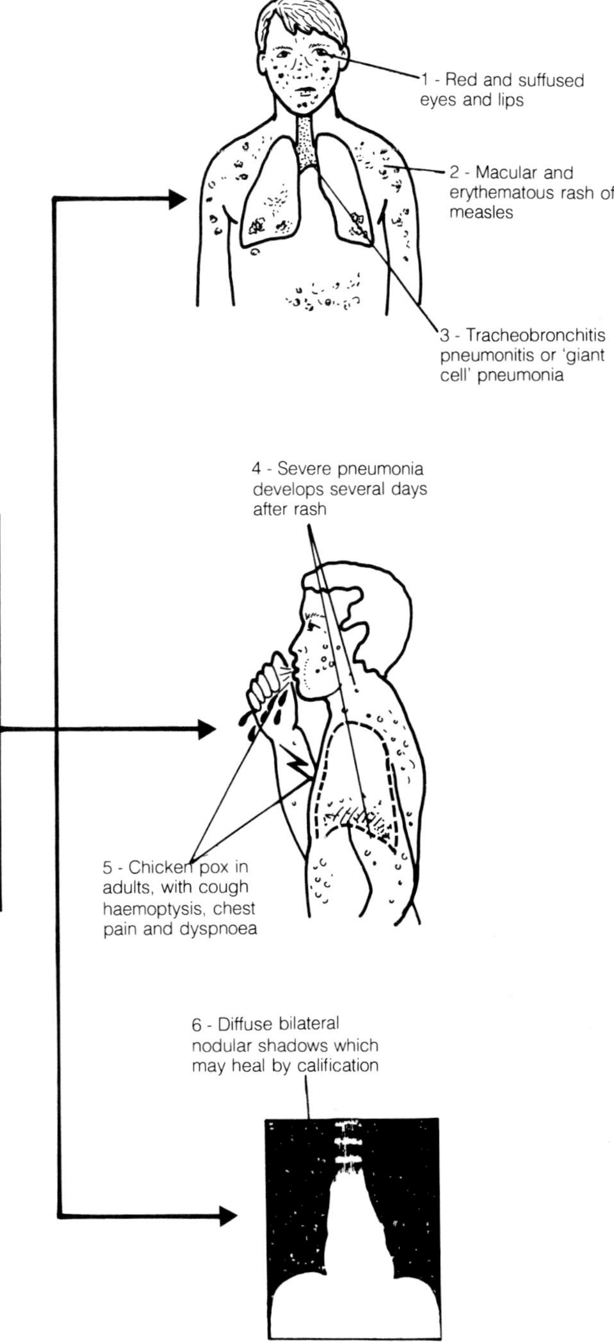

The role of antiviral chemotherapy (and steroids) in severe cases remains on clinical trial, but adenine arabinoside and acycloguanosine show promise.

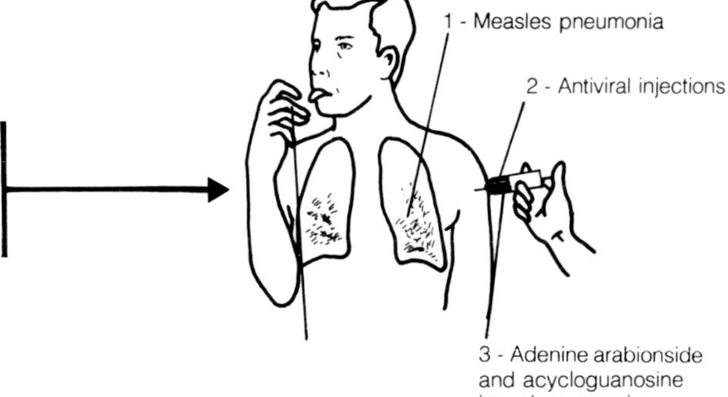

Cytomegalovirus causes both primary infections of the lungs and can be reactivated – particularly in immunosuppressed patients (e.g. bone marrow or renal transplant recipients). The disease is typically a widespread bronchopneumonia or interstitial pneumonia associated with systemic features including pyrexia, generalised lymphadenopathy and hepatosplenomegaly.

In transplant recipients, CMV infections occur 2 weeks –2 months post-transplant and are diagnosed from serology. Adenine arabinoside, interferon, acycloguanosine are under trial, but more effective drugs (such as trifluorothymidine derivatives) have so far proved too toxic. CMV pneumonia remains a serious malady in the immunosuppressed.

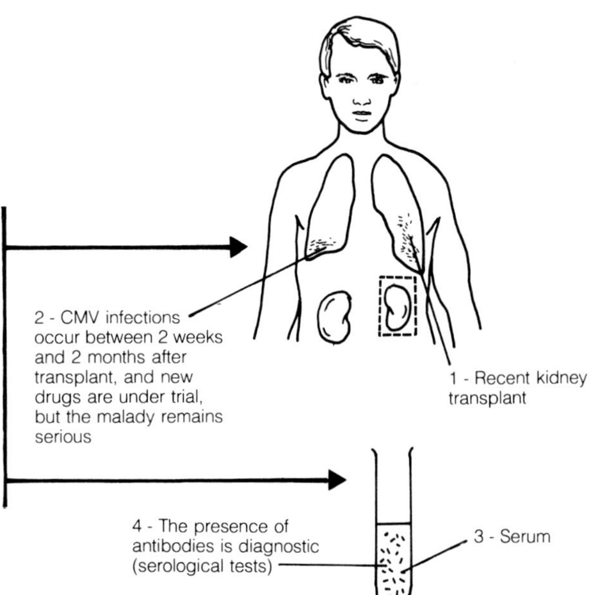

FUNGAL AND PROTOZOAL PNEUMONIAS

Aspergillus fumigatus may cause a severe necrotising pneumonia usually in already sick patients. The pneumonia is severe and almost always accompanied by some irreversible lung damage which is not infrequently extensive with large cavities forming. Sputum staining and culture gives the diagnosis. Amphotericin B intravenously is the most effective agent but is often inadequate and the illness fatal.

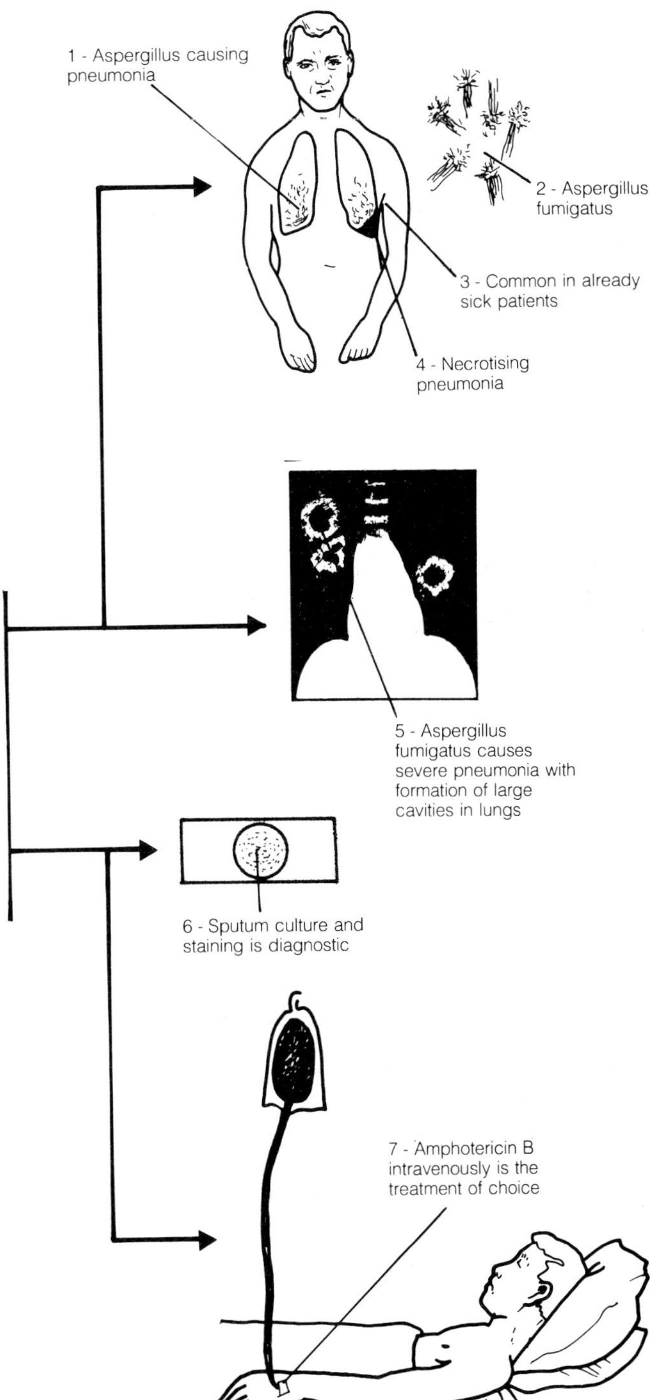

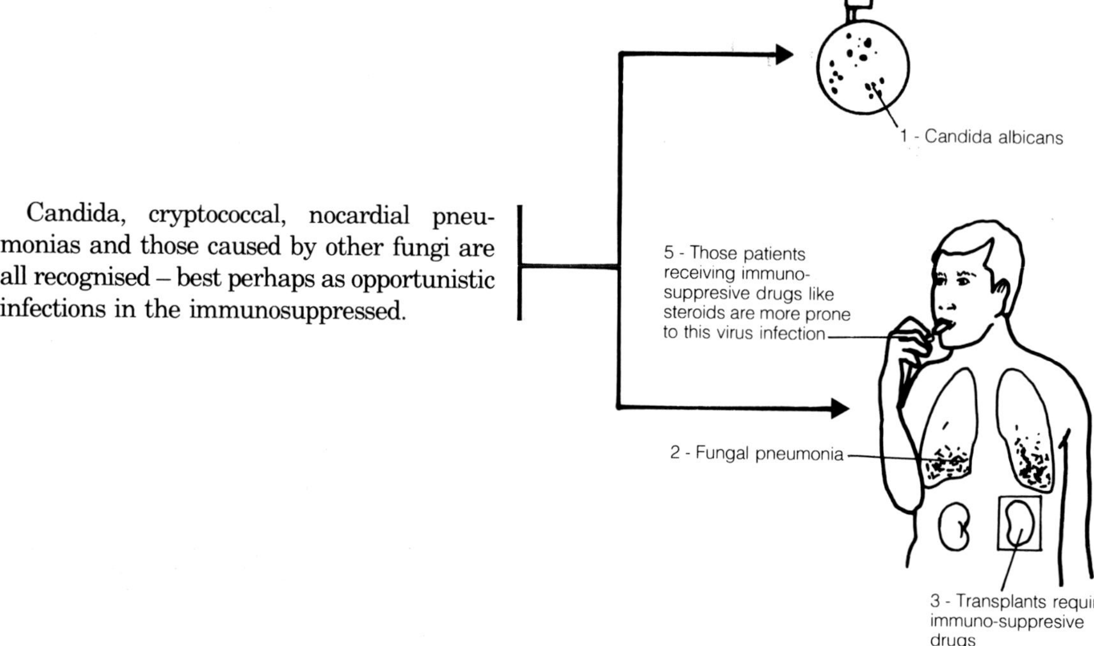

Candida, cryptococcal, nocardial pneumonias and those caused by other fungi are all recognised – best perhaps as opportunistic infections in the immunosuppressed.

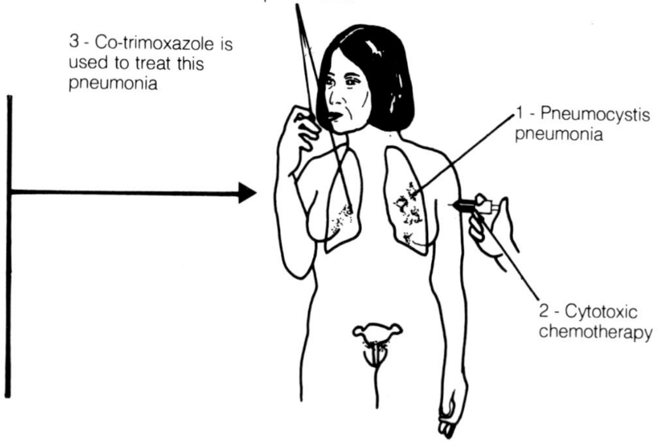

Pneumocystis carinii is an opportunist protozoan causing a pneumonia – not uncommonly seen in oncologic practice amongst patients with cancer and on cytotoxic chemotherapy (both predisposing). Co-trimoxazole is an effective agent.

Pneumocystis pneumonia is becoming an increasingly important first manifestations of the Acquired Immunodeficiency Syndrome (AIDS).

ASPIRATION PNEUMONIA

This inhalation pneumonia is recognised as a separate illness although it may be caused by one of many pathogens. It is caused by aspiration of mucus, saliva, food, foreign bodies etc into the distal bronchial tree, with inadequate cough reflex. It may be secondary to oral or dental infection, neuromuscular disease imparing swallowing or coughing, laryngal or oesophageal disease, general debility or post-anaesthetic.

Once material or secretions have pooled – and this usually occurs in the basal regions of the lungs – secondary infection occurs and a widespread bilateral basal bronchopneumonia may occur or the disease may localise to one site with a segmental pneumonia, or suppurate to form a lung abscess here.

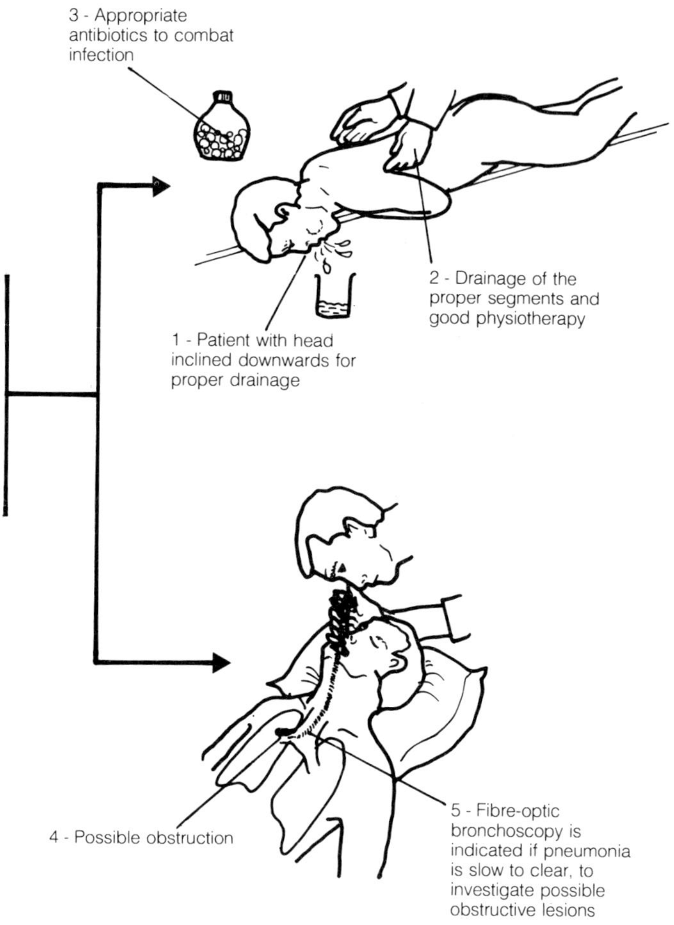

Treatment depends on drainage of the involved segments obtained by good physiotherapy, and appropriate antibiotics. If such pneumonia is slow to clear from one site, a fibre-optic bronchoscopy may be indicated to search for an endobronchial lesion causing obstruction.

LUNG ABSCESS

A lung abscess may follow on from an unresolving pneumonia – particularly those caused by staphylococci, Gram negative rods and anaerobic bacteria:

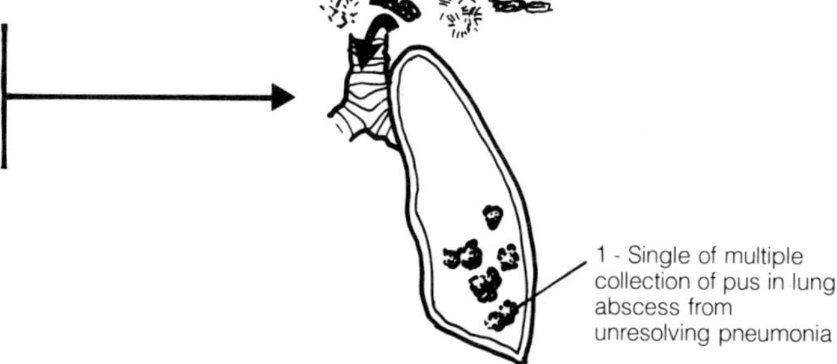

it localises as one or multiple collections of pus. However, there are other causes and these include suppurative infection of a recent pulmonary infarct, (usually caused by a septic embolus), or suppuration distal to an endobronchial obstruction such as a foreign body or carcinoma. In the tropics, the trans-diaphragmatic spread of an amoebic liver abscess may lead to localised lung suppuration; indeed any subpleural abscess may "point" similarly.

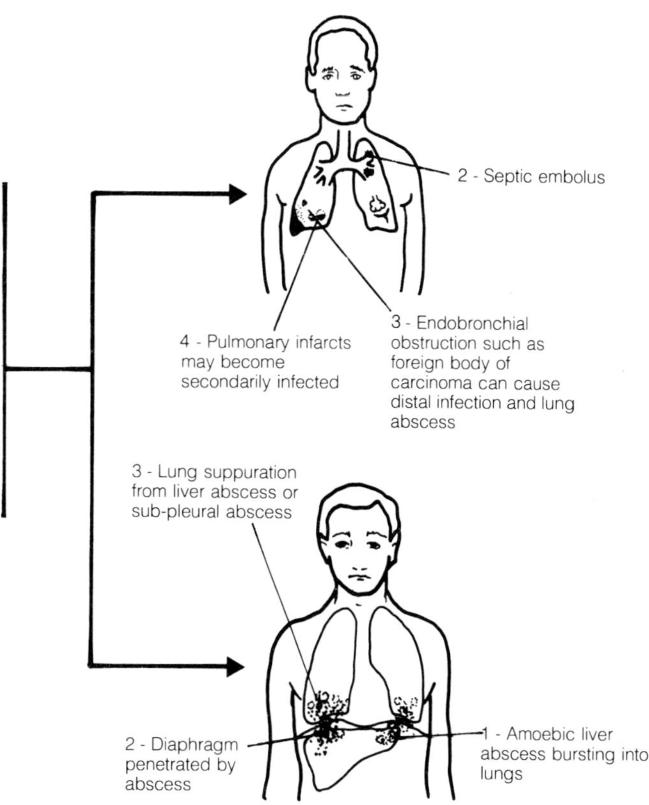

The patient is systemically ill with typically a high swinging fever and perhaps pleuritic chest pain. There is a marked polymorphonuclear leucocytosis. The patient coughs up large quantities of purulent sputum and the breath is foul (halitosis). The chest signs vary but there

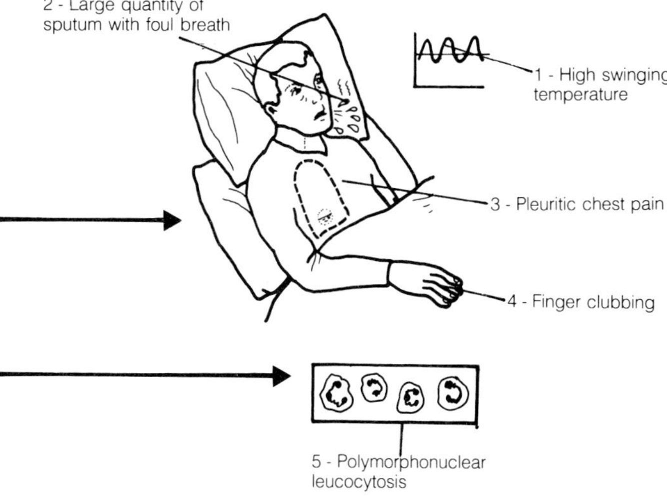

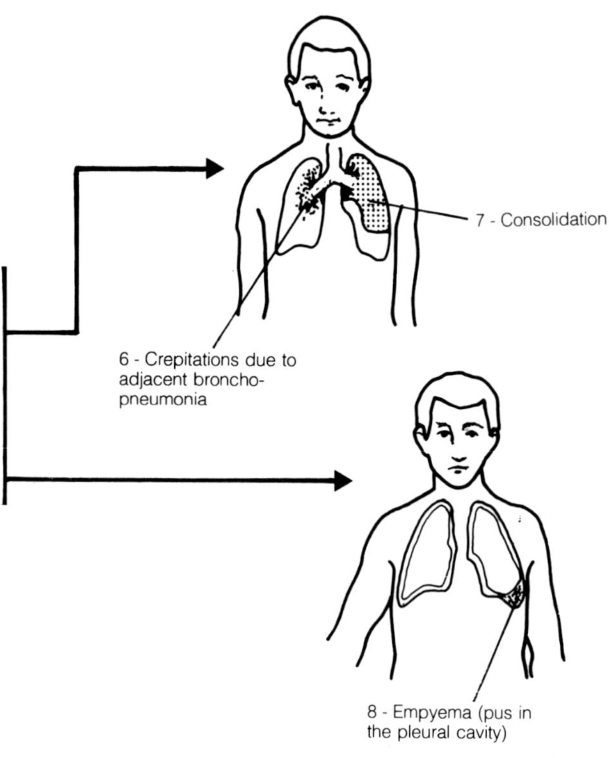

may be the signs of consolidation over the area and perhaps further afield with crepitations, due to adjacent broncho-pneumonia. Unchecked, that diagnostically helpful accompaniment of chest suppuration – finger clubbing, develops. Spread to the pleural space leads to **empyema.**

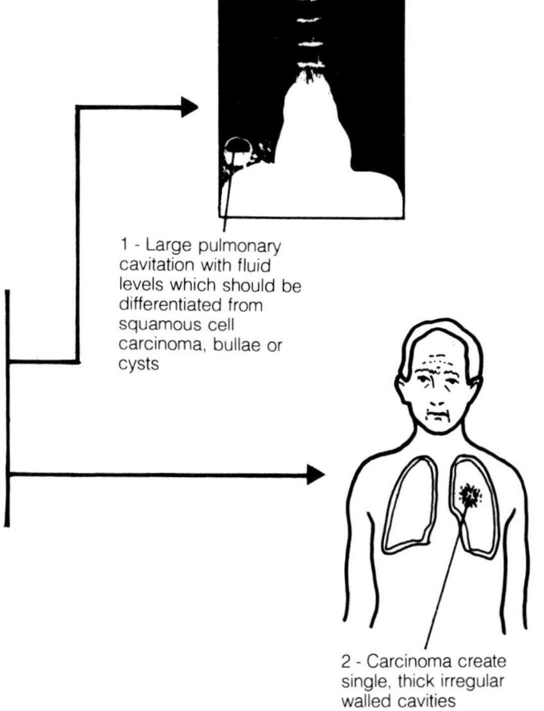

The chest X-ray reveals pulmonary cavitation with fluid levels, the differential diagnosis of which can only be secondarily infected cavitating squamous carcinoma, bullae or cysts. Carcinomas tend to create single, thick and irregular walled cavities – thicker than acute primarily infective abscesses.

Treatment comprises ridding the patient of any endobronchial obstruction (which necessitates bronchoscopy – usually rigid) followed by physiotherapy with postural drainage and intensive systemic antibiotics, as appropriate. In the absence of endobronchial obstruction, this treatment is usually successful. If treatment fails and the suppuration remains localised, surgical resection must be considered.

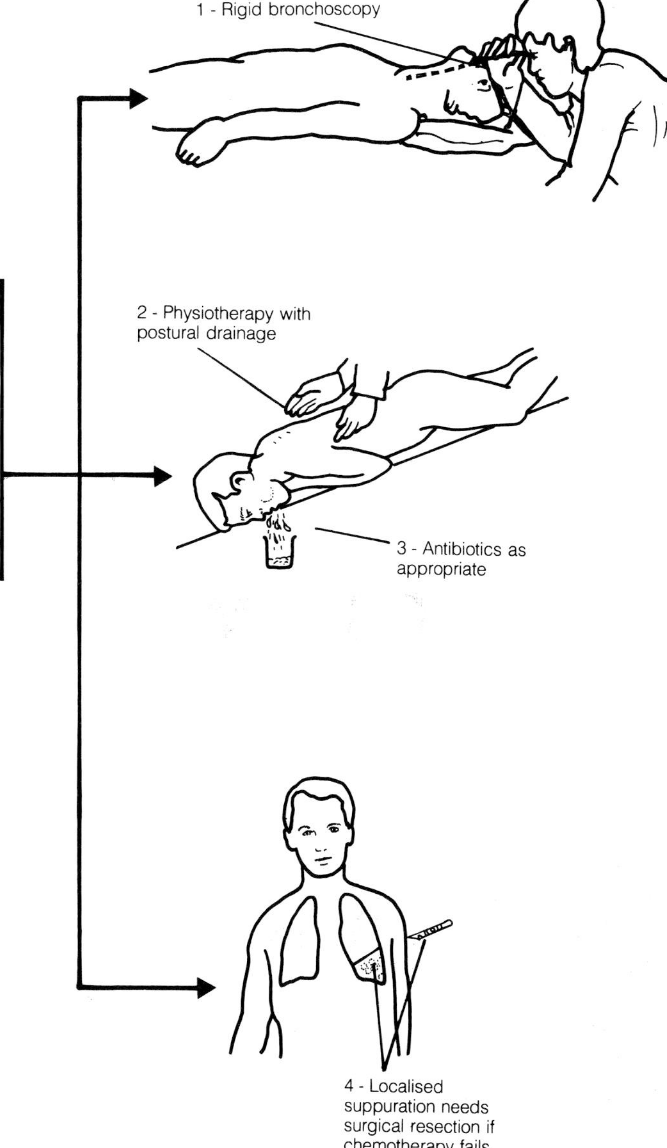

BRONCHIECTASIS

Bronchiectasis means dilatation of the bronchi. It may be secondary to previous bronchial obstruction or chronic infection, particularly in childhood, or congenital maldevelopment of the bronchi or atresia. The widened bronchi may be dilated in cylindrical (tubular), saccular (cystic) or fusiform (spindle) formations, but all have impaired ciliary function.

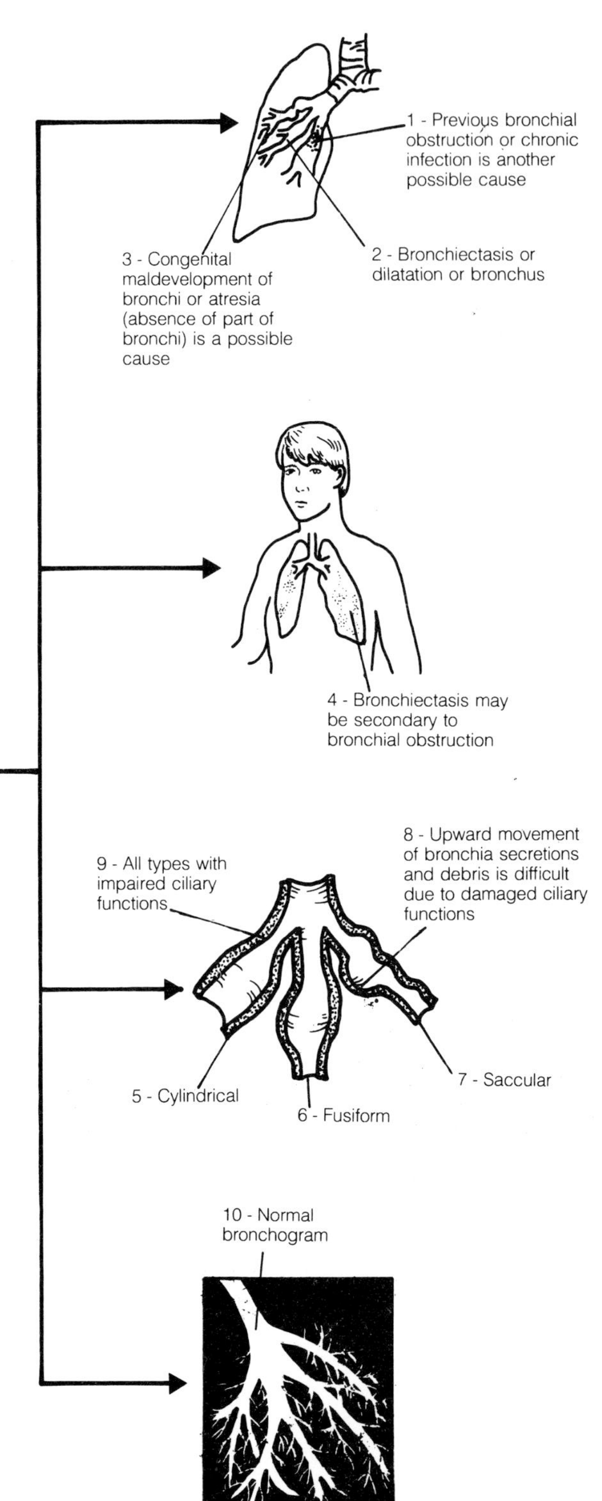

Bronchography

11 - Gross saccular
bronchiectasis

12 - Proximal
bronchiectasis

Thus the upward transport mechanism for bronchial secretions and debris is deficient – and conditions are ripe for perpetual infection.

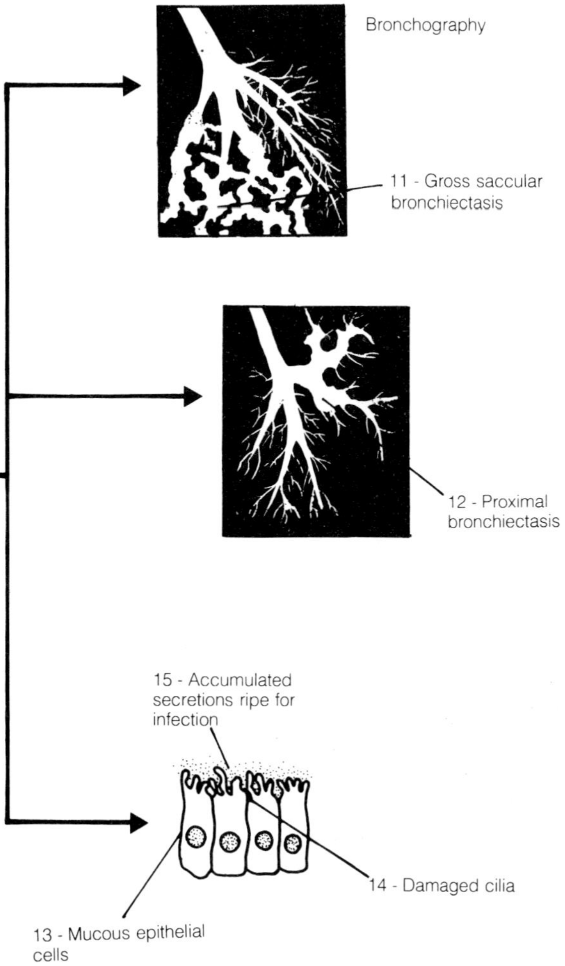

15 - Accumulated
secretions ripe for
infection

14 - Damaged cilia

13 - Mucous epithelial
cells

The conditions that are commonly associated with bronchiectasis are cystic fibrosis (mucoviscidosis), immunodeficiency diseases (e.g. agammaglobulinaemia, selective IgA deficiency, chronic granulomatous disease), and diseases of poor ciliary activity (Kartagener's syndrome).

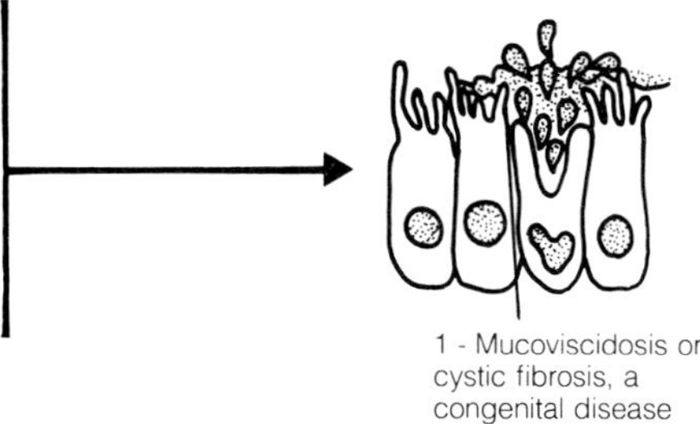

1 - Mucoviscidosis or
cystic fibrosis, a
congenital disease

The clinical problem in bronchiectasis is a great difficulty in eradicating infection from bronchiectatic areas, and the periodic relapse of infection in these lung areas with fever, systemic upset and copious production of purulent sputum with, of course, the potential for greater damage to the lung with each infective exacerbation.

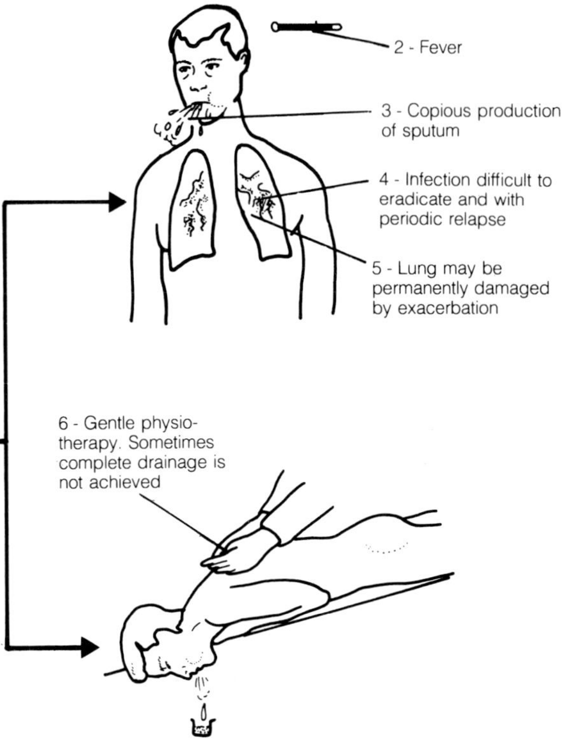

Physical examination reveals an unwell, clubbed patient with halitosis, possibly dyspnoea and even cyanosis if the disease is widespread. Chest examination will reveal the changes of consolidation, collapse or fibrosis, and coarse crepitations will almost invariably be present.

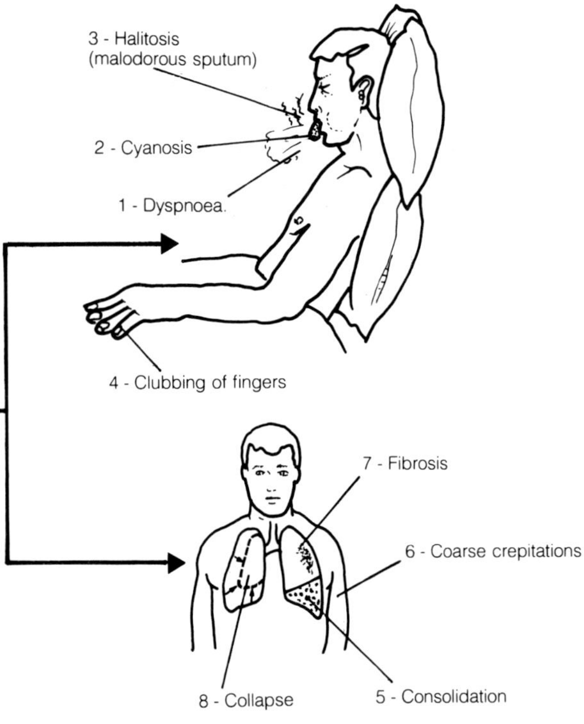

The chest X-ray may show many things. Bronchiectasis is commoner in the lower zones (unless post-tuberculous) and tubular shadows caused by dilated bronchi full of secretions may be visible. Ring shadows, perhaps with fluid levels, may be seen in saccular bronchiectasis. Adjacent and associated atelectasis or patchy bronchopneumonic areas of consolidation may be seen. After treatment, in the latent period between infective exacerbations, increased linear markings are still usually apparent in the affected lung areas. The **diagnosis** of bronchiectasis is made radiologically by bronchography, in which a radio-opaque aqueous suspension is gently injected through the crico-thyroid membrane to coat the bronchial walls and demonstrate their contours on X-rays.

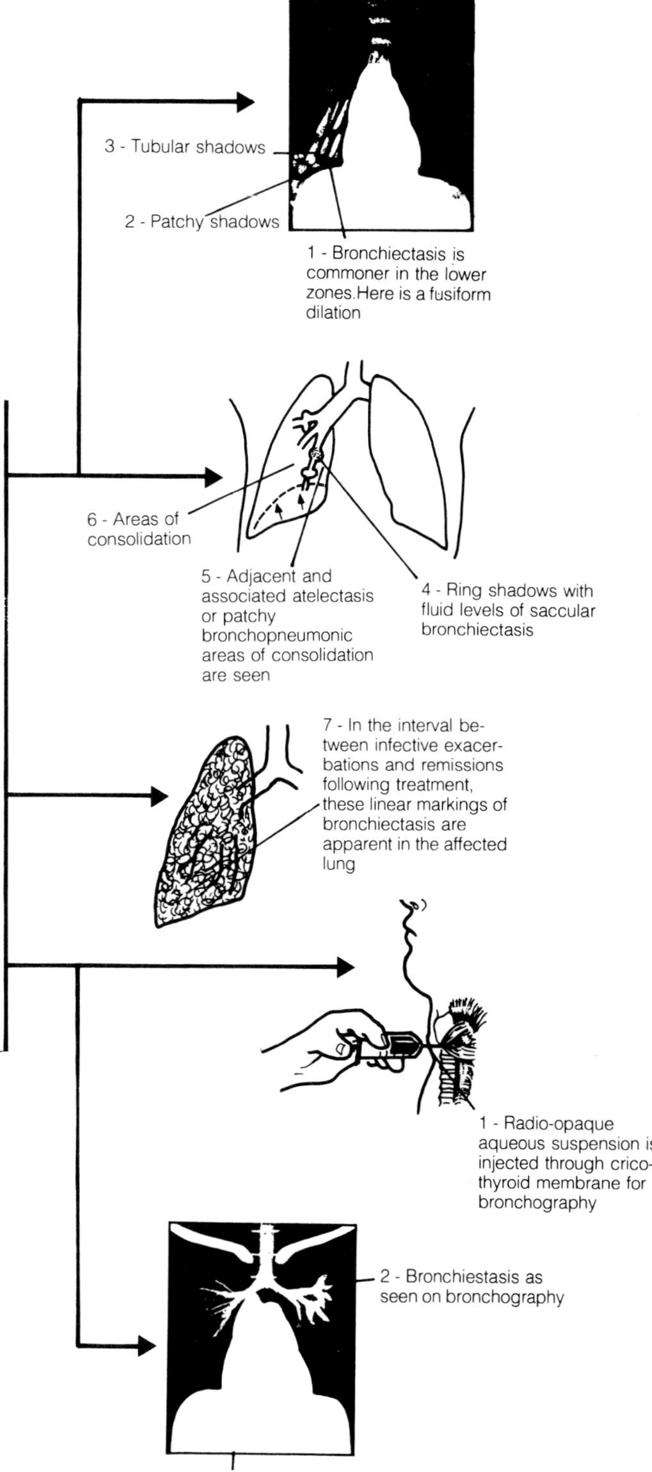

Regular, twice daily, 10 minute spells of postural drainage and chest percussion during postural (gravity) drainage are important methods of ridding secretions, as is also the "huffing" (forced expiration and coughing) technique. For acute infective episodes, the patient must have immediate access to antibiotics – to be taken as soon as the sputum production increases in volume and purulence. The exact antibiotics depend on the individuals but, for example, in patients with cystic fibrosis it is important to cover H. influenzae with amoxycillin 250-500 mg oral q.d.s., and Staphylococcus with flucloxacillin 500 mg oral q.d.s. and to watch for another evil pathogen: Pseudomonas may require periodic intravenous aminoglycoside and carbenicillin therapy.

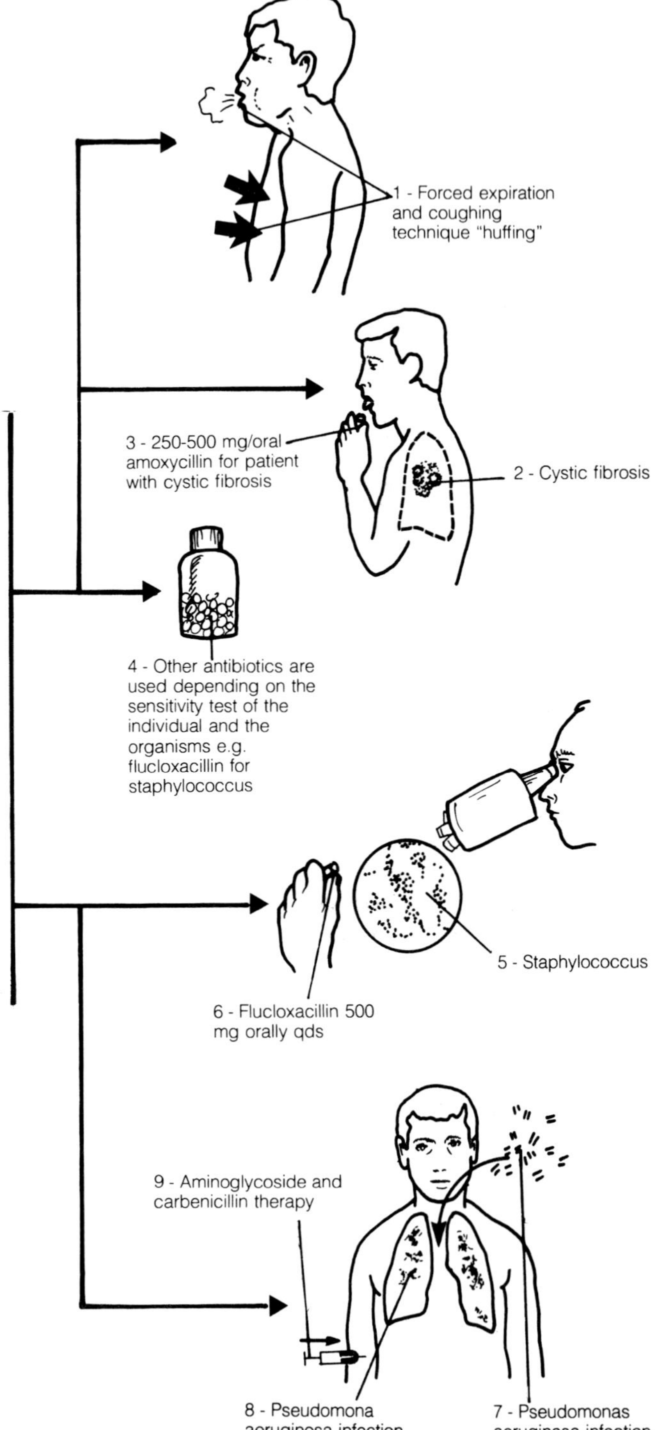

If infective episodes occur many times each year, then prophylactic antibiotics are indicated, at least in winter, A simple tetracycline regime (doxycycline 100 mg/day) is probably as good as any unless the patient is known to harbour a particular, resistant pathogen, when other and perhaps cycling courses of antibiotics may be appropriate.

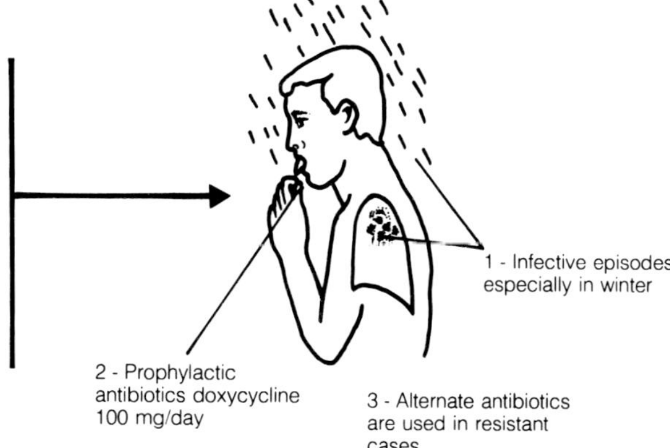

Surgical resection of bronchiectatic lung areas is indicated if the bronchiectasis is confined to one discrete lung area, or if the clinician deems one area to be the major "trouble-spot" from which recurrent infections originate and put further lung areas at greater risk. The increased vascularity with bronchopulmonary anastomoses that occur in bronchiectatic lung areas, render the patient liable to quite severe haemoptyses and uncontrollable haemoptyses is an indication for surgery (although therapeutic embolisation is an alternative). Superinfection of a bronchiectatic segment by an aspergilloma has also caused us to resect this lung area.

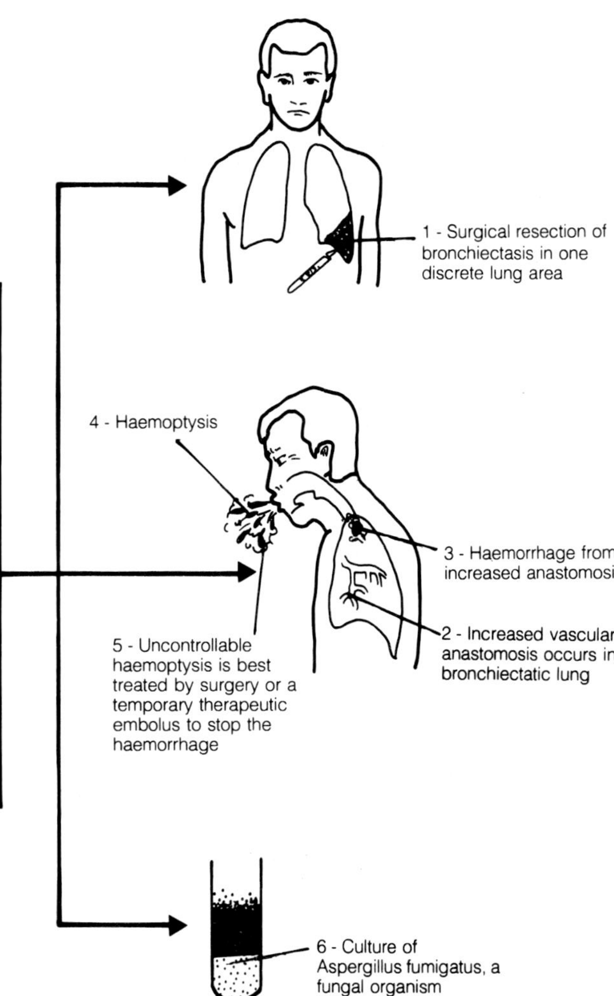

PULMONARY TUBERCULOSIS

Pulmonary tuberculosis (T.B.) remains one of the most specific, communicable diseases on a world scale, resulting .in nearly 3 million deaths annually, the vast majority in developing countries. In England and Wales the incidence is a fraction of that at the turn of this century with an annual notification of 15×10^{-5} and a disproportionately large contribution to that figure comes from the Asian immigrant population. Many risk factors

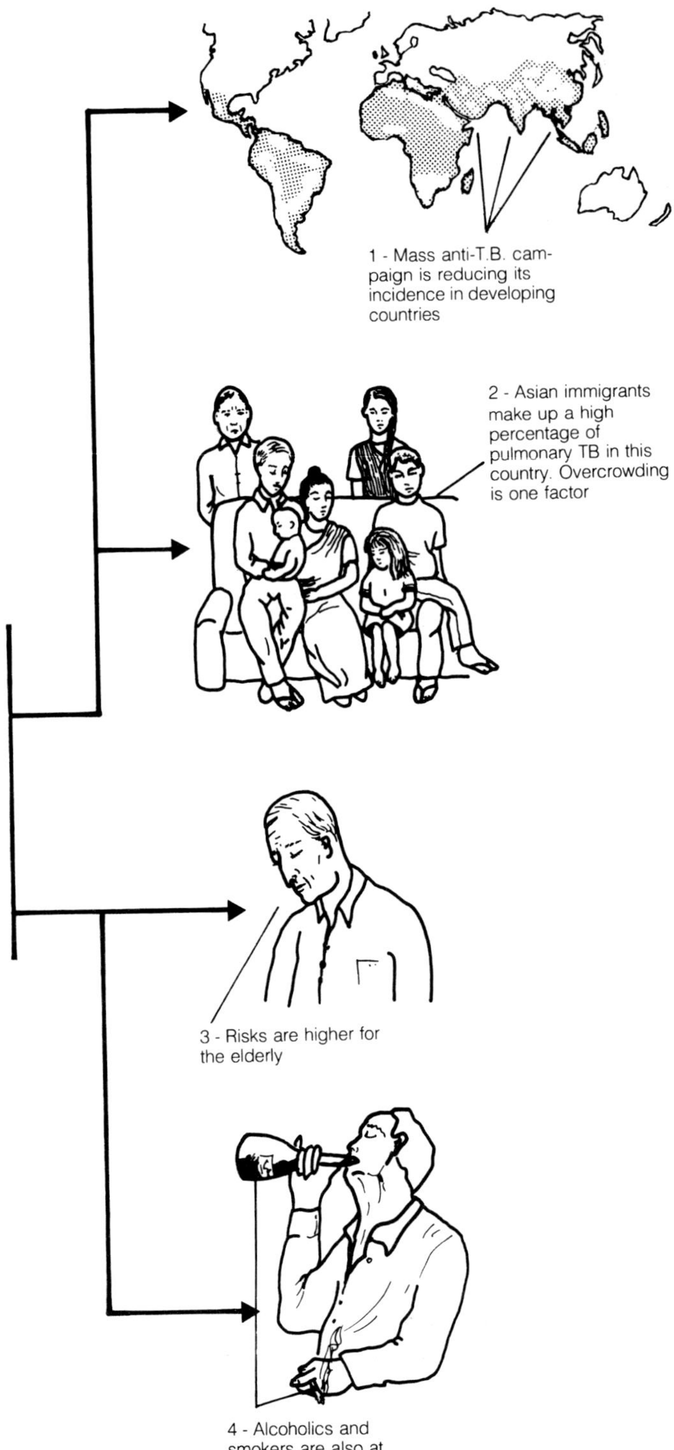

1 - Mass anti-T.B. campaign is reducing its incidence in developing countries

2 - Asian immigrants make up a high percentage of pulmonary TB in this country. Overcrowding is one factor

3 - Risks are higher for the elderly

4 - Alcoholics and smokers are also at high risk

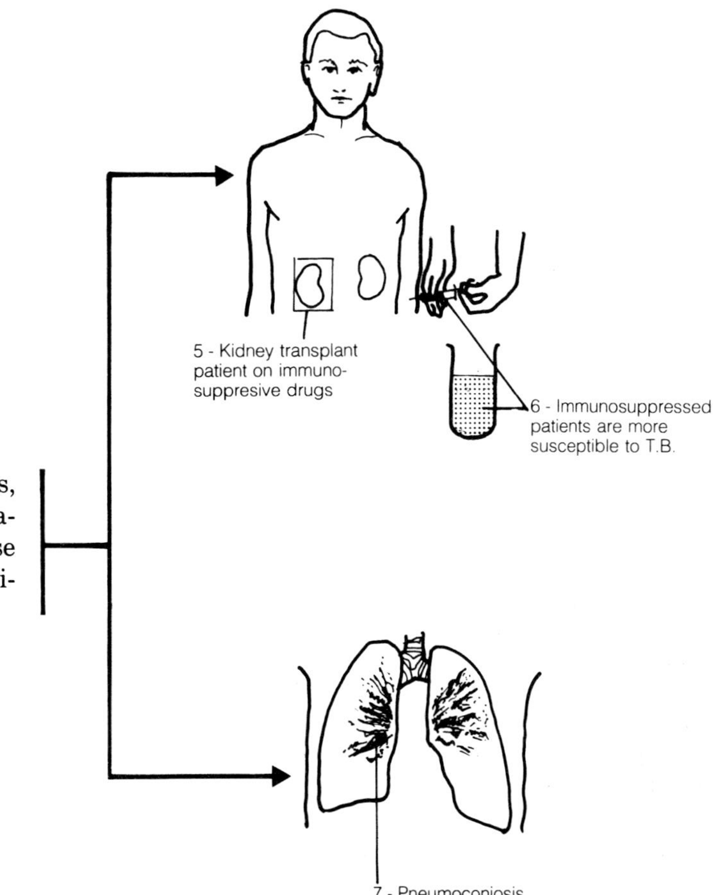

exist: close crowding of many individuals, the elderly, the immunosuppressed, diabetics, alcoholics, smokers, and those with pneumoconioses, (particularly silicosis) are all at greater risk.

Mycobacterium tuberculosis (M.tb) is a non-motile, non-sporing, aerobic, Gram + ve bacillus, which tends to aggregate with other bacilli into "serpentine cords". Its

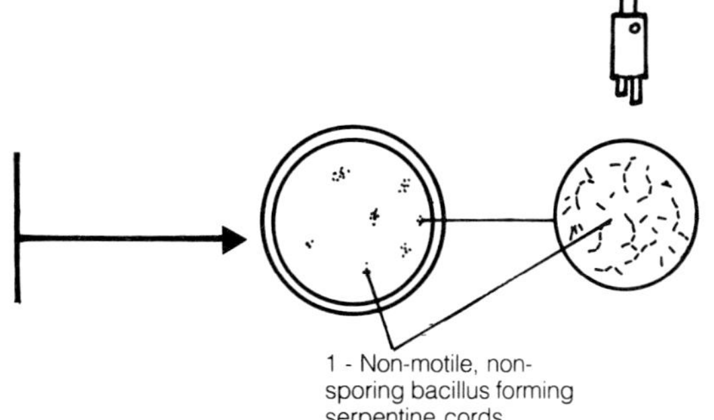

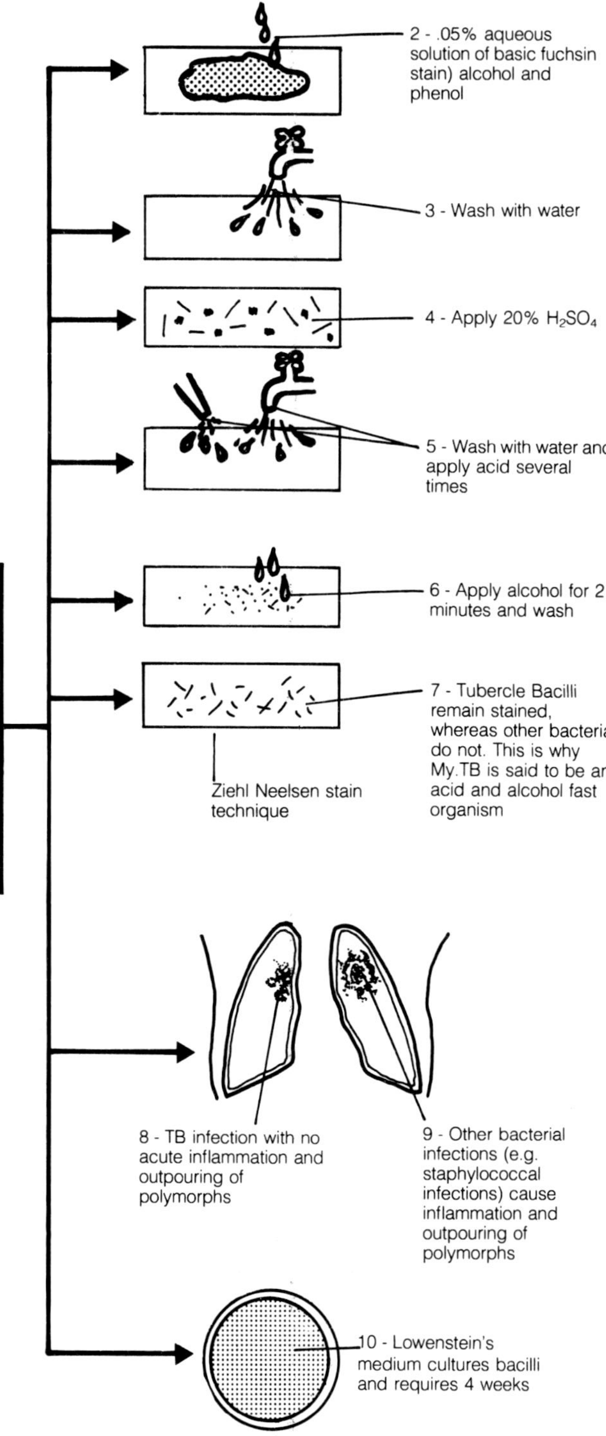

waxy outer coat makes the Gram stain difficult and it is better stained by the Ziehl Neelsen technique. The organism requires an enriched medium (e.g. Lowenstein's medium) to grow *in vitro* and takes approximately 4 weeks to produce a recognisable colony. When M.tb infects the human, there is not the acute inflammatory outpouring of polymorphs that accompanies many bacterial pathogens:

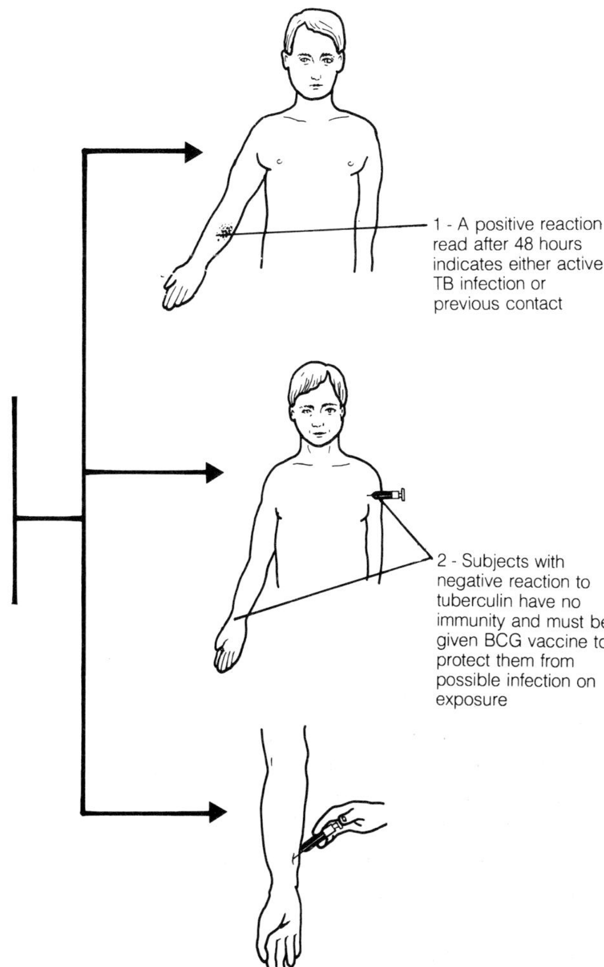

M.tb engenders a type IV cell-mediated immune response that we test for in the tuberculin test. This test develops earlier and is stronger if the patient has had a TB infection before and recently: for this reason we need to distinguish primary from post-primary TB.

The **micropathology** of a typical M.tb proliferative lesion needs also to be mentioned in these general introductory remarks as these "tubercles" are the hallmark of the disease and can occur anywhere in the body: M.tb is a classic example of intracellular parasitisation of the macrophage system. Having infected tissue

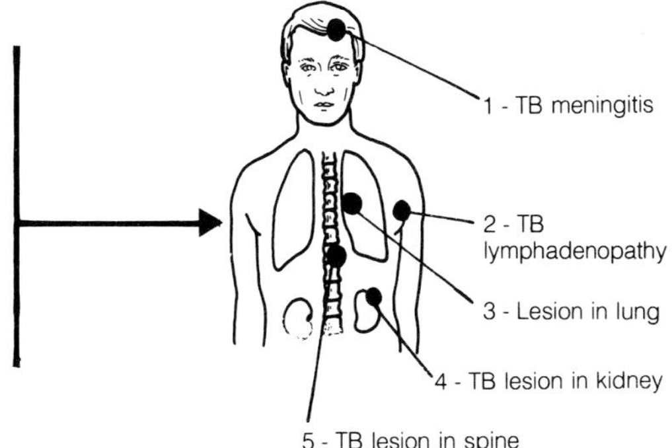

macrophages and after a latency of a few days the intracellular M.tb starts dividing rapidly as a tissue reaction/immune reaction (of the Type IV or cell-mediated type) to M.tb occurs. This includes vascular changes and a mononuclear leucocyte invasion with a compartmentalising of the M.tb infective focus. When fully developed, this compartmentalised **"tubercle"** comprises a variable outer "wall" of fibrous tissue inside which is a corona of reactive lymphocytes "attending" larger epithelioid, macrophages and giant cells (typically with a horseshoe appearance of their multiple nuclei – **Langhans cells**) and a central, amorphous/structureless area of necrosis – **caseative necrosis**.

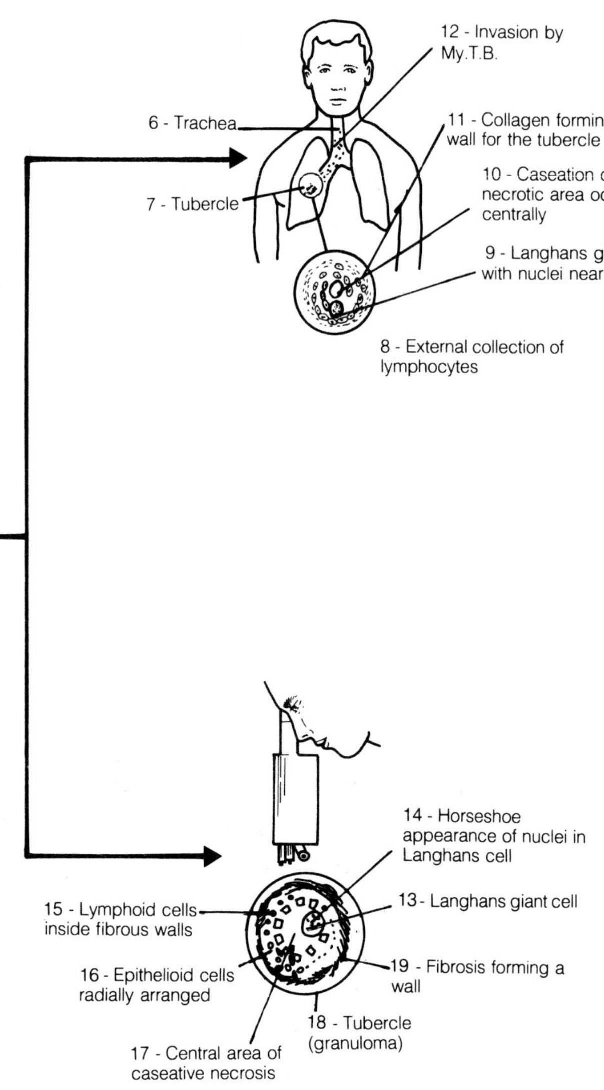

Such tubercles can arrest and remain static for years or, under immune conditions unfavourable to the host, enlarge and liquefy, due to massive proliferation of M.tb and a tuberculous abscess (with septicaemic potential) develop. Thus depending on the "resistance" of the patient, humans have the ability to localise T.B. and retard the multiplication of My.tb for many years, or the disease may progress due to unchecked multiplication of My.tb and death result from disseminated M.tb within a few weeks of diagnosis.

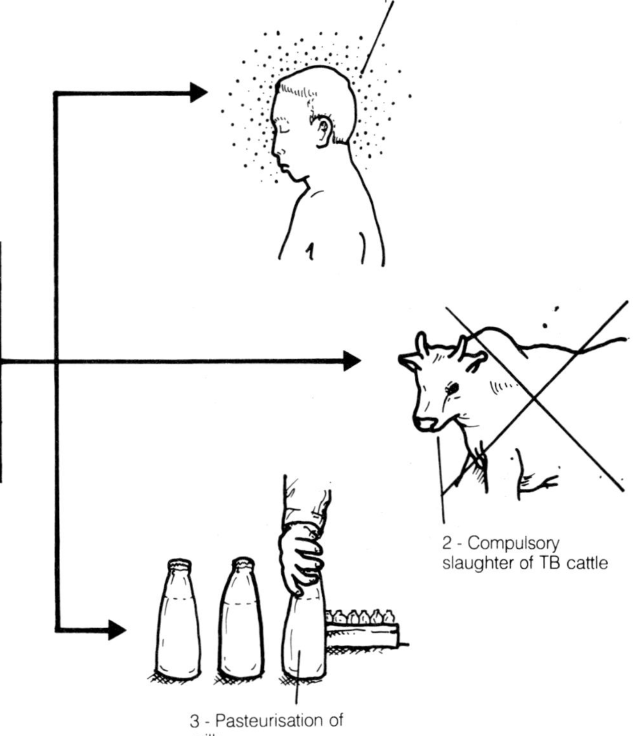

Man is the major source of My.tb and infection is spread by inhaled droplets. Following compulsory slaughter of tuberbulous cattle, bovine strains have largely disappeared from developed countries and the continued pasteurisation of milk is an important means of eliminating this oral route of human infection.

Despite the uncertainty of progression of T.B., there is a pattern or sequence of events that follows pulmonary infection:–

Primary Pulmonary T.B. –Primary T.B. is a disease of patients who have not experienced M.tb before and have no tuberculin (the cellular antigen for the Type IV reactivity) sensitivity. It is most commonly seen in children. The pulmonary infection consists of two components. The lung component is often sub-pleural, involves any lobe and is often small (the Ghon focus).

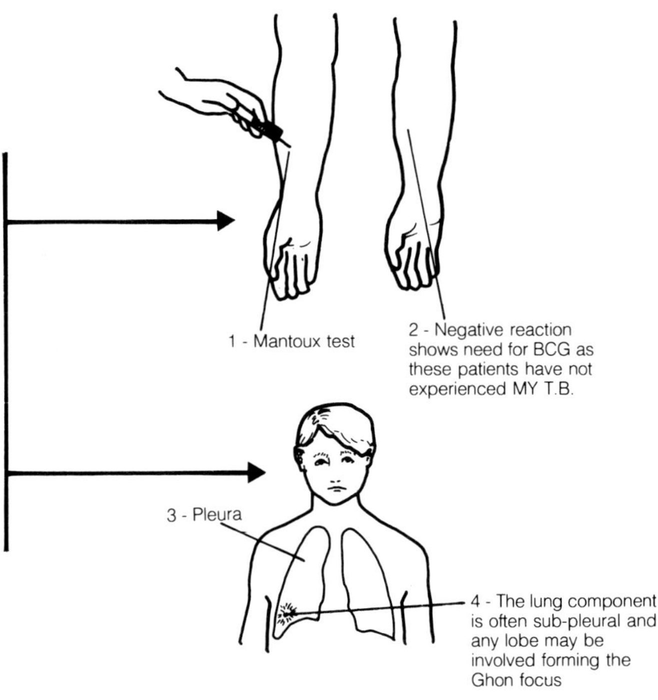

Lymphatic spread to the hilar nodes engenders disproportionately large hilar lymphadenopathy. It is at this stage (and up to a couple of months after the infecting inoculum) that the tuberculin skin test becomes positive. The systemic upset at this time is frequently minor

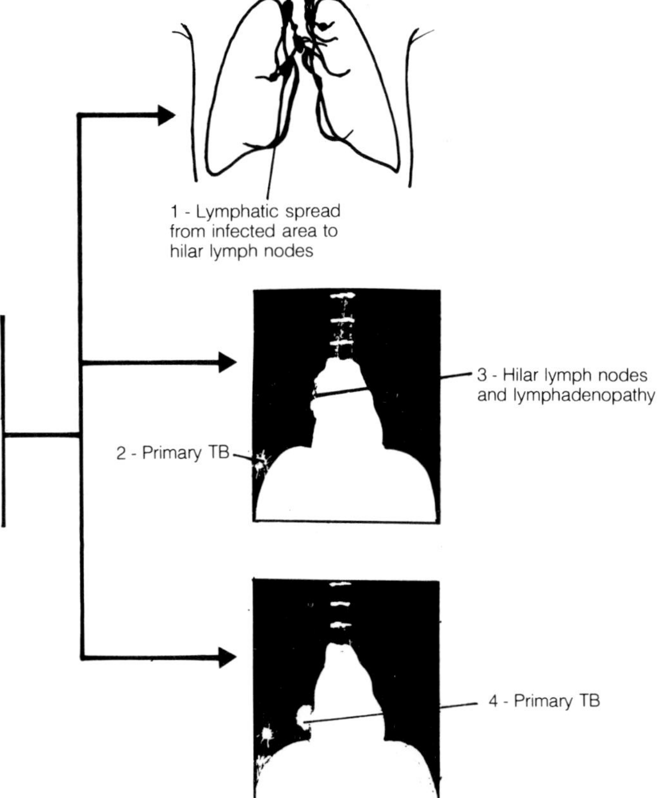

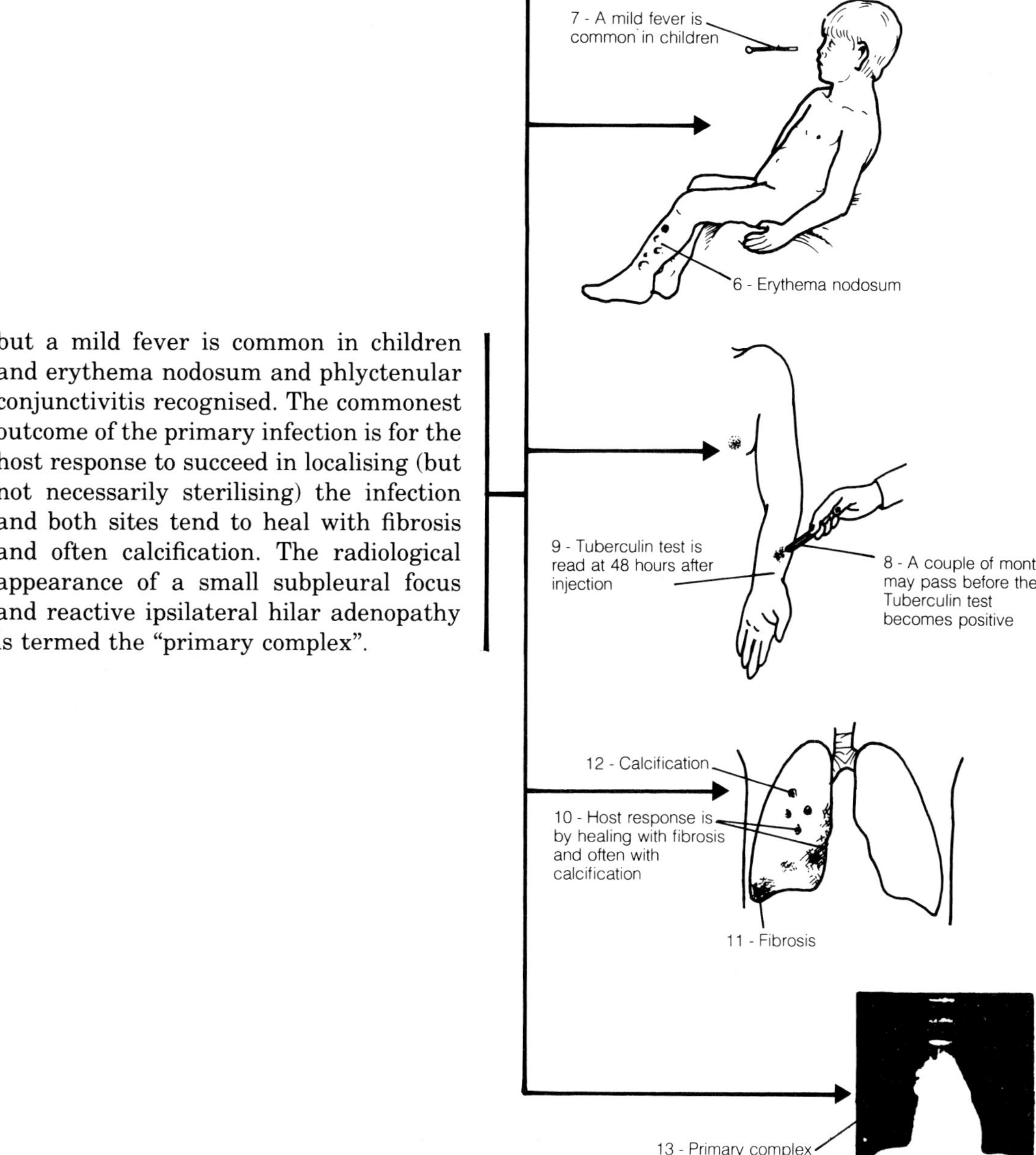

but a mild fever is common in children and erythema nodosum and phlyctenular conjunctivitis recognised. The commonest outcome of the primary infection is for the host response to succeed in localising (but not necessarily sterilising) the infection and both sites tend to heal with fibrosis and often calcification. The radiological appearance of a small subpleural focus and reactive ipsilateral hilar adenopathy is termed the "primary complex".

However, healing is not the only possible outcome. Progression of the lung component tends to be most commonly encountered in adolescents and young adults. The pace is often slow and even episodic with enlargement of the **Ghon focus**, cavitation and later spread to other parts of the lung as a T.B. bronchopneumonia. **Pleural involvement** may lead to pleural effusion, usually within 3-6 months of infection. Progression in the lymph nodes tends to be a feature of primary T.B. in young children.

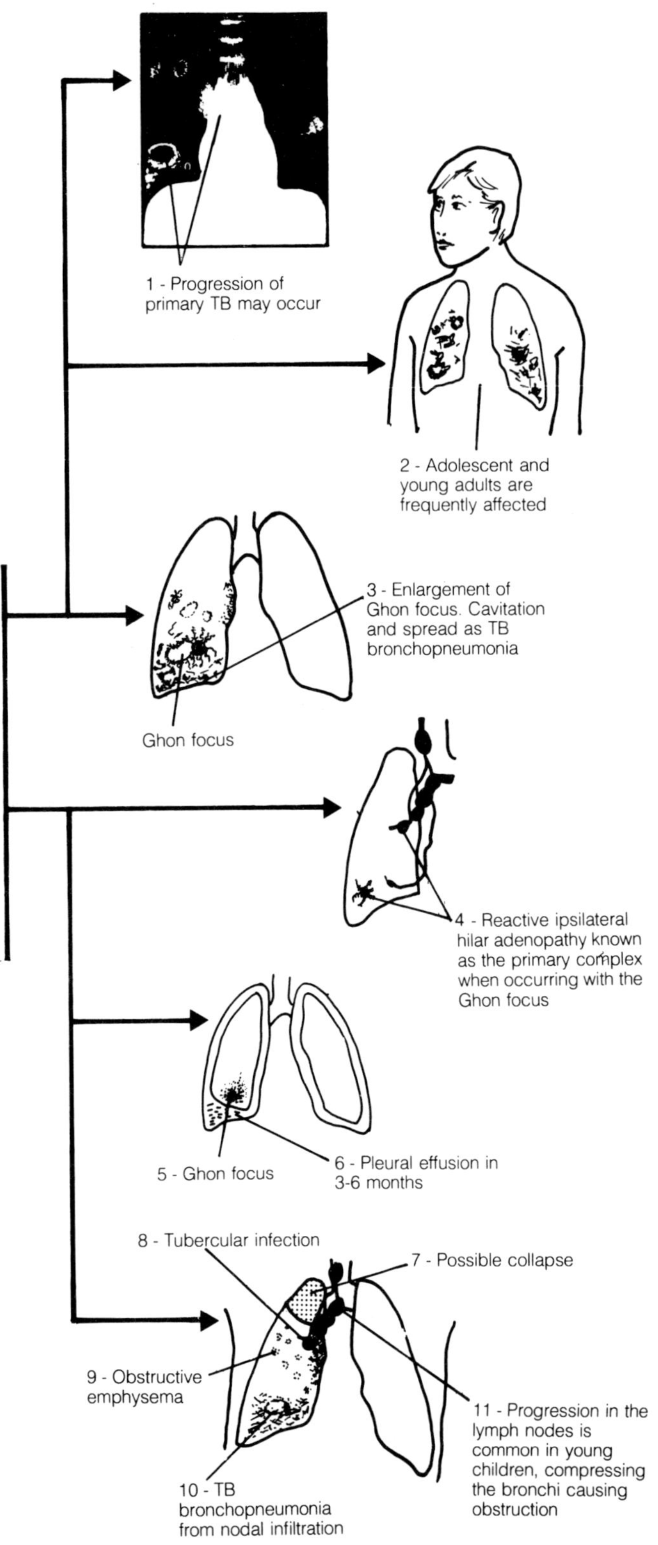

Firstly, this may lead to mechanical compression of bronchi with obstructive emphysema, collapse or bronchopneumonia (perhaps due to M.tb itself if the nodes have eroded the bronchial wall) distal to the site of compression (most commonly affecting the middle lobes).

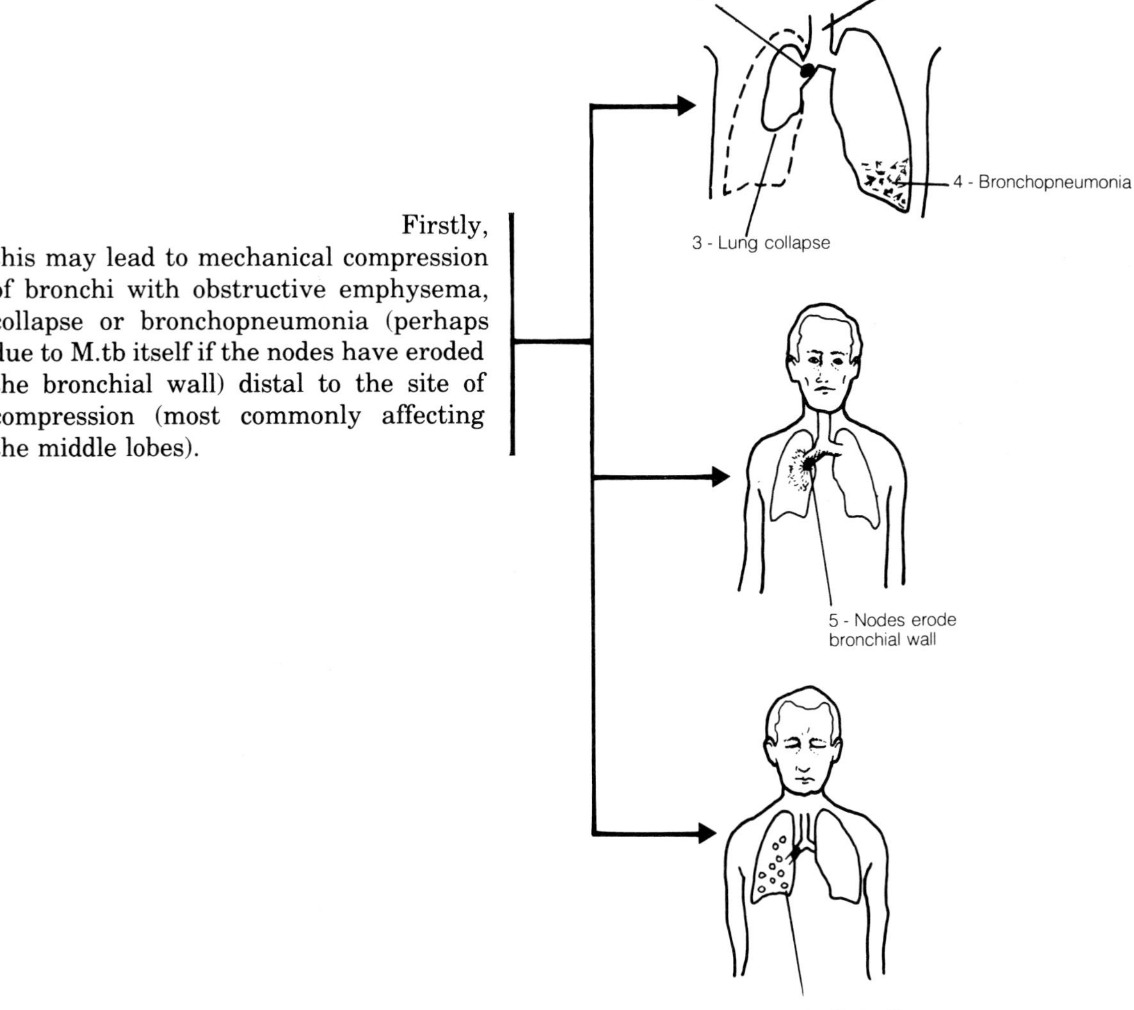

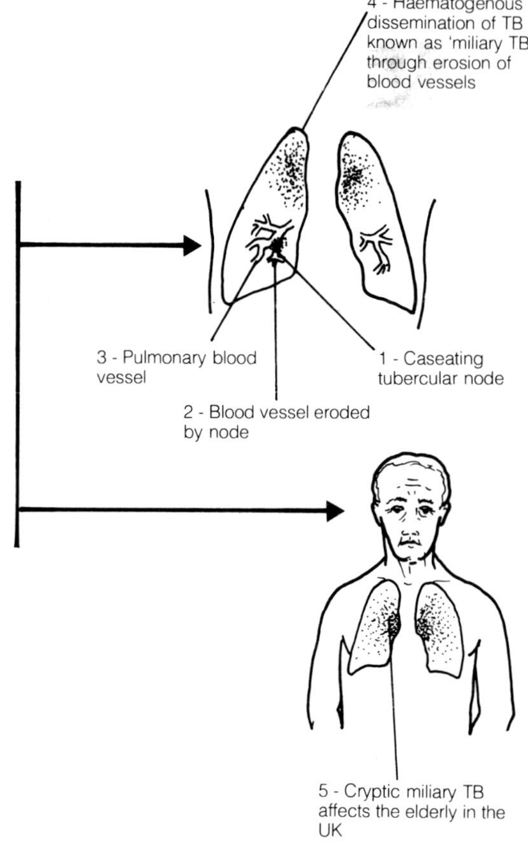

Secondly, there is a great risk of an enlarging caseating node eroding a blood vessel and causing haematogenous dissemination of T.B. at this time. In the past, "miliary T.B." due to this phenomenon was most commonly seen in youngsters at about this time in the disease, (although in the U.K. at present miliary T.B. is becoming commoner as a more occult and insidious phenomenon, – cryptic miliary T.B., in elderly subjects with post-primary T.B.).

Miliary T.B. – In unchecked primary T.B., about 1 in 20 young children and a slightly lower percentage of older subjects will develop this catastrophic form of septicaemic spread within the first year of infection. In its classical form, the systemic disturbance develops rapidly and becomes profound with drenching sweats and a high remittent or intermittent pyrexia.

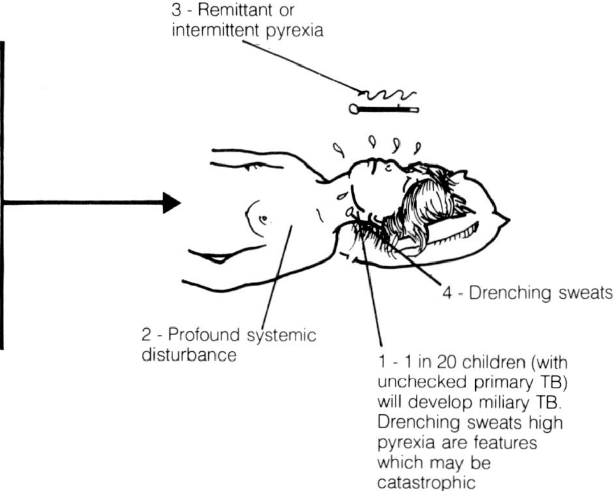

Peripheral blood leucocytosis is often absent. The disease is due to many foci of T.B. (tubercles) developing in all the major viscera, and the physical signs are variable although fine crepitations may be audible in the chest and mild hepatosplenomegaly may occur. Development of tubercles in the choroid of the eyes is visible on retinoscopy in 40% of patients and a search for these choroidal tubercles is important diagnostically. Similarly a chest X-ray which shows multiple, small, discrete nodules throughout both lung fields (out of proportion to the relative paucity of physical signs) is also important diagnostically.

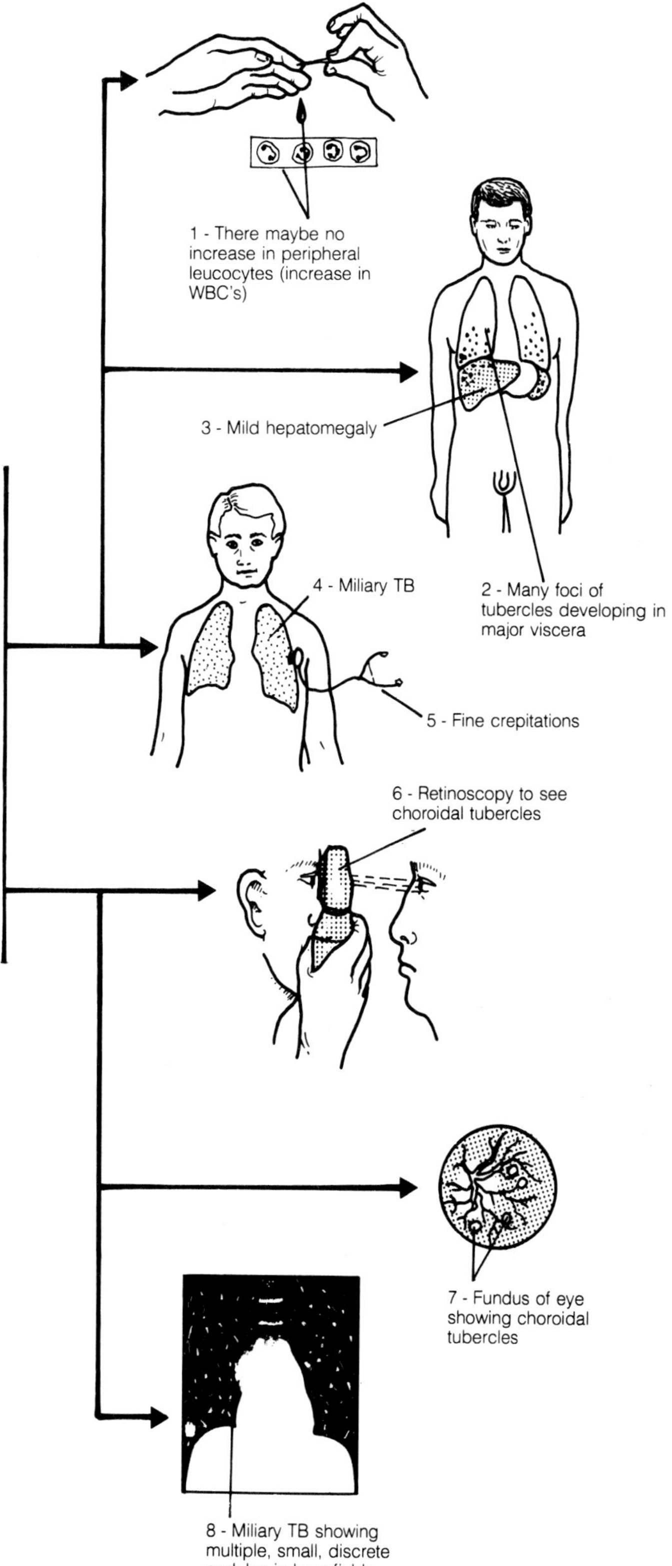

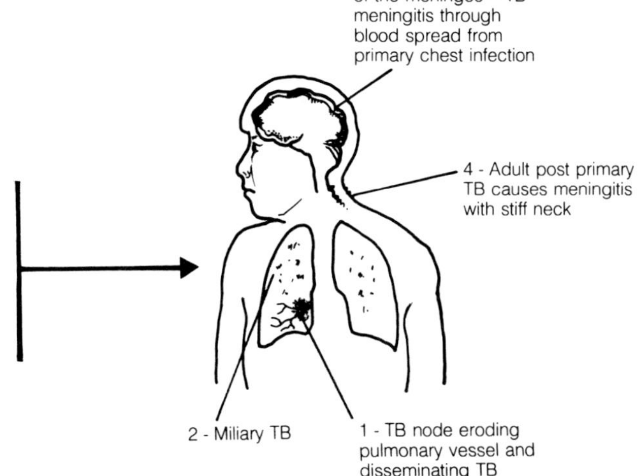

The **diagnosis** is confirmed by Z.N. staining (and much later culture) of sputum, urine, bone marrow or liver biopsy specimens and the urgent introduction of chemotherapy is needed.

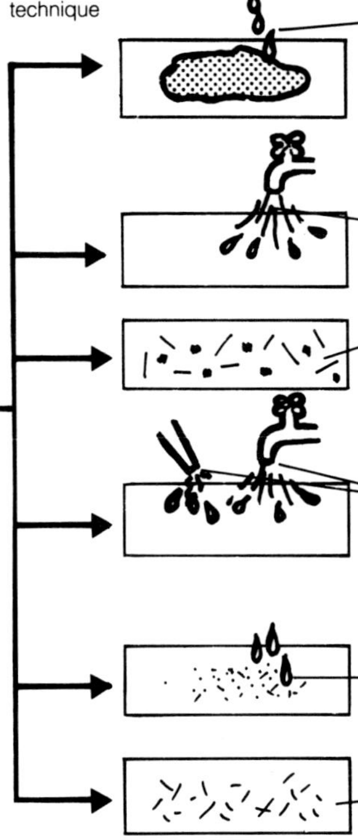

TUBERCULOUS MENINGITIS

T.B. meningitis is also an early complication of haematogenous spread of primary T.B. and may be a part of miliary T.B: it is also a feature of adult/post primary T.B. where the clinical features of meningism are often more clear cut. In children with T.B. meningitis the symptoms may be vague with listlessness and irritability, but vomiting, deteriorating conscious level or photophobia even without classic signs of meningism should be enough to indicate a lumbar puncture.

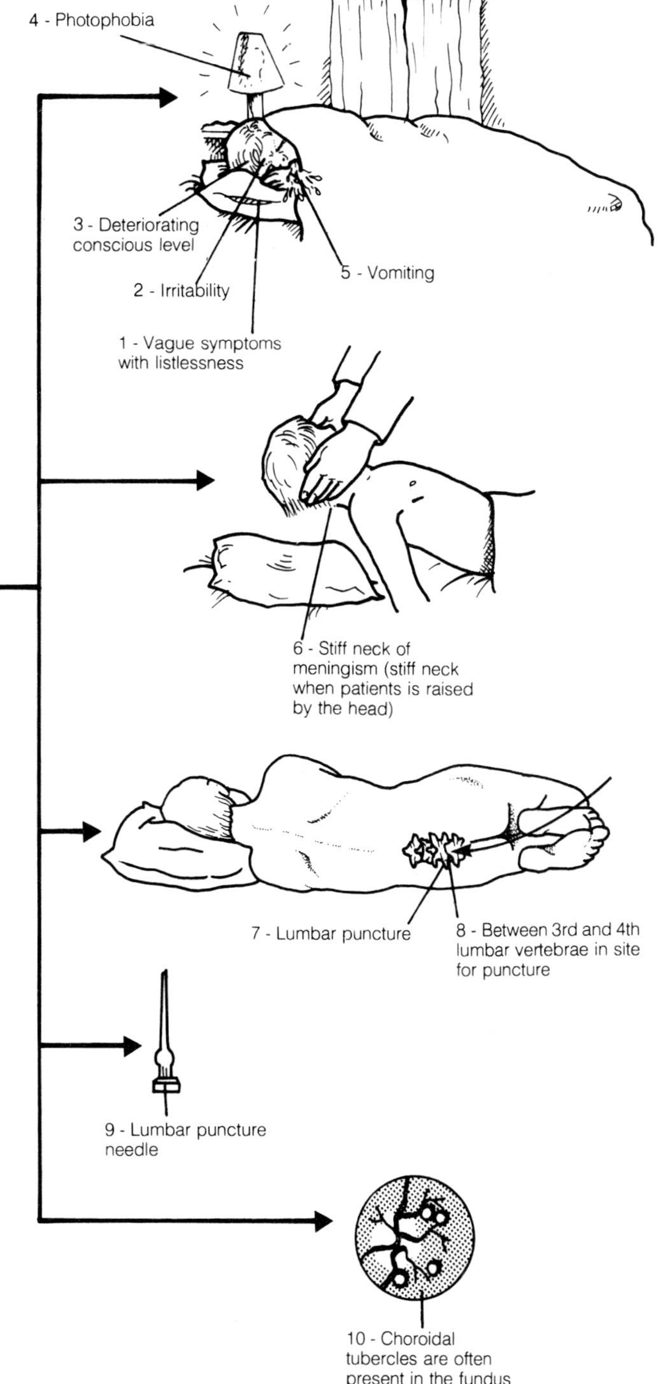

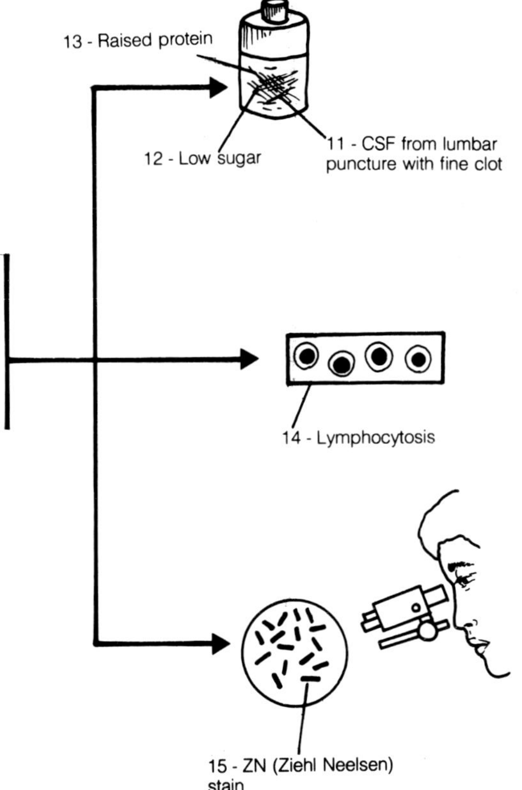

Choroidal tubercles are often present also. A lumbar puncture often shows a clear CSF, perhaps with a fine clot, a raised protein, a low sugar and a lymphocytosis Z.N. staining may be diagnostic whilst culture takes 4 weeks.

Treatment should not be delayed even in the absence of a positive smear if other features point to the diagnosis. Treatment is systemic. The role of intrathecal therapy is controversial but it is safe to give an initial course of streptomycin (10-50 mg per dose according to age) or isoniazid (10-50 mg per dose according to age) may be added for 10 injections.

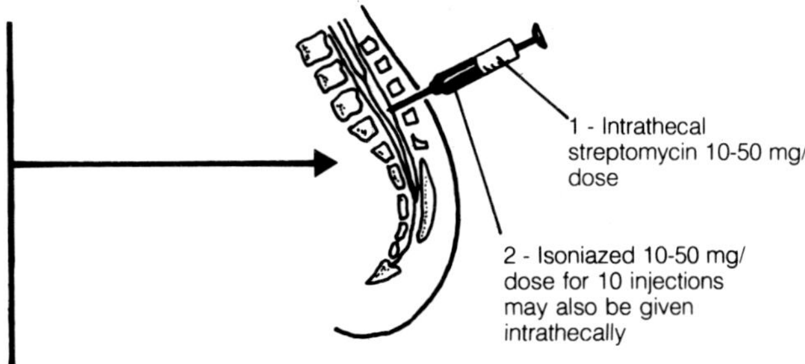

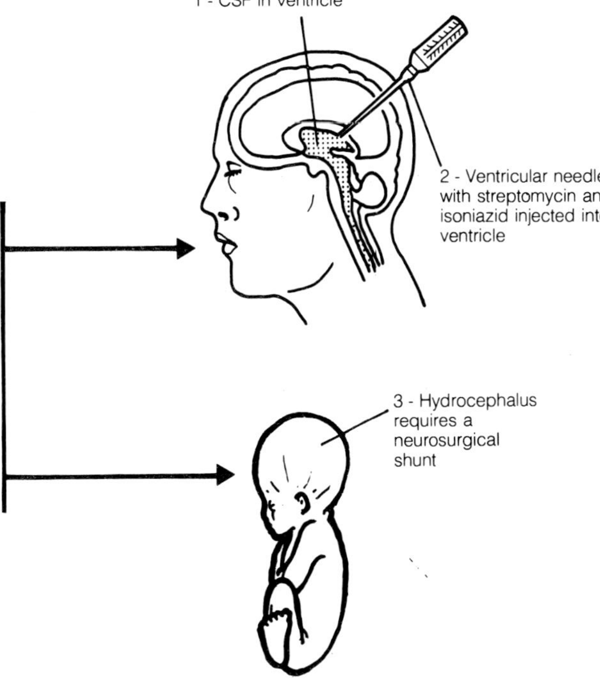

If there is evidence of a block of CSF pathways, intraventricular injections may be required. Systemic pyrazinamide gives high CSF levels and many clinicians would add this to standard initial systemic therapy. The role of corticosteroids in reducing meningeal inflammatory blocks to CSF circulation is controversial and best left to experts. Hydrocephalus may necessitate a neurosurgical shunt.

POST-PRIMARY TUBERCULOSIS

Post-primary T.B. may be due to the progression of the primary lesion but is much more commonly due to reactivation (perhaps many years later) of the primary lesion; uncommonly, it is due to re-infection. The "pace" of post-primary T.B.

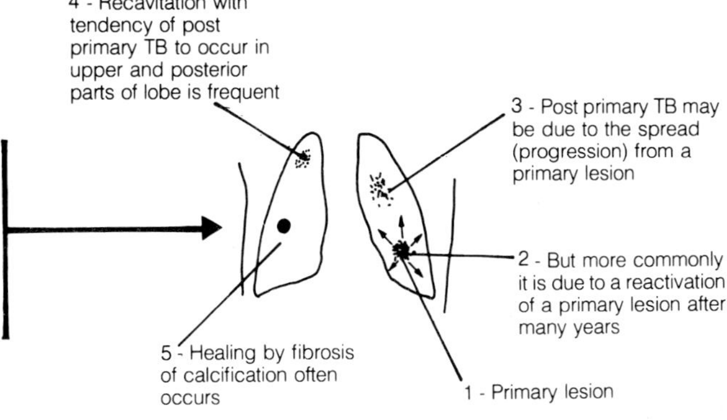

(the rate of progression, extent and spread and degree of healing by fibrosis) differs enormously from individual to individual.

There is a definite predilection for post-primary T.B. to occur in the upper lobes

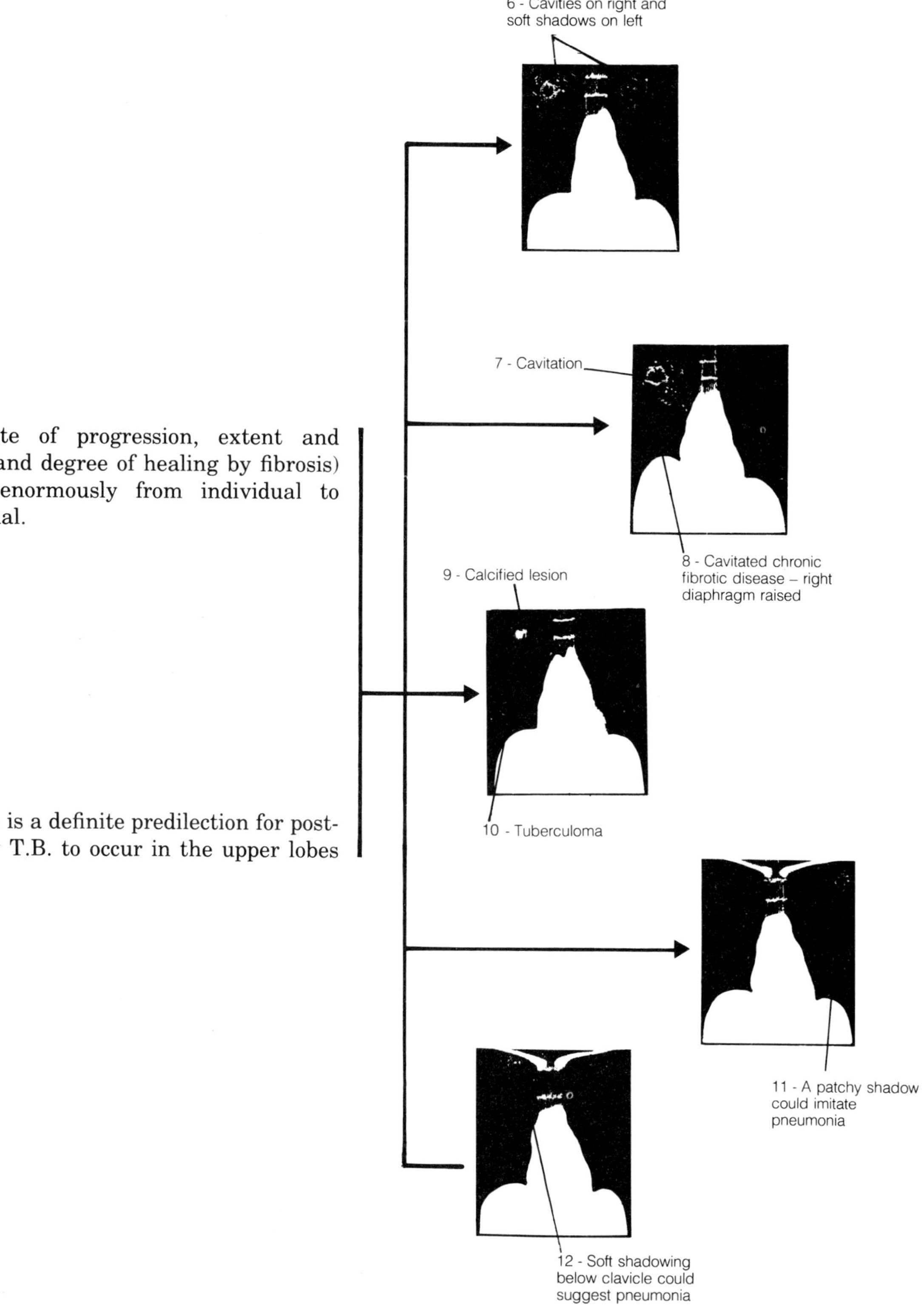

and posterior parts of the lungs; it is often bilateral and the hilar lymph node component is small or minimal. The tuberculous areas slowly enlarge, destroying lung upon which the disease encroaches – the pathological lesion is typical and caseating tuberculomatous histology is seen with cavitation and variable fibrosis.

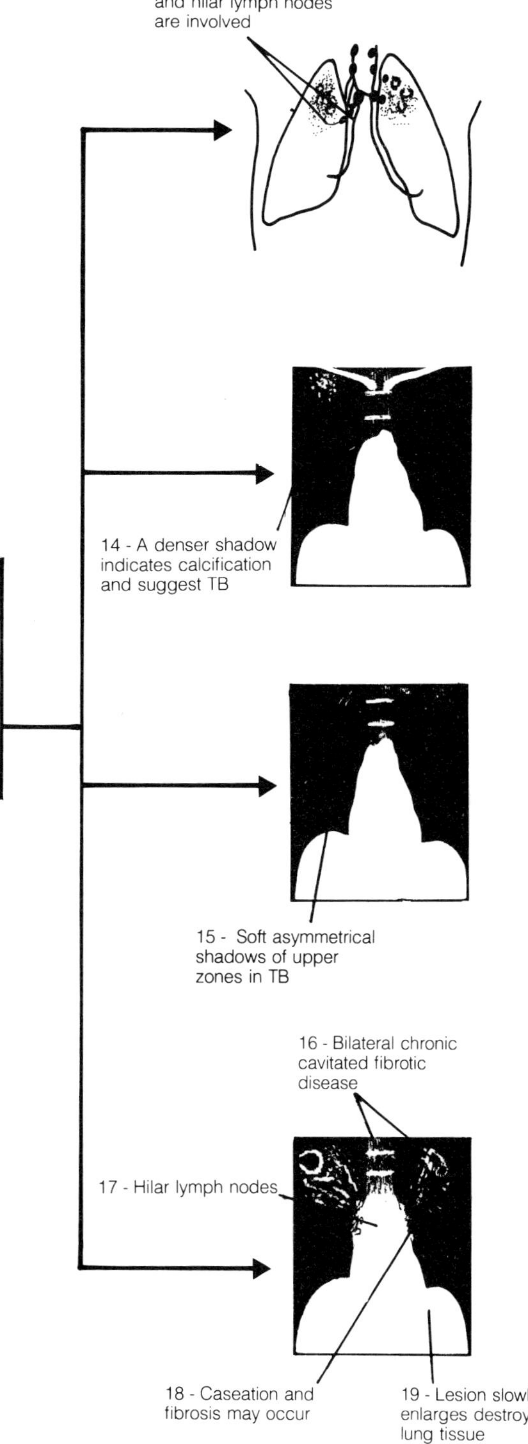

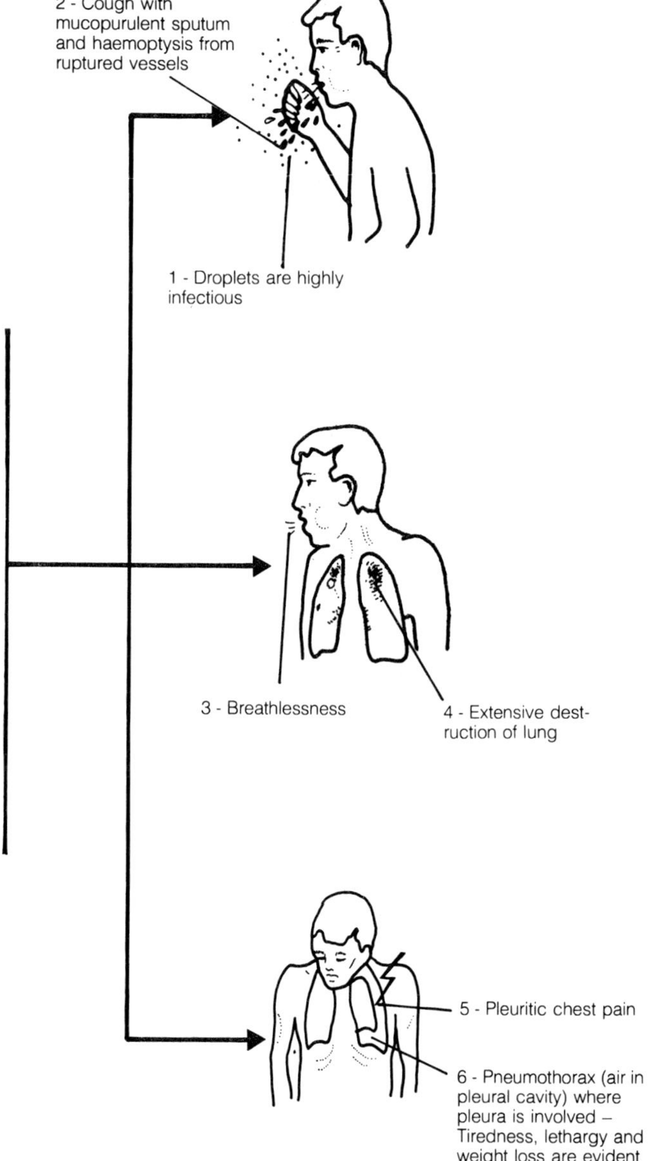

The clinical onset is usually insidious with **cough** productive of mucoid (and later mucopurulent) sputum with haemoptysis caused by blood vessel erosion often bringing the patient to clinical attention. The patient is highly infectious at this stage. **Breathlessness** may be a symptom if lung destruction is extensive. **Pleuritic chest pain** may be a feature if the pleura becomes involved and a pneumothorax may occur under these circumstances. Systemic symptoms of tiredness, lethargy and weight loss are usually present but often have been present for some months. Nevertheless, it is "general ill-health" that brings some patients to the doctor.

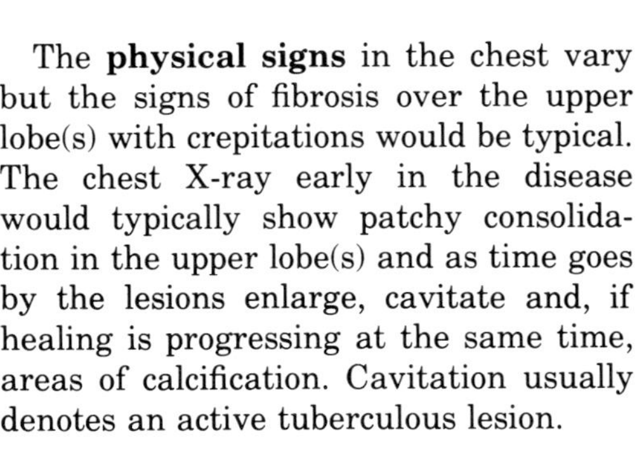

The **physical signs** in the chest vary but the signs of fibrosis over the upper lobe(s) with crepitations would be typical. The chest X-ray early in the disease would typically show patchy consolidation in the upper lobe(s) and as time goes by the lesions enlarge, cavitate and, if healing is progressing at the same time, areas of calcification. Cavitation usually denotes an active tuberculous lesion.

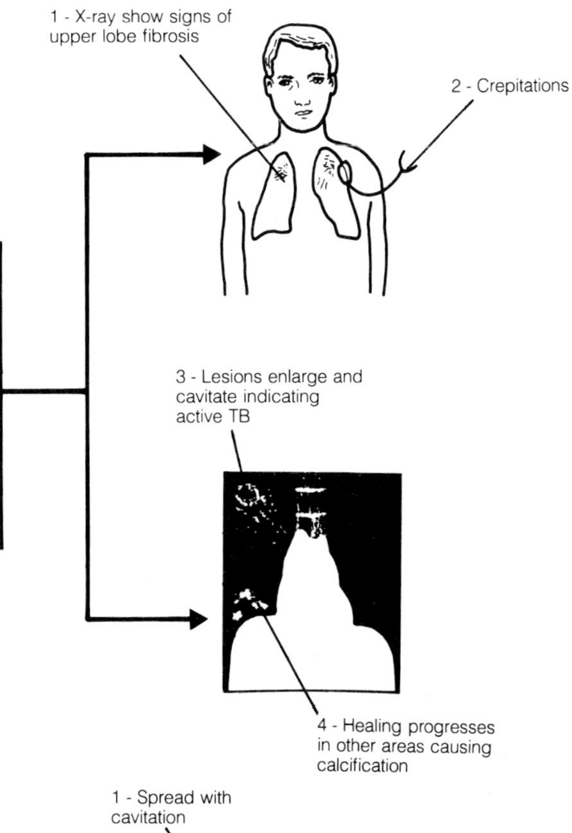

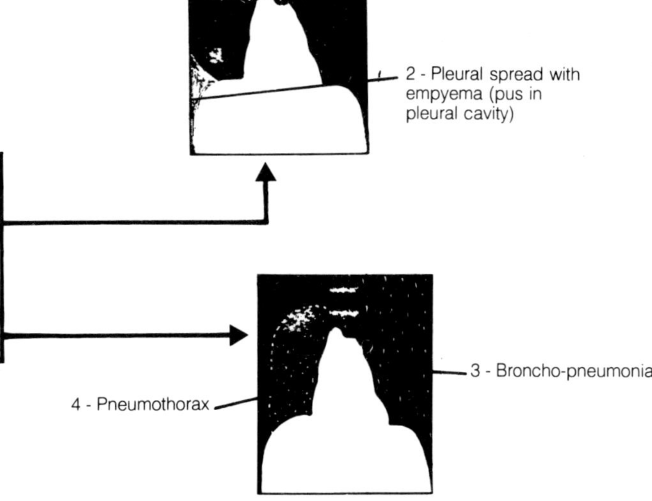

The disease may progress in the chest with T.B. bronchopneumonia, or pleural spread with pleurisy, empyema or pneumothorax. Tuberculous laryngitis may occur from infected sputum. Swallowing of infected sputum may lead to gastrointestinal T.B., particularly in those with low gastric acidity. A cicatrising tuberculous mass in the ileum or ileo-caecal region is a well-recognised site of localisation of the disease leading to diarrhoea, malabsorption or obstruction, but other sites include tuberculous ischio-rectal abscesses and fistula-in-ano.

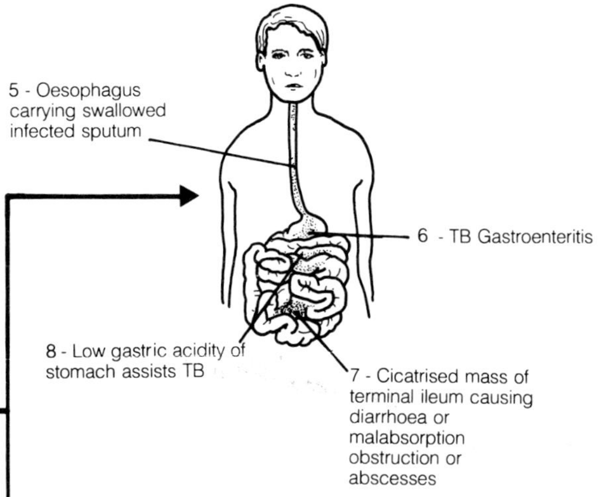

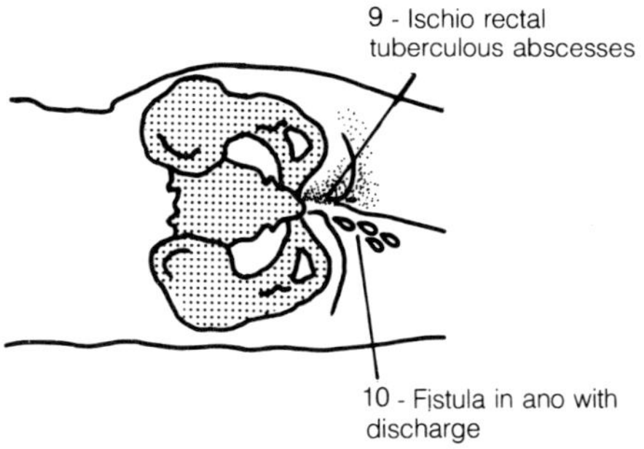

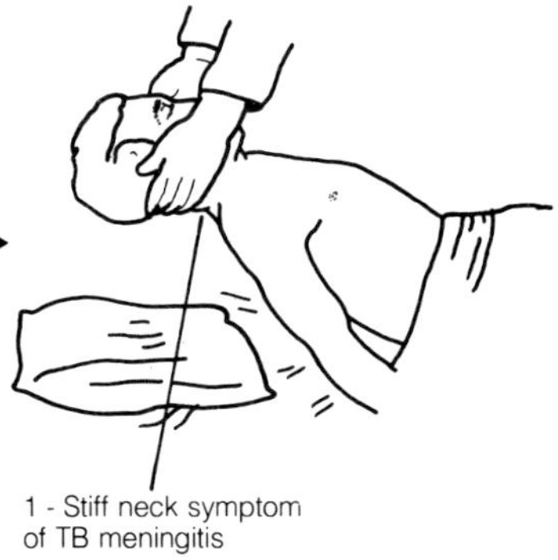

Haematogenous dissemination may lead to meningitis (see above), peritonitis, **epididymo-orchitis** or **fallopian tube** infection with tubal abscess. Tuberculous spread to the **adrenal glands** is a recognised cause of Addison's disease.

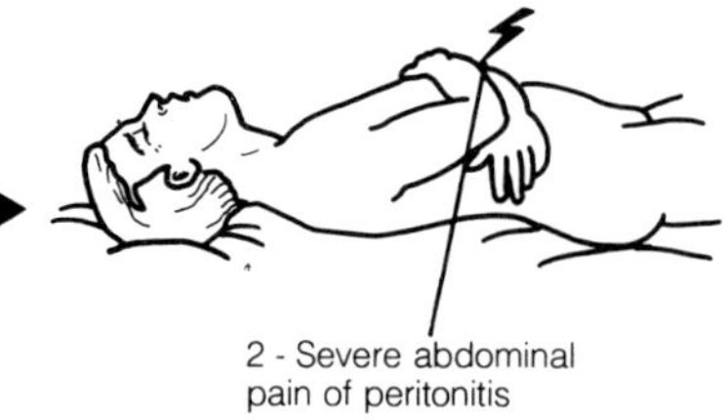

Pericarditis may be due to direct spread of the chest lesion or **haematogenous spread**; not only is the acute pericarditis very serious but the healing with fibrosis of the chronic cases leads to constriction of the pericardium.

Haematogenous spread to **bones and joints** is important to recognise. The typical clinical picture is of a pale, warm (i.e. without the signs of acute inflammation), "boggy" joint with some pain on movement and marked wasting of the surrounding muscles which may be in spasm. The **synovial thickening** is marked although the effusion may only be moderate in size.

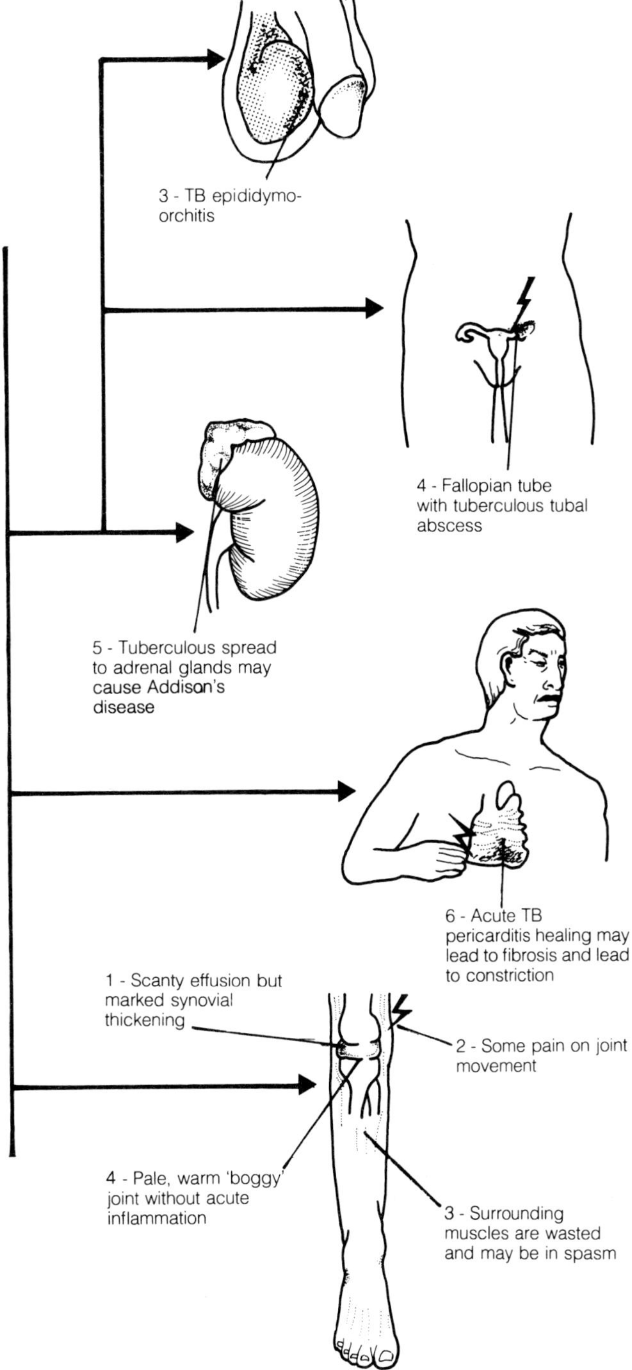

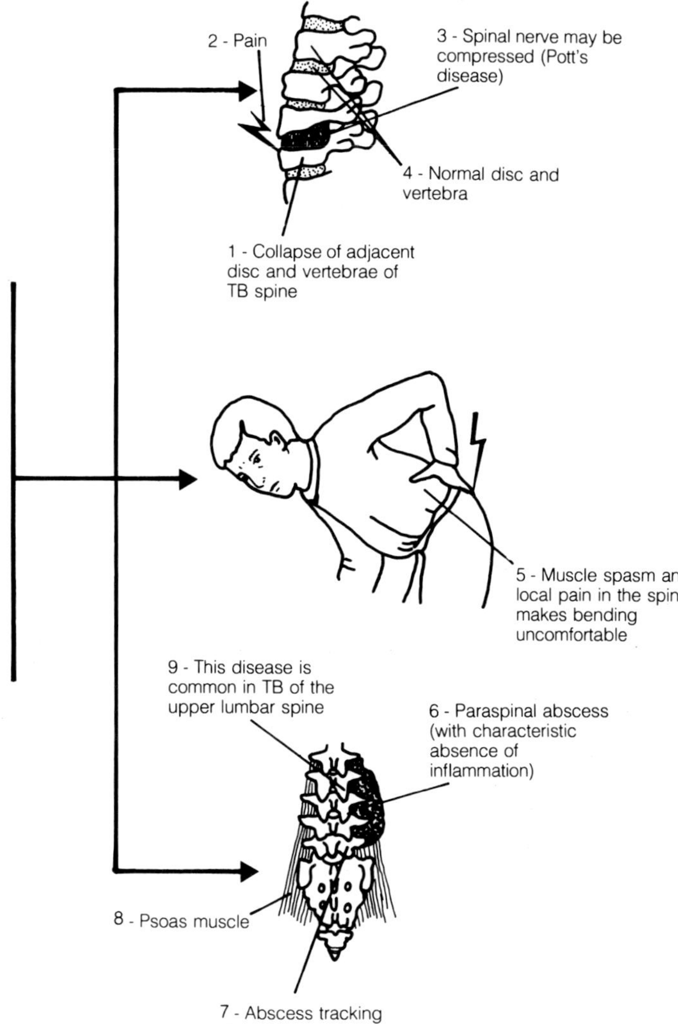

In the **spine,** muscle spasm and local pain makes bending uncomfortable from an early stage. The **spinal disease** may involve several adjacent vertebrae and discs which may collapse with production of pain, a gibbus and even spinal compression, (Pott's disease). A **paraspinal "cold abscess"** (so called because, once again, there are none of the signs of acute inflammation) may form and track downwards in the psoas sheath; (the disease is most common in the upper lumbar spine).

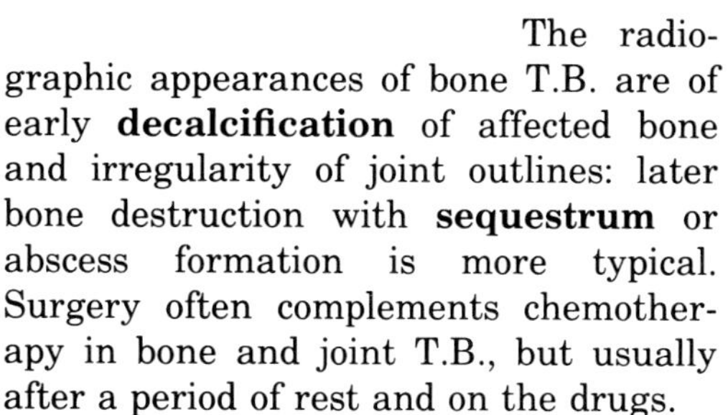

The radiographic appearances of bone T.B. are of early **decalcification** of affected bone and irregularity of joint outlines: later bone destruction with **sequestrum** or abscess formation is more typical. Surgery often complements chemotherapy in bone and joint T.B., but usually after a period of rest and on the drugs.

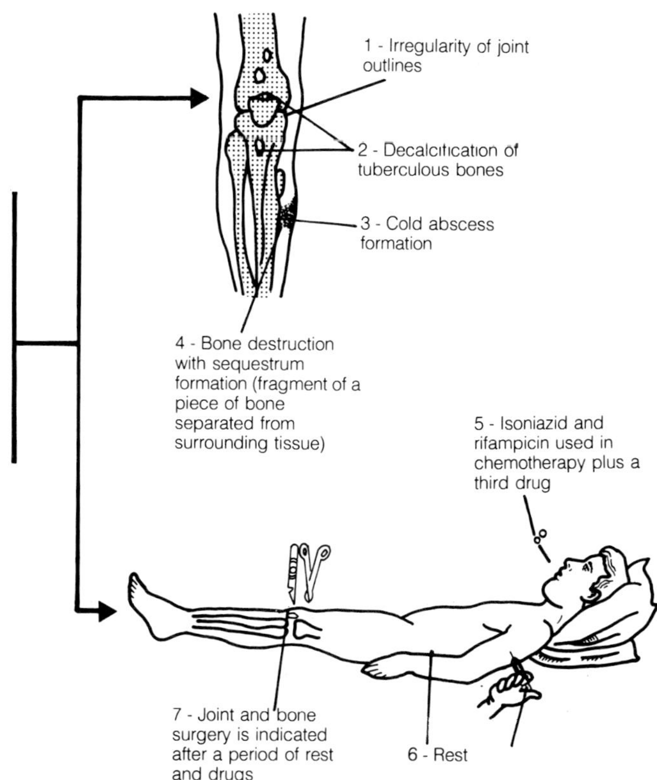

Genito-urinary T.B. is also caused by haematogenous spread. It is commoner in men and is often advanced before recognised clinically because renal pain does not occur early and haematuria is also often a late occurrence. An increased

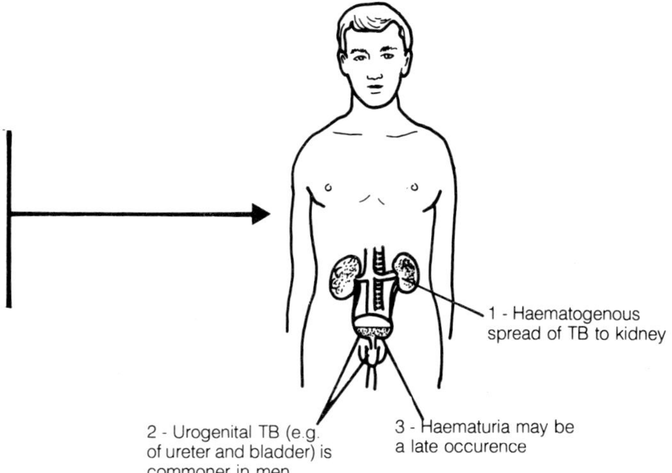

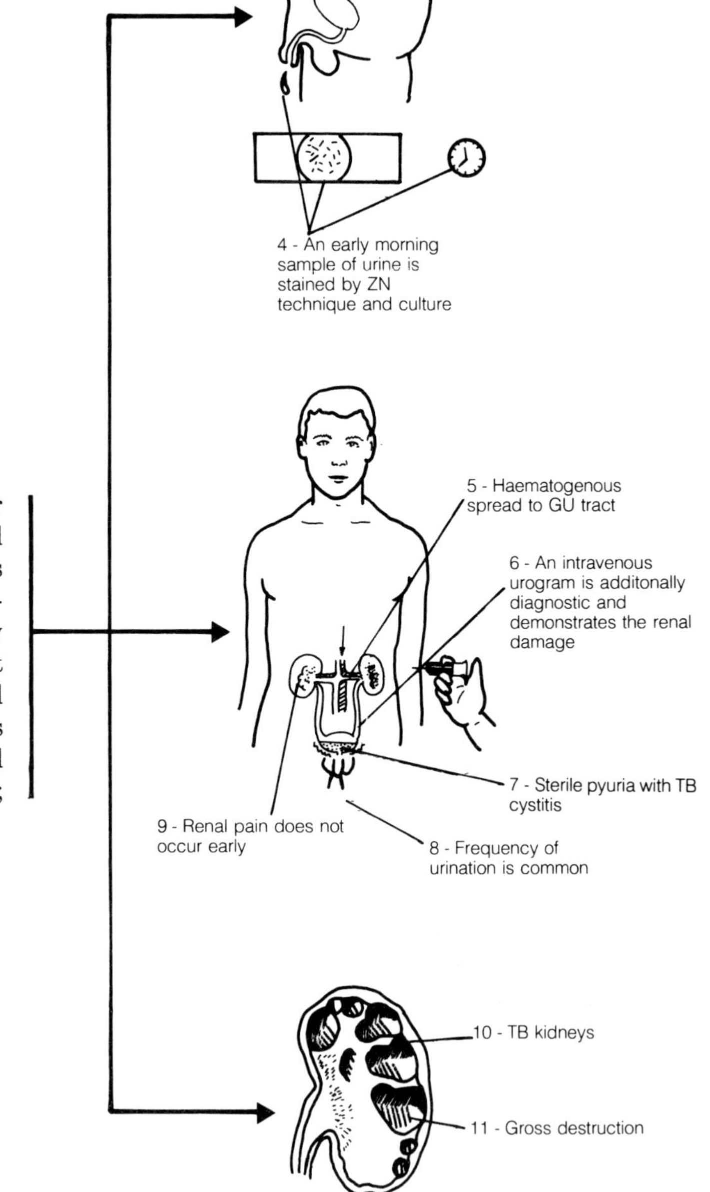

frequency of micturition occurs earlier and may lead to investigation, or spread of M.tb with the production of tuberculous cystitis and a "sterile" pyuria may produce presentation symptoms. An early morning urine specimen with the deposit stained by Ziehl Neelsen technique and cultured, together with an intravenous urogram (IVU) give the **diagnosis** and demonstrate the degree of renal damage;

the serum creatinine or creatinine clearance assess overall renal function. **Surgery** may be required to complement chemotherapy in the management of this form of T.B.

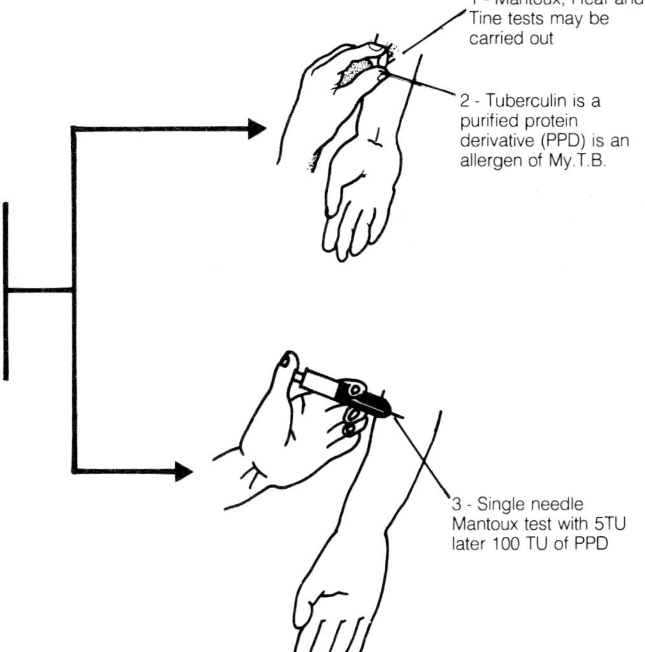

Extrapulmonary T.B. is commoner in ethnic groups from the Indian subcontinent.

TREATMENT OF T.B.
Prophylaxis: –

The **Tuberculin Reaction** and BCG Vaccination – The tuberculin test (Mantoux, Tine, Heaf techniques) all measure the immune response to tuberculin or purified protein derivative (PPD) – the major allergen of M.tb The multipuncture

Heaf test makes six needle punctures intradermally through a drop of PPD (containing 100,000 tuberculin units (T.U.)/ml) and this simple test elicits the same reactivity as a Mantoux test with 5 T.U. followed by 100 T.U. of PPD. The Heaf test is read at 48-96 hours and the reaction graded 1-4. Children with strong reactivity require chemoprophylaxis as they have recently been infected whilst strong reactivity in adults requires at least very close follow up with chest X-rays.

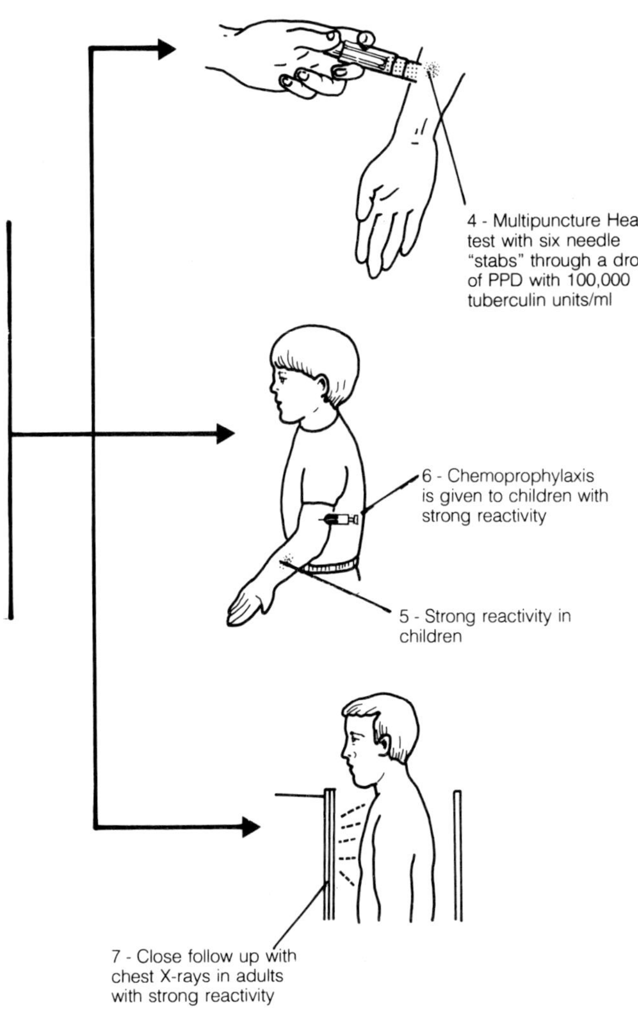

Tuberculin negative reactors should be given Bacille-Calmette-Guérin (BCG) vaccination. In developing countries, BCG vaccination is a cheap and important method of preventing T.B., which should be used widely in infants. It is not completely protective but gives perhaps 80% protection for 15 years. The need to

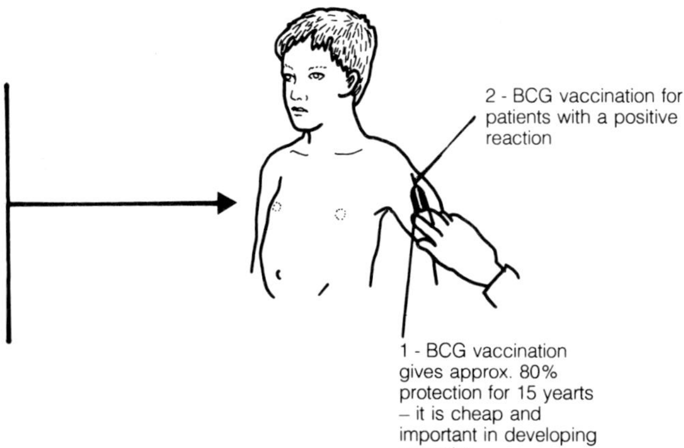

continue BCG vaccination of all school children in countries with falling incidences should be kept under review but is still recommended for tuberculin negative, 13 year olds in the U.K. An intradermal injection (which latterly can be given by a multiple puncture or jet technique) of the freeze-dried vaccine gives the best results. A **papule** (or small ulcer) at the site of injection, within 7-14 days, indicates successful vaccination. **Complications** are rare but include a local ulcer, abscesses or regional lymphadenopathy – all slow to heal.

Chemoprophylaxis – Isoniazid 5 mg/Kg/day is usually recommended in strong tuberculin reactors in children, recent tuberculin converters of any age or patients with known past T.B. (perhaps only from changes on their chest X-ray) who require prolonged immunosuppressive therapy (steroids, azathioprine, cancer therapy).

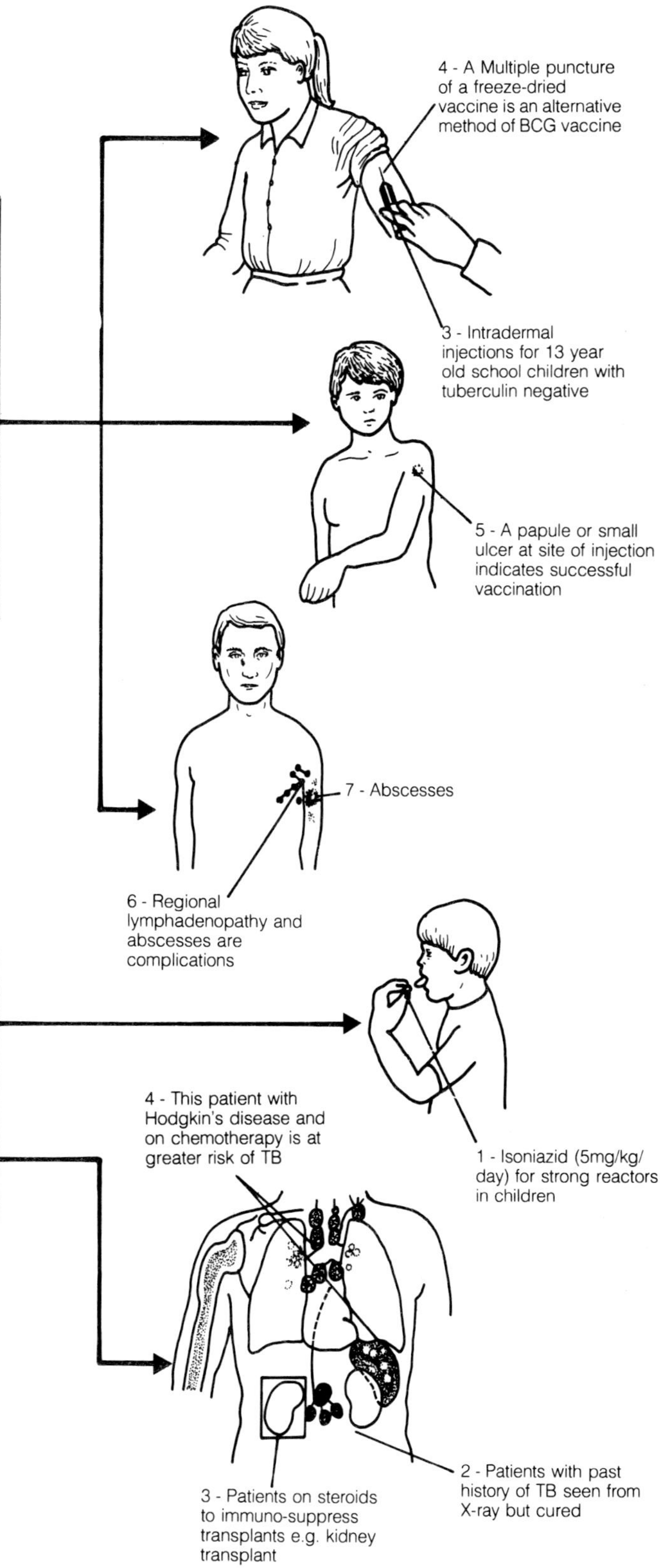

Therapy of Established T.B. – A nine month course of rifampicin and isoniazid supplemented by a third drug (ethambutol or streptomycin) for the first two months is now standard chemotherapy *(see table)* and the sputum should quickly revert to negative for M.tb. Combined preparations are acceptable in this context. Poor patient compliance in tablet taking for this long period is a major problem in some communities, not least because drug toxicities and hypersensitivity reactions are common. Minor **gastrointestinal upset** is very common and may be assisted by tablet taking with meals.

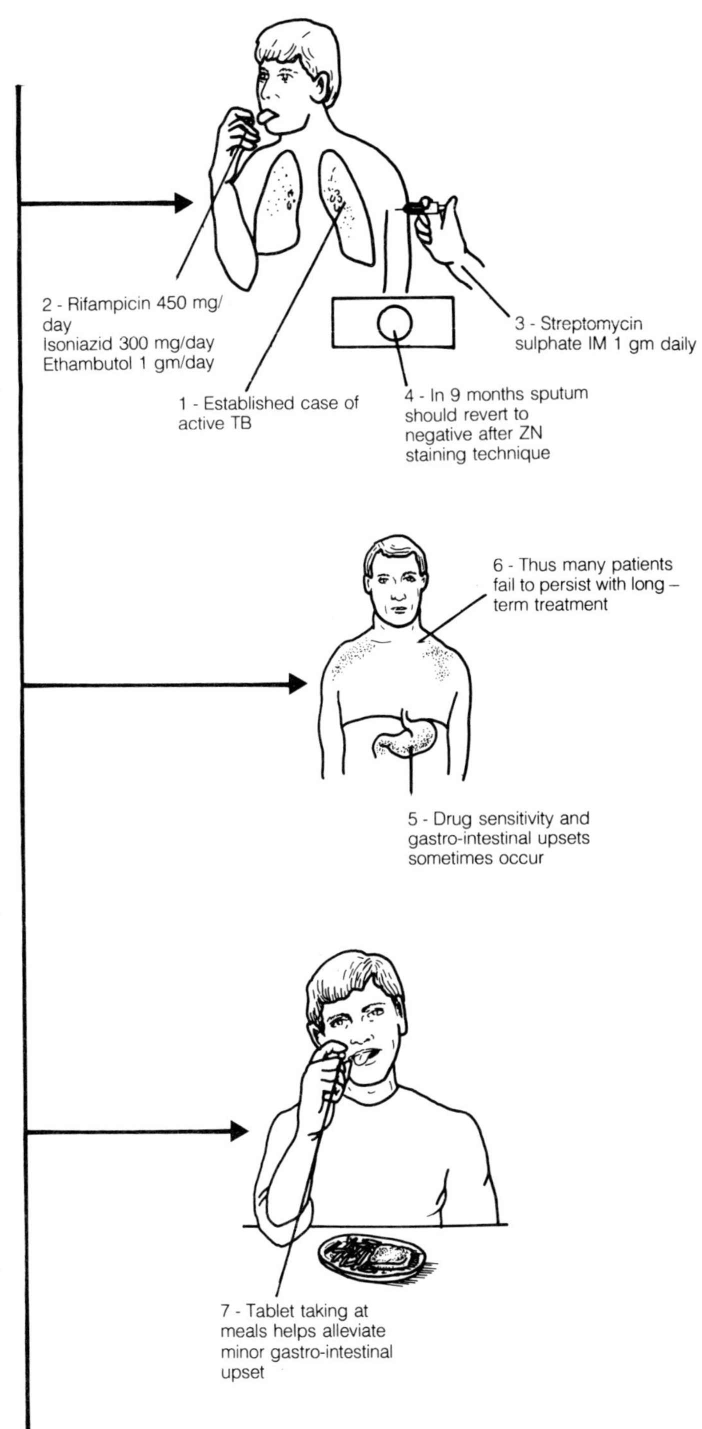

ANTITUBERCULOUS CHEMOTHERAPY

Drug	Dose	Side Effects
Isoniazid	Adult: 300mg/day Child: 10mg/kg/day	Sensitivity reactions Hepatitis, Neuropathy
Rifamipicin	Adult: (<55kg): 450mg/day (>55kg): 600mg/day Child: 20mg/kg/day	Hepatitis, Pink urine Possibly weakly teratogen May antagonise contraception, Thrombocytopenia (rare)
Ethambutol	Adults only: 15mg/kg/day	Optic neuropathy
Streptomycin	Adult: 0.75–1.0g/day I.M. Child: 30mg/kg/day (max 1g)	Sensitivity reactions Vestibular damage
Para-amino salicylic acid (PAS)	Adult: 12g/day in two doses Child: 200mg/kg/day	Gastrointestinal intolerance Hypersensitivity reactions
Pyrazinamide (Used as a first line drug by some)	Adults only: 20-35mg/kg/day in 3 doses (max 3g/day)	Hepatitis

Hepatitis is an important toxicity of rifampicin but can also be caused by isoniazid and pyrazinamide; a transient **rise in liver transaminases** is not necessarily the harbinger of a full blown hepatitis and treatment may proceed with careful monitoring. A cutaneous flushing and pruritus may occur with rifampicin but does not require the drug to be discontinued; however, the rare cases of thrombocytopenia with the drug should be taken very seriously and the drug stopped. **Paraesthesiae** and "burning sensations" in hands and feet may precede an isoniazid induced peripheral neuropathy; this may be ameliorated by pyridoxine supplements. Patients should have a formal ophthalmologic opinion before starting ethambutol and any visual symptoms should be taken seriously – either by stopping the drug or dose reduction (even

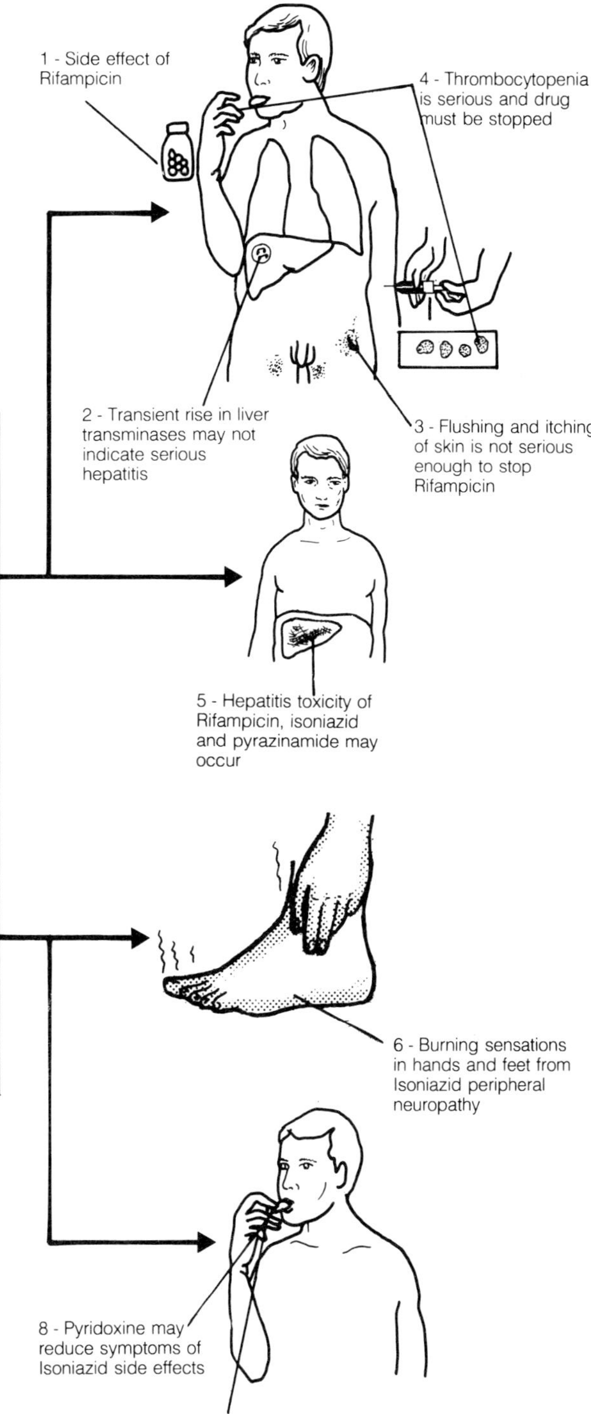

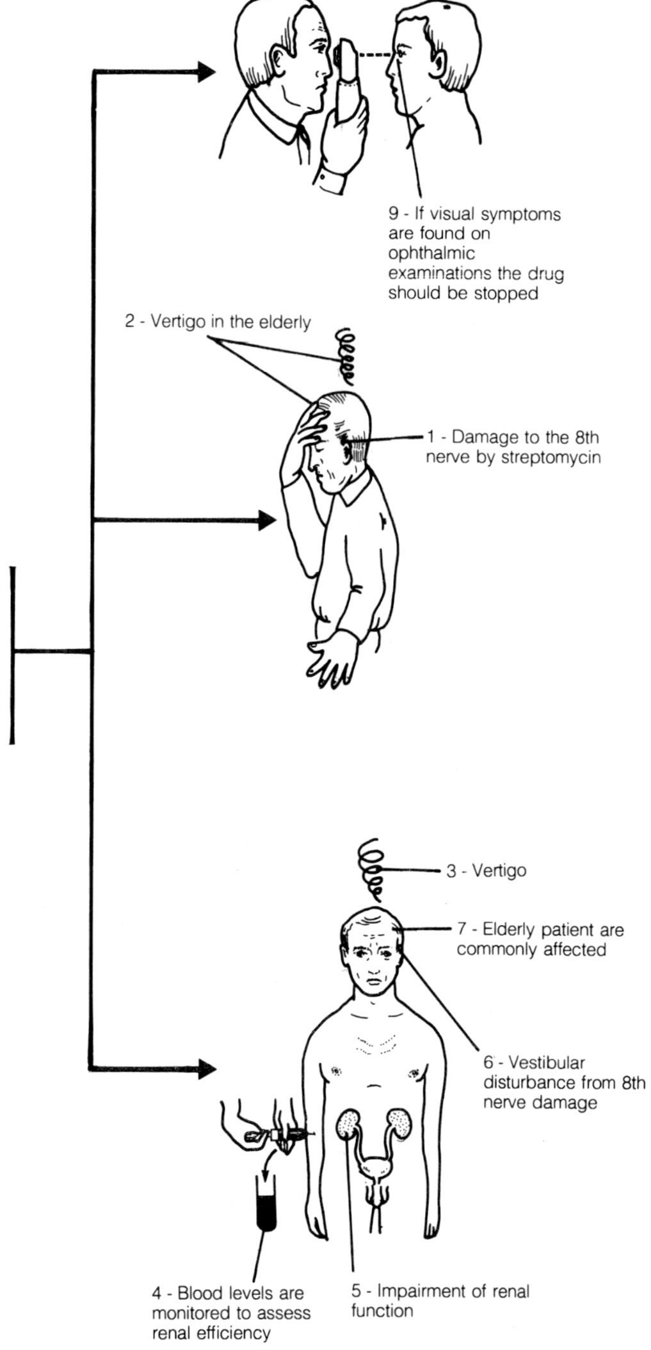

if temporary). The **vestibular toxicity** of streptomycin may be heralded by vertigo and is more likely to occur in the elderly and those with impairment of renal function: blood levels must be monitored in these patients.

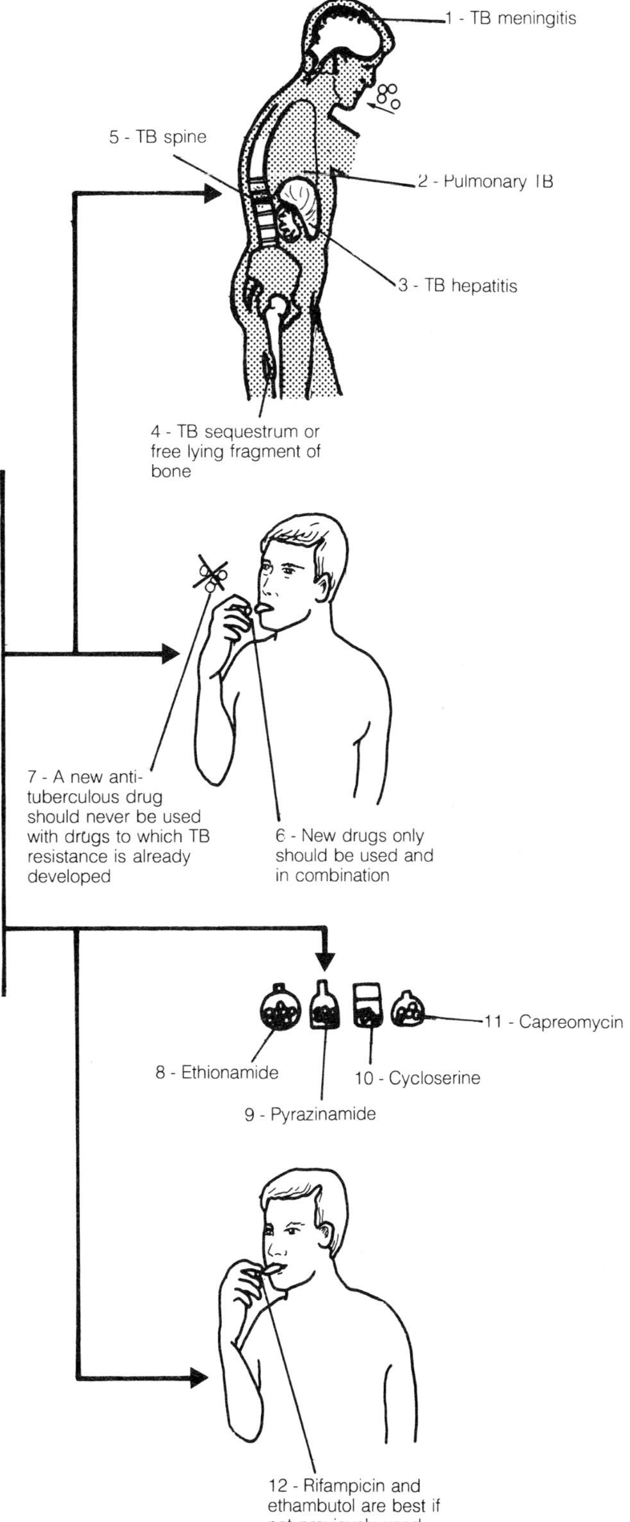

Patients with **massive disease** or bulk disease in sequestered sites (e.g. Pott's disease) may receive pyrazinamide added as a fourth drug initially and treatment may be more prolonged than 9 months. **Drug resistance** is a problem in populations where good standard multiple agent chemotherapy is not practised. Drug regimens for resistant disease must be carefully thought out and should never comprise the addition of a single drug to a previously unsatisfactory regimen. Rifampicin and ethambutol are the best drugs if they have not already been given and ethionamide, prothionamide, pyrazinamide, cycloserine and capreomycin may have a place.

Surgery has been mentioned in the treatment of some cases of bone and genito-urinary T.B. It is rarely required in pulmonary T.B. except when an open, albeit healed, cavity becomes secondarily infected by the opportunist fungus: aspergillus which may grow to form a fungus ball or mycetoma in the cavity. Surgical drainage of an empyema is another indication.

1 - Test tube culture of aspergillus fumigatus

2 - Aspergillus forming a fungus ball of mycetoma requires surgery

3 - Surgery is indicated in urogenital and bone TB — sometimes

4 - Surgical drainage of an empyema

5 - Aspergillus may grow to form a fungus ball.

The use of **corticosteroids** in the therapy of T.B. was controversial but there are now some well worked out indications where corticosteroids combined with chemotherapy are of benefit: in critically ill tuberculous patients and at times where a rapid reduction of inflammation is important (e.g. ocular, pleural, pericardial exudates) or abscess with critical compressive symptoms. Steroids are also used in the treatment of severe drug hypersensitivity during therapy – indeed, steroids and drug hyposensitisation may both be used to allow continuance of a particular drug in "difficult cases" of T.B.

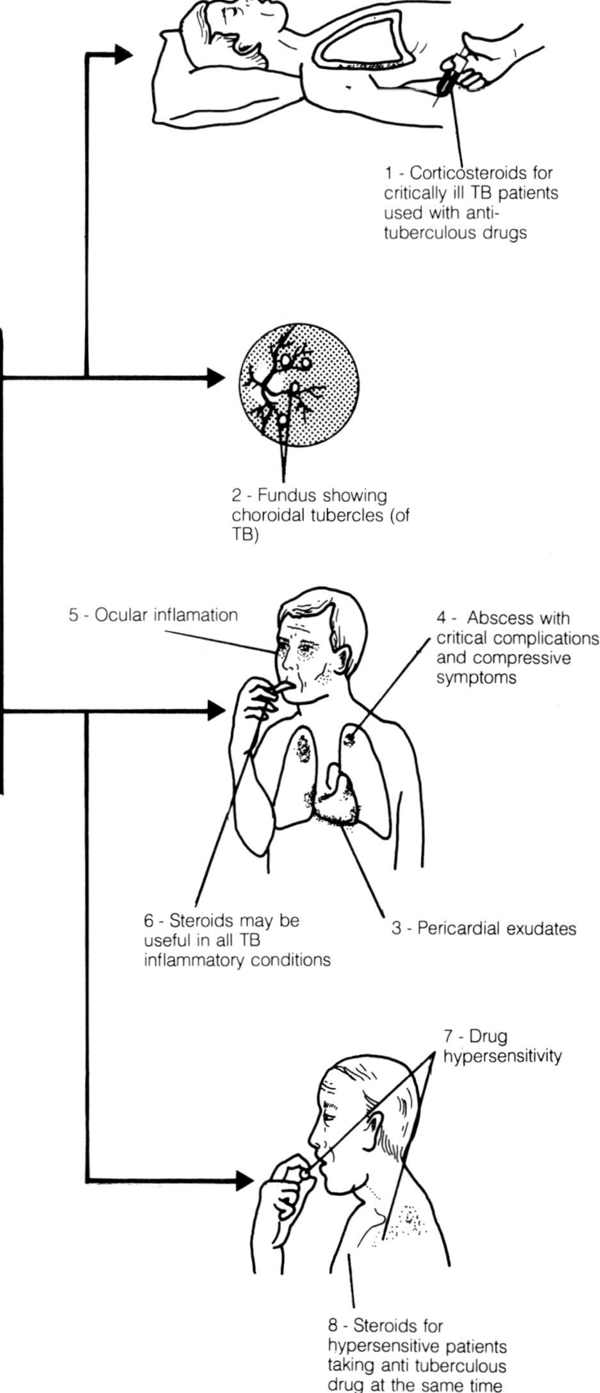

FUNGAL INFECTIONS

Fungal lung infections tend to be opportunistic, infecting those immunosuppressed or debilitated. Aspergillus fumigatus is perhaps the commonest example. This fungus, spread by air-borne spores, flourishes in healed tuberculous cavities, bronchiectatic segments, pulmonary infarcts etc. Usually the infection remains localised perhaps as a fungal ball (the aspergilloma or mycetoma) in these diseased areas, but in the immunosuppressed, the disease may spread to become a life-threatening, necrotising pneumonia; septicaemia may follow. If the sputum does not contain the fungus, rising serum precipitin titres may give the diagnosis.

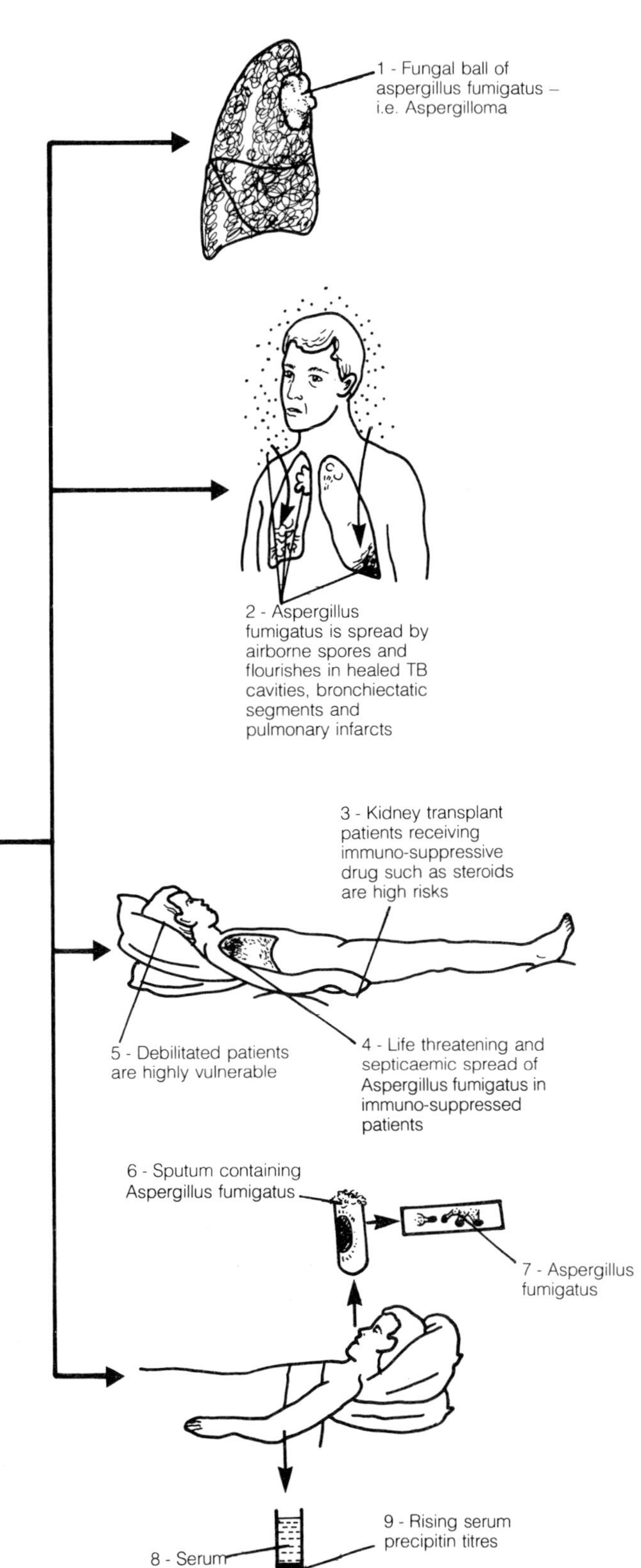

Allergic bronchopulmonary aspergillosis is a separate syndrome affecting atopic asthmatics, comprising recurrent areas of pulmonary shadowing on chest X-ray accompanying mild systemic and chest symptoms sometimes with the expectoration of brown, cylindrical and bronchial shaped "plugs". The peripheral blood shows an eosinophilia. This is a type III immunological reaction to aspergillus. The fungus may be found histologically in the brown plugs, and skin testing will be positive (for type I and III reactions).

Infections with Nocardia asteroides, Cryptococcus neoformans and Mucorales sp. are occasionally encountered in the U.K., and, in the U.S.A., Histoplasma capsulatum, Blastomycosis dermitididis and Coccidioides immitis cause granulomatous disease (in certain respects like T.B.) and are endemic in some areas.

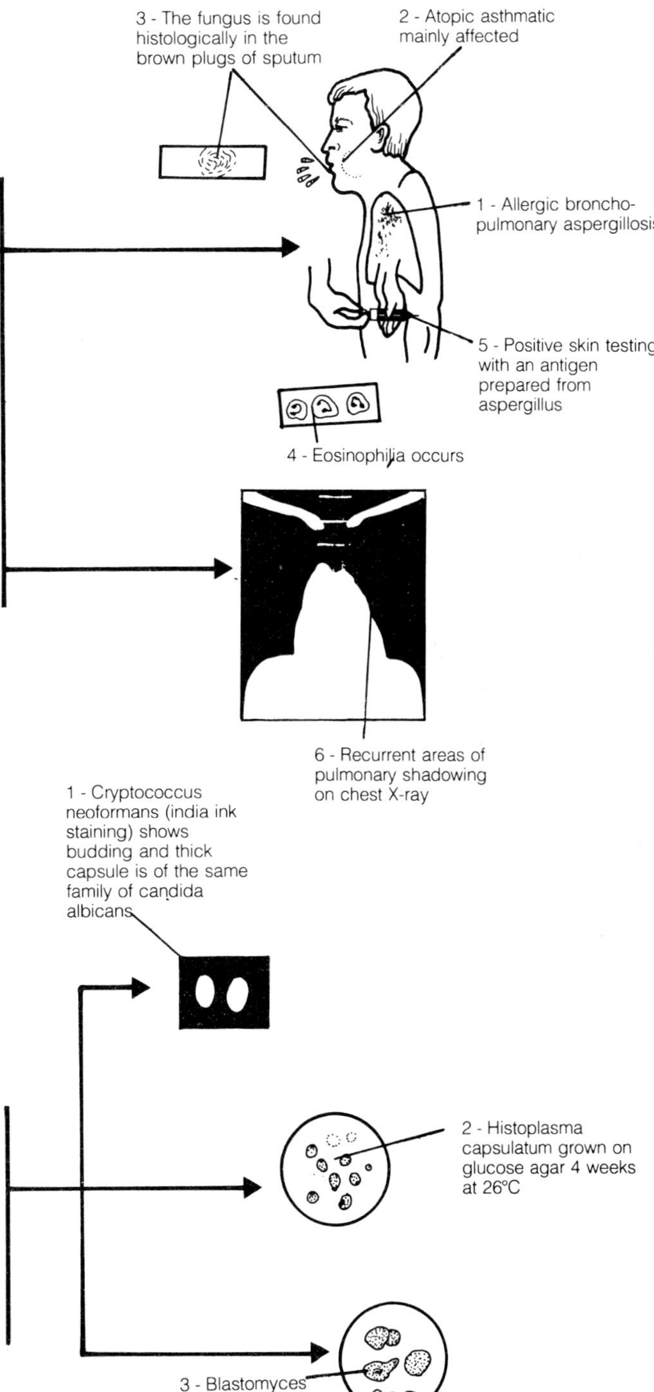

Candida albicans is a normal commensal of the skin and alimentary tract which can dominate the local flora under certain conditions (e.g. diabetes mellitus, Cushing's syndrome, patients on broad spectrum antibiotics) causing moniliasis ("thrush"). In debilitated or immunosuppressed agents, candida may spread to the lower respiratory tract – pulmonary candidiasis.

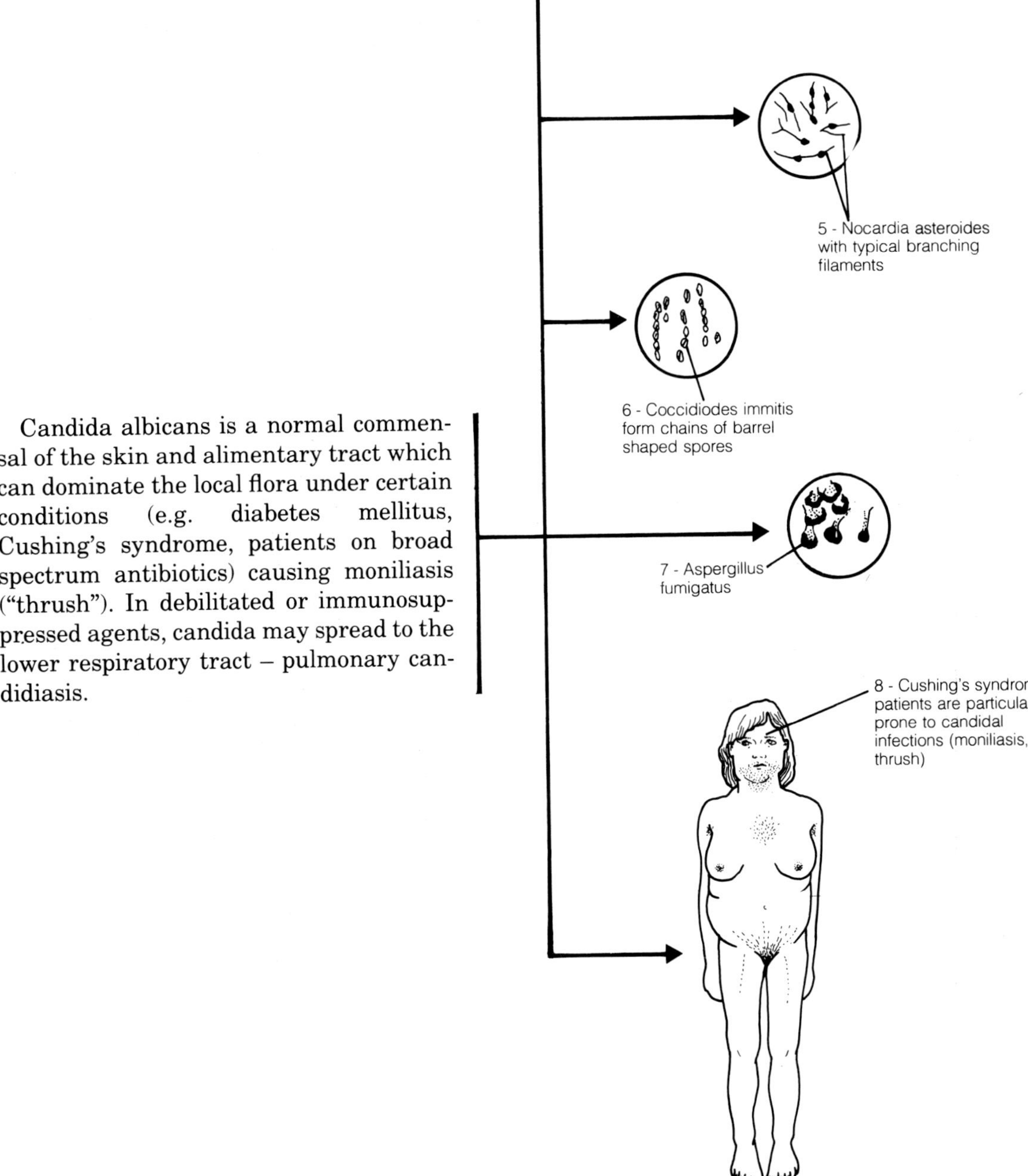

Treatment:– Nystatin is a safe topical anti-candidal therapy. Amphotericin B, and newer antifungal agents for systemic therapy have potentially serious side effects and need to be given by carefully controlled administration. 5-Fluorocytosine is less effective but active against Candida and Cryptococcus; clotrimazole is orally active against many fungi.

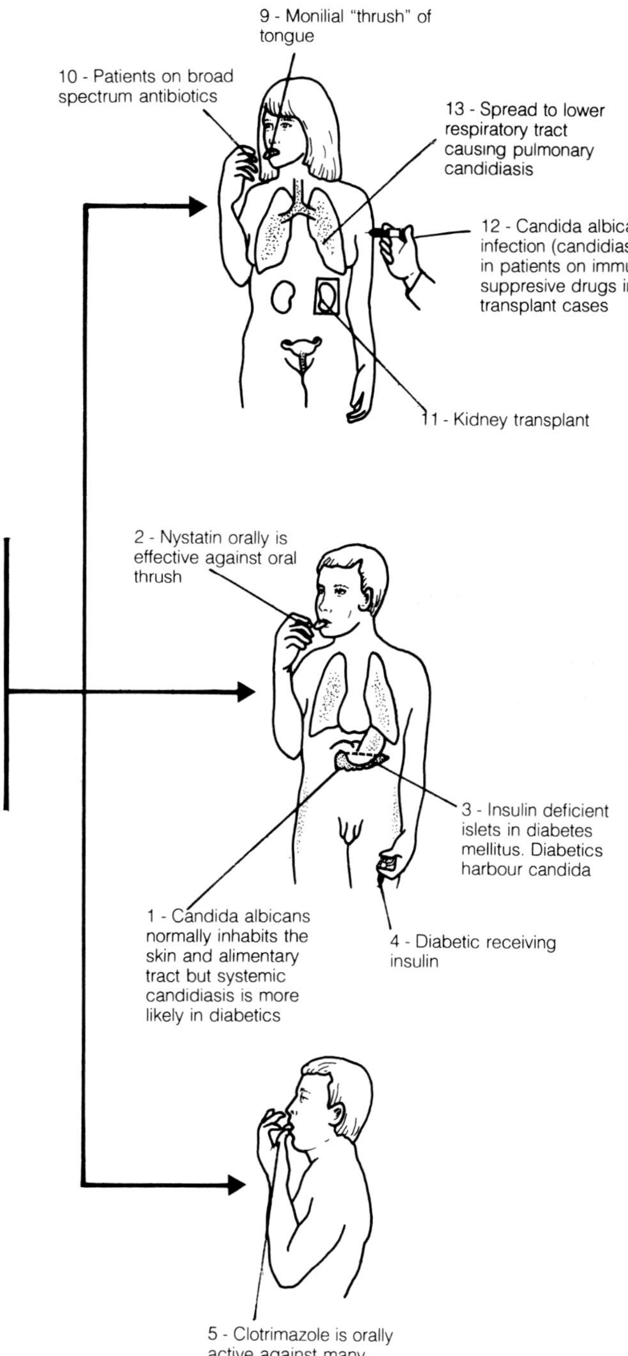

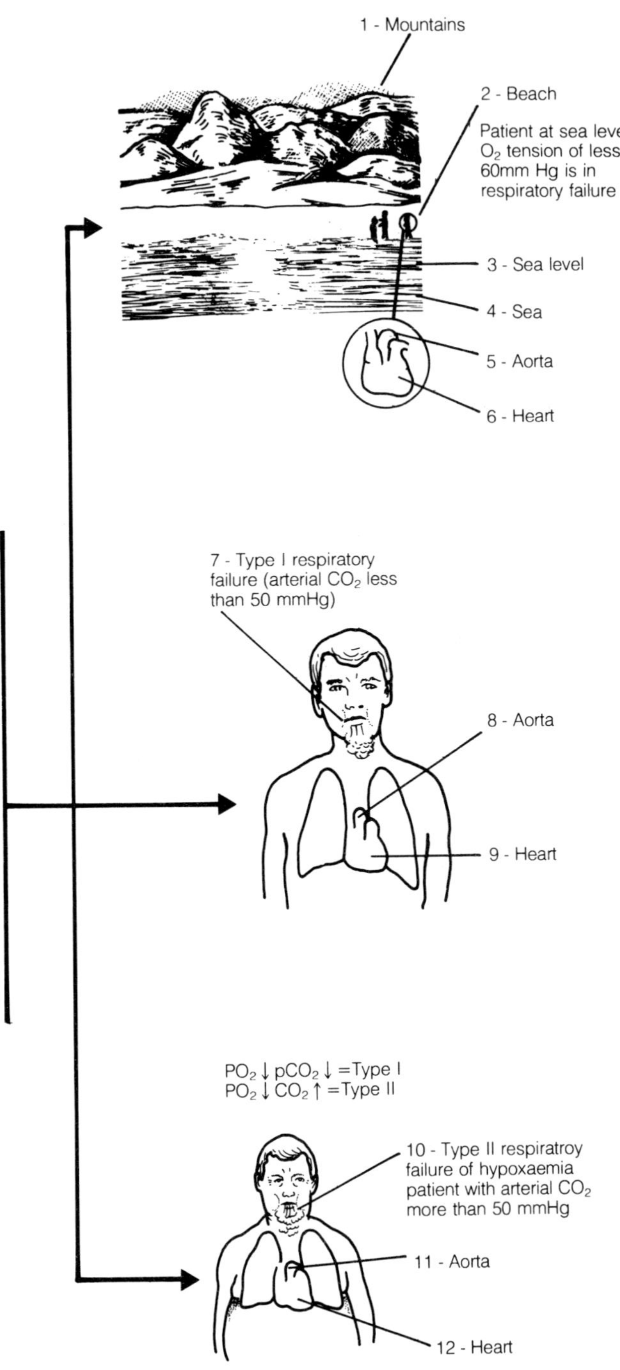

RESPIRATORY FAILURE

If a patient breathing air at sea level has an arterial oxygen tension of less than 8.0 kPa (60 mmHg) then he is in respiratory failure. He is usually centrally cyanosed. Two types of respiratory failure are recognised; the first (Type I respiratory failure) refers to hypoxaemic patients with an arterial $PaCO_2$ of below 6.6 kPa (50 mmHg), the second (Type II respiratory failure) refers to hypoxaemic and hypercapnic patients – with an arterial $PaCO_2$ of more than 6.6 kPa. In the early pages of this chapter, it has already been described how a ventilation/perfusion (V/Q) imbalance in certain lung regions can lead to type I gas tensions.

Type I respiratory failure (normal $PaCO_2$) is seen typically with severe restrictive lung disease due to widespread lung fibrosis (e.g. fibrosing alveolitis) oedema (e.g. left ventricular failure) or infiltration (e.g. lymphangitis carcinomatosa) – all producing stiff, non-compliant lungs. The failure is treated by increasing the inspired oxygen tension, which is quite safe to do, as retention of CO_2 is not a risk. A face mask (e.g. MC mask) delivering 60% O_2 at 6 litres per minute would be typical treatment. Pre-terminally, type I respiratory failure gives way to type II when, due to exhaustion and the very widespread nature of the disease process, the arterial $PaCO_2$ rises.

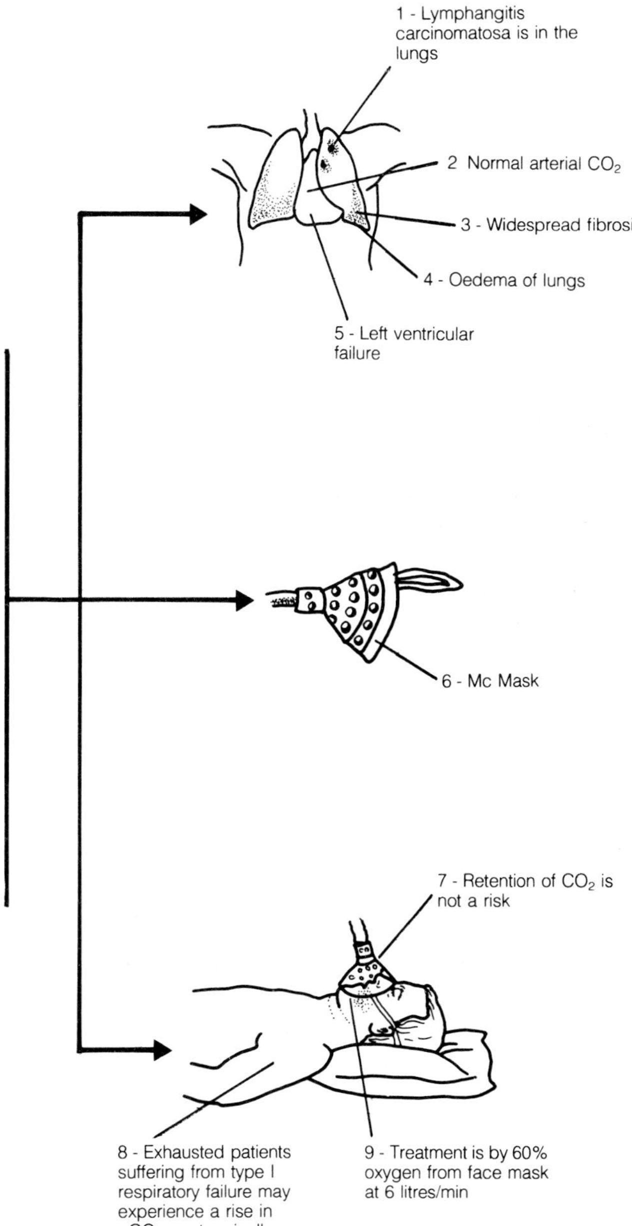

Type II respiratory failure (with raised $PaCO_2$) is typically encountered in patients with severe obstructive ventilatory defects throughout both lungs e.g. chronic obstructive airways disease – COAD.

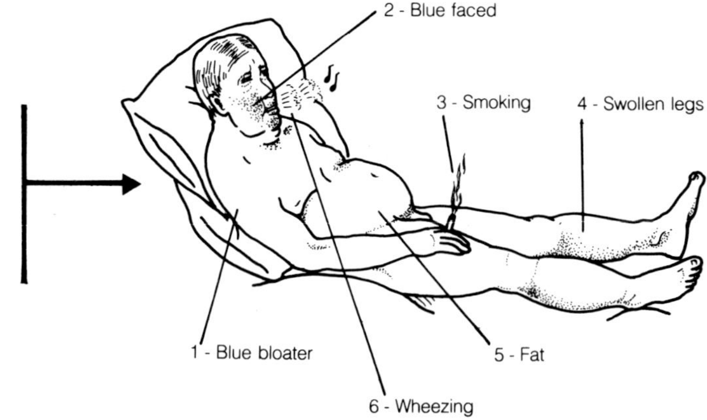

However, this type of ventilatory failure is also seen where there is reduced ventilatory movement e.g. due to central depression of respiratory centre, neuromuscular disease as in polyneuritis, poliomyelitis or myasthenia gravis, flailing chest due to severe chest trauma. The

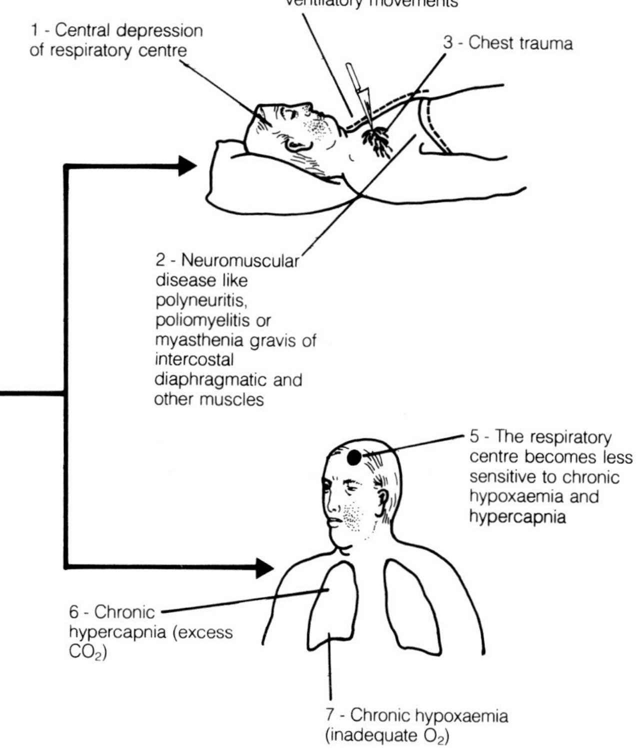

addition of chronic hypercapnia to the chronic hypoxaemia of COAD may lead to confusion, restlessness, a warm periphery, a bounding pulse with dilated peripheral veins, and a mild tremor of the outstretched hands, and perhaps headache and papilloedema due to raised intracranial pressure. The combination of a low PaO_2 and high $PaCO_2$ normally exerts a strong central stimulus for added respiratory effort, but with chronic hypercapnia the respiratory centre becomes insensitive to the high $PaCO_2$ and down regulated as regards response to hypoxia.

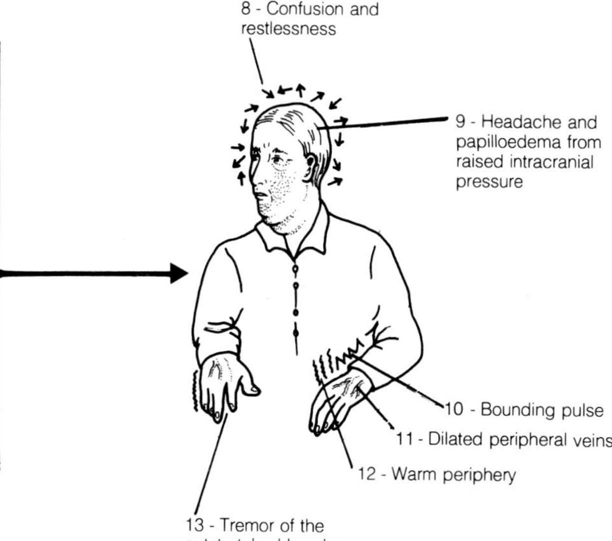

Under these circumstances, the medical administration of high tensions of inspired oxygen or of sedatives may lead to decreased respiratory effort and hypercapnic coma or even death. **Treatment of type II** respiratory failure is with controlled oxygen therapy – that implies close monotoring of arterial gas tensions whilst modestly enriching the inspired air with

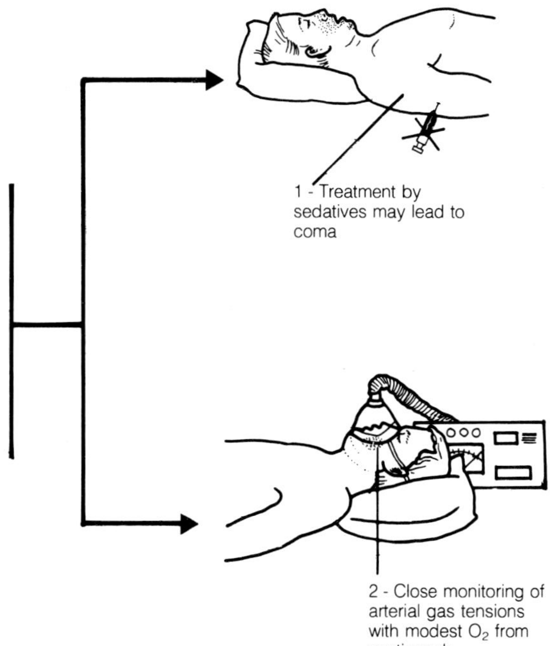

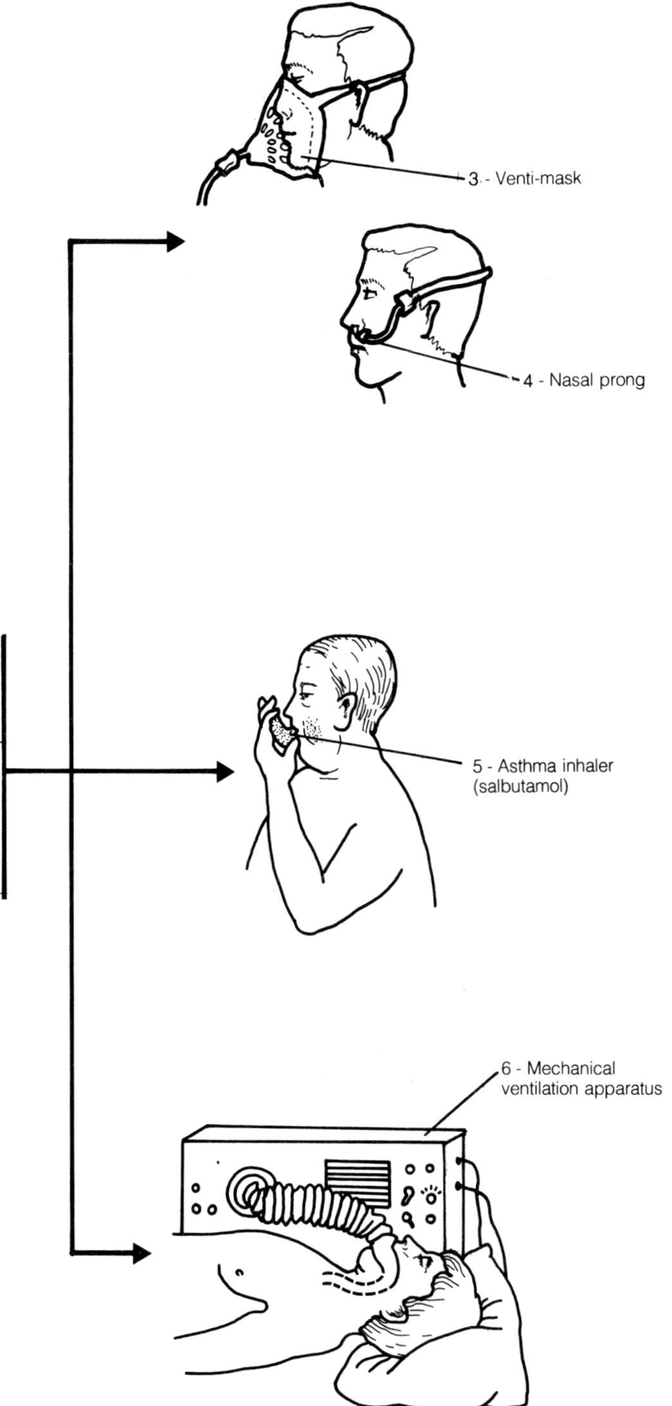

oxygen (e.g. 24%, 28% or 35% oxygen inspired via a Venti-mask or nasal prongs). In addition specific treatment aimed at the underlying cause of the failure is implemented (e.g. suction clearance of airways, antibiotics, or anti-asthma therapy etc). If all these measures fail to improve the blood gases then mechanical ventilation is required.

CHRONIC OBSTRUCTIVE AIRWAYS DISEASE (COAD)

COAD is the "Englishman's disease" as WHO figures show that chronic bronchitis and emphysema – the main components—are commonest in the U.K. However, all industrial societies with cold, wet winters suffer to some extent and also other communities with a high prevalence of cigarette smoking and atmospheric pollution.

Chronic Bronchitis – Chronic bronchitis is defined clinically as the persistent daily expectoration of mucoid, (muco-purulent or at times purulent) sputum for at least three months of three consecutive years, and not due to a localised bronchiectatic lung region. This clinical picture arises from the basic pathological process viz. bronchial mucus gland hyperplasia – often at the expense of the normally continuous, beating, cilial carpet. The cough of the chronic bronchitic is the effort at improving the deficient muco-ciliary clearance process.

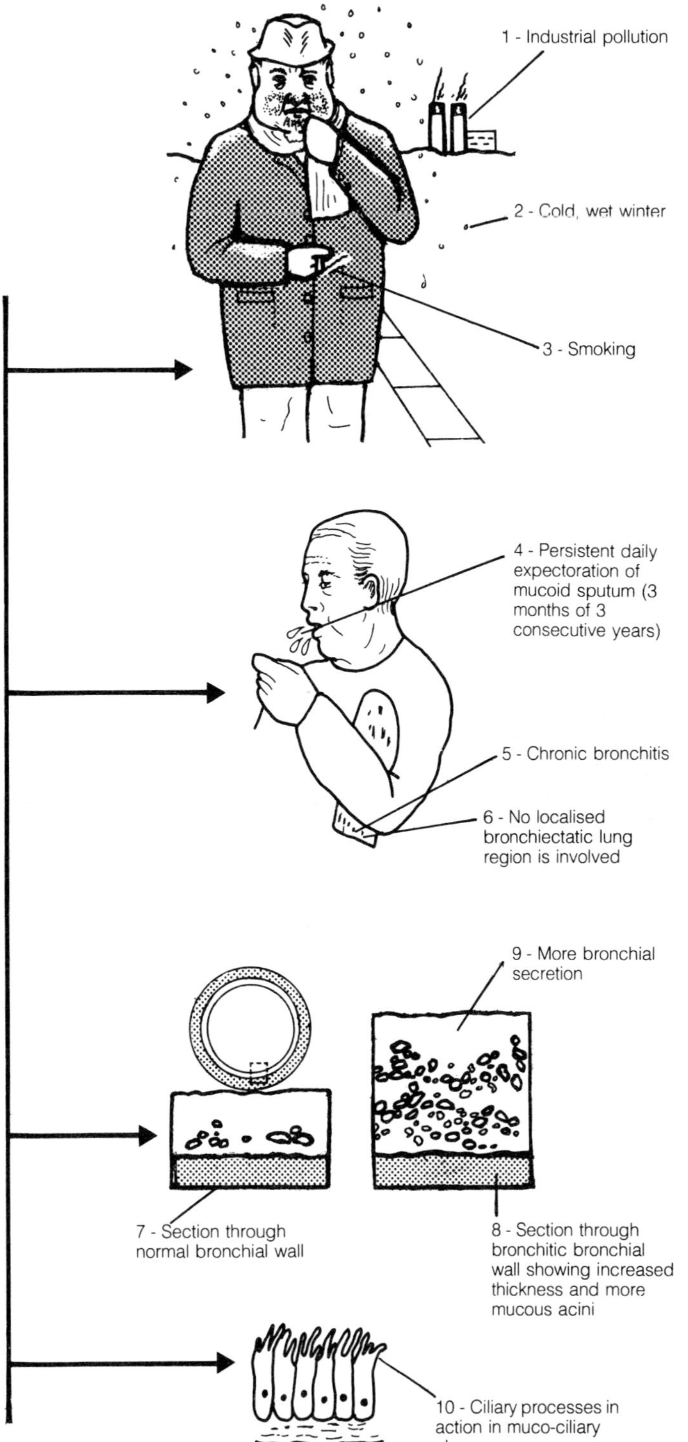

The early clinical picture is of a "smoker's cough" with sputum, usually with acute infective exacerbations in winter when the sputum becomes more purulent and the patient may notice some wheeze or shortness of breath on exertion. After a period of years, shortness of breath on exertion becomes noticeable at all times and on less effort (as the patient's FEV_1 and PEFR fall indicating the diffuse airways obstruction. The FEV_1/FVC ratio is below 70%). In severe cases, winter-exacerbations become life-threatening as the patient is admitted to hospital with severe bronchopneumonia and attendant right sided heart failure (**cor pulmonale**).

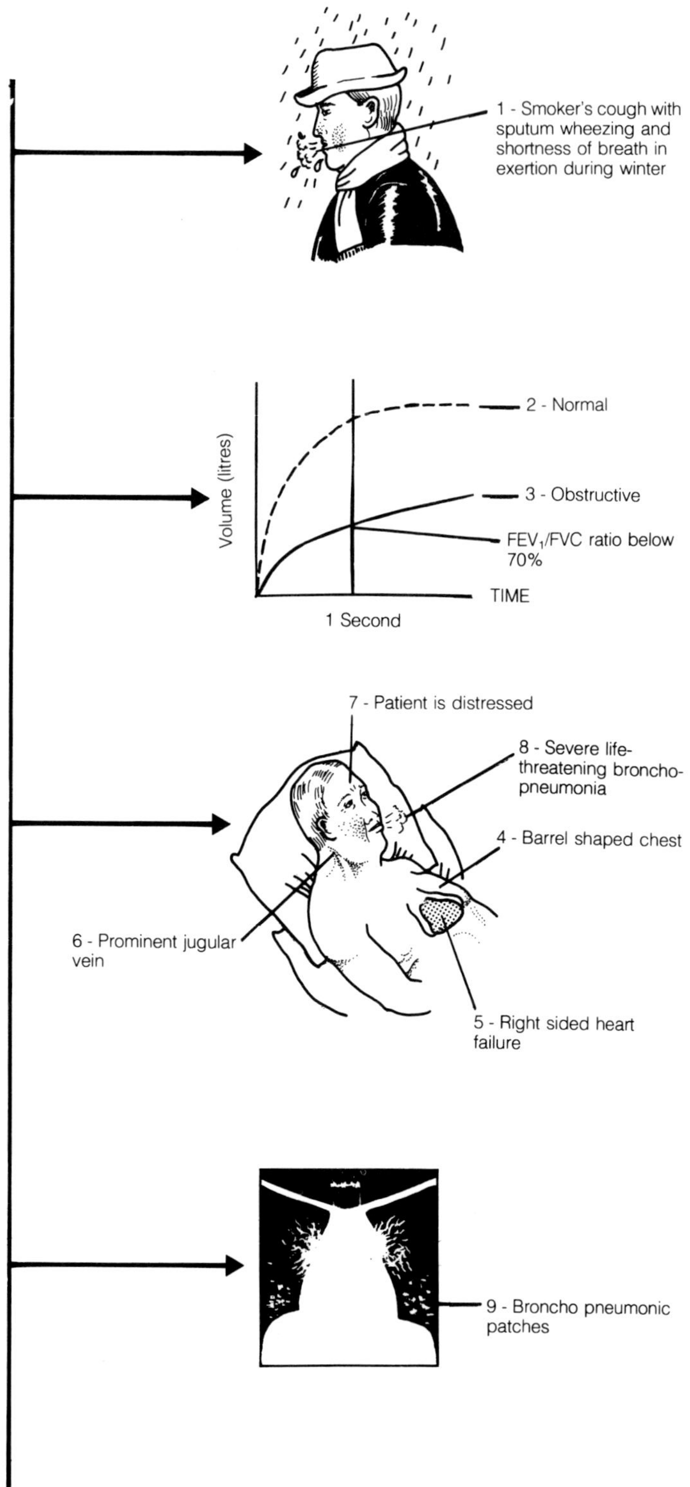

Such a patient typically a smoking, urban living man presents cyanotic and confused (due to hypoxaemia and hypercapnia), barrel chested (due to an emphysematous element) and oedematous (due to cor pulmonale). Professor Dornhurst coined the descriptive nickname for such patients: "Blue Bloaters". The auscultatory signs are of diffuse bilateral rhonchi and perhaps scattered crepitations. The chest X-ray will reveal any bronchopneumonic patches and any emphysema but is not diagnostic for chronic bronchitis. If there is cor pulmonale, cardiomegaly and engorged pulmonary vessels may be apparent (c.f. emphysema).

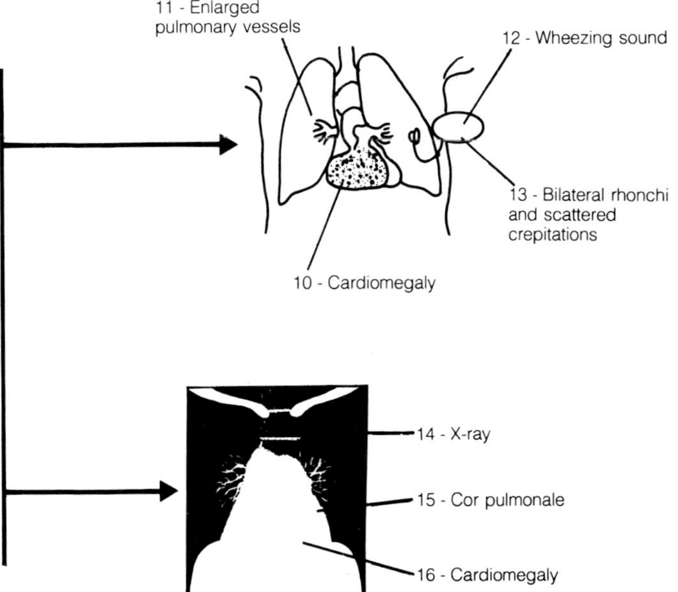

Treatment starts at the early stages. Patients should be advised to give up smoking and in an ideal world move to a sunny climate! They must keep warm in winter and avoid cold and fog. Influenza vaccination in autumn is advisable and a bottle of broad spectrum antibiotic against the commonest pathogens – pneumococcus and H. influenzae—should be available to the patient to initiate as soon as an exacerbation occurs e.g. amoxycillin, tetracycline, co-trimoxazole.

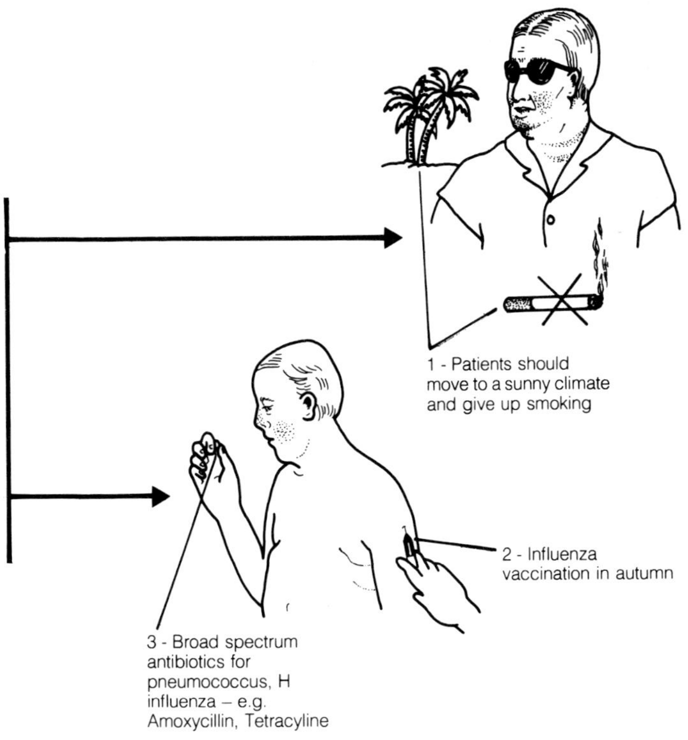

Selective bronchodilators e.g. salbutamol inhalers, help to reduce bronchospasm and are worthwhile. In an acute exacerbation, intravenous aminophylline (500 mg intravenously over five minutes) may be useful together with controlled oxygen therapy and physiotherapy. Diuretics are first therapy for cor pulmonale.

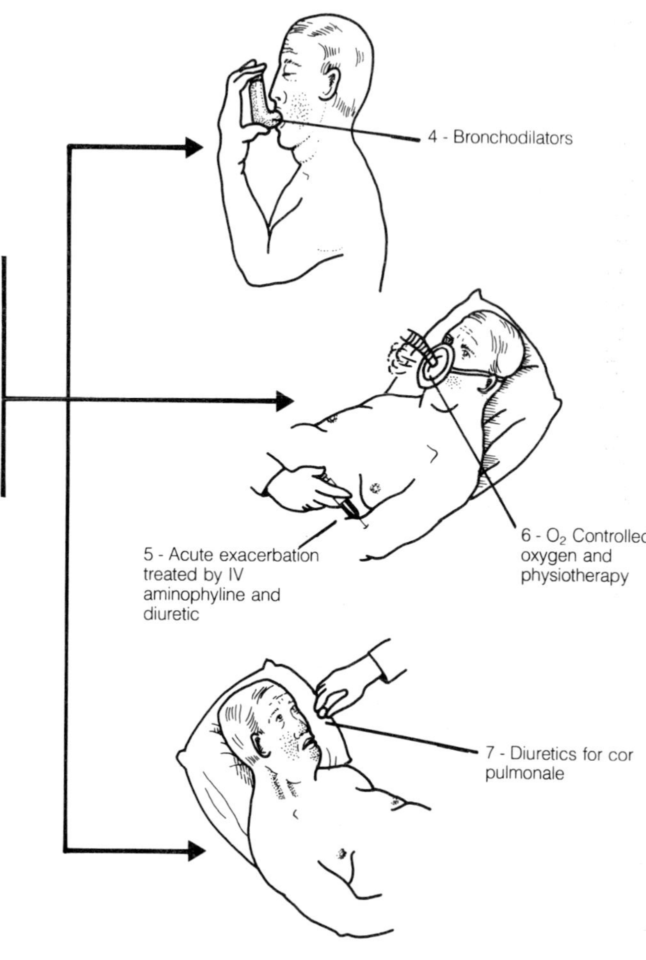

Oral steroids or inhaled beclomethasone may be worthy of a trial to detect chronic asthmatics with COAD. The spirometry is assessed before and after a seven day trial of prednisolone (10 mg. q.d.s.). One is looking for a 20% improvement of FEV_1: such an improvement justifies a maintenance (lower) steroid dose. Mucolytic agents do not have an established place in the management of chronic bronchitis.

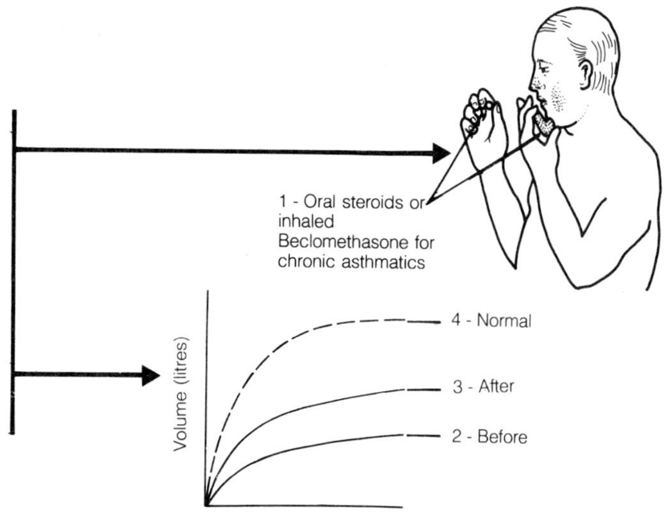

Emphysema is defined as pathological dilatation of air space distal to the terminal bronchioles. Emphysema almost always accompanies chronic bronchitis but it may also occur as a primary lung disease. It is commonly believed but not proved that the widespread bronchial/ bronchiolar obstructive narrowing of chronic bronchitis leads to distal air trapping in the acini with pathological dilatation. However, emphysema itself causes weakening of the walls of respiratory bronchioles which collapse early in expiration exacerbating any existing obstructive lung disease.

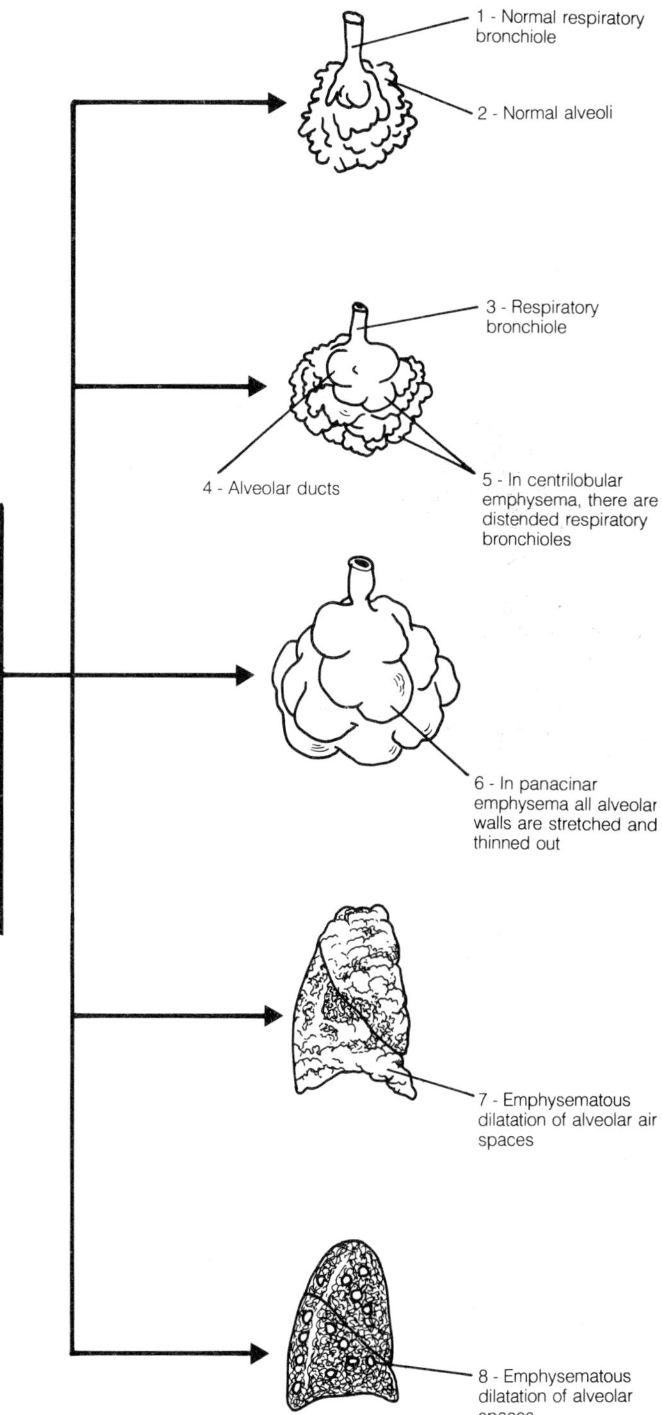

The emphysema sufferer may exhale through "pursed lips" in order for back pressure to prevent this collapse. The consequences of these pathologically dilated air spaces are an over-expanded chest due to lungs with a high TLC, high RV and high RV/TLC ratio. The patient uses the accessory muscles of respiration to breathe and the breath sounds over the over-expanded chest are diminished although the percussion note is resonant, (often resoundingly resonant, including over the area of normal cardiac dullness).

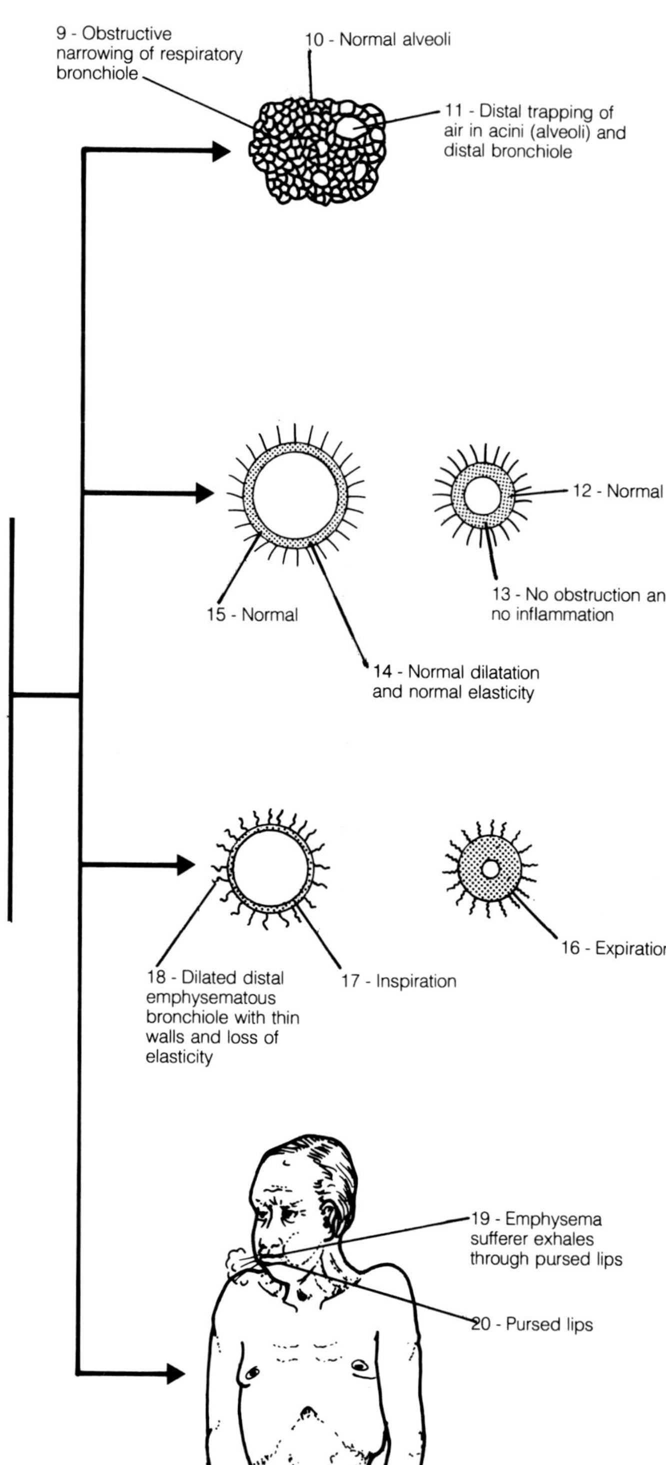

The chest X-ray demonstrates the hyper-inflated lungs by the low and flattened diaphragm and horizontal ribs; the heart appears long and thin and there is a reduction in the more distal pulmonary vascular markings as one attempts to trace the very full central vessels out radially from the hila.

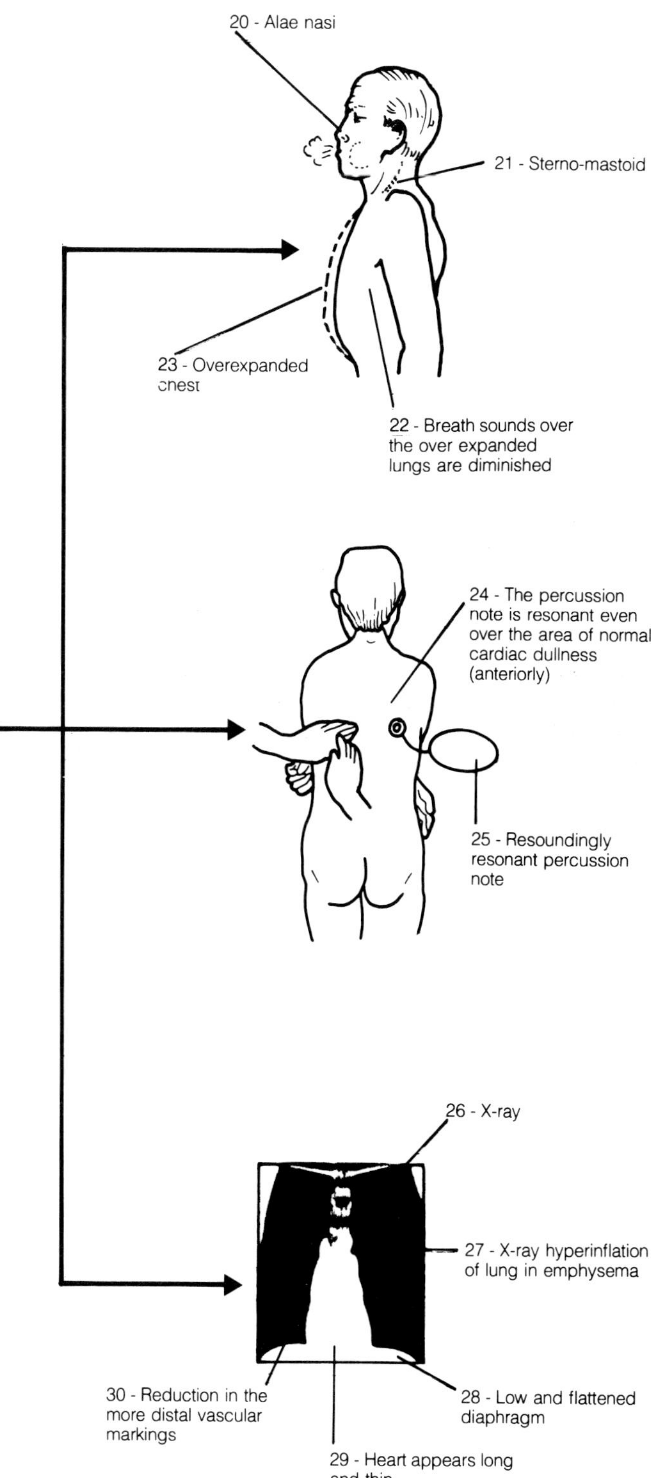

There are few conditions which can be confused with chronic bronchitis and emphysema and if treatment is directed to the former at an early stage, the COAD may be self-limiting. However, chronic adult asthma must be remembered as a possible contributing element and the degree of reversible airways obstruction at a non-infected time should be assessed by lung function tests. Should a patient with COAD become suddenly more breathless two possible diagnoses should be suspected. The first is the formation of a giant bulla. This is a cystic emphysematous space that may blow up, "balloon fashion" and compress adjacent functioning lung tissue. The bulla is often seen on a chest X-ray as demarcated by a line shadow and it may require surgical removal.

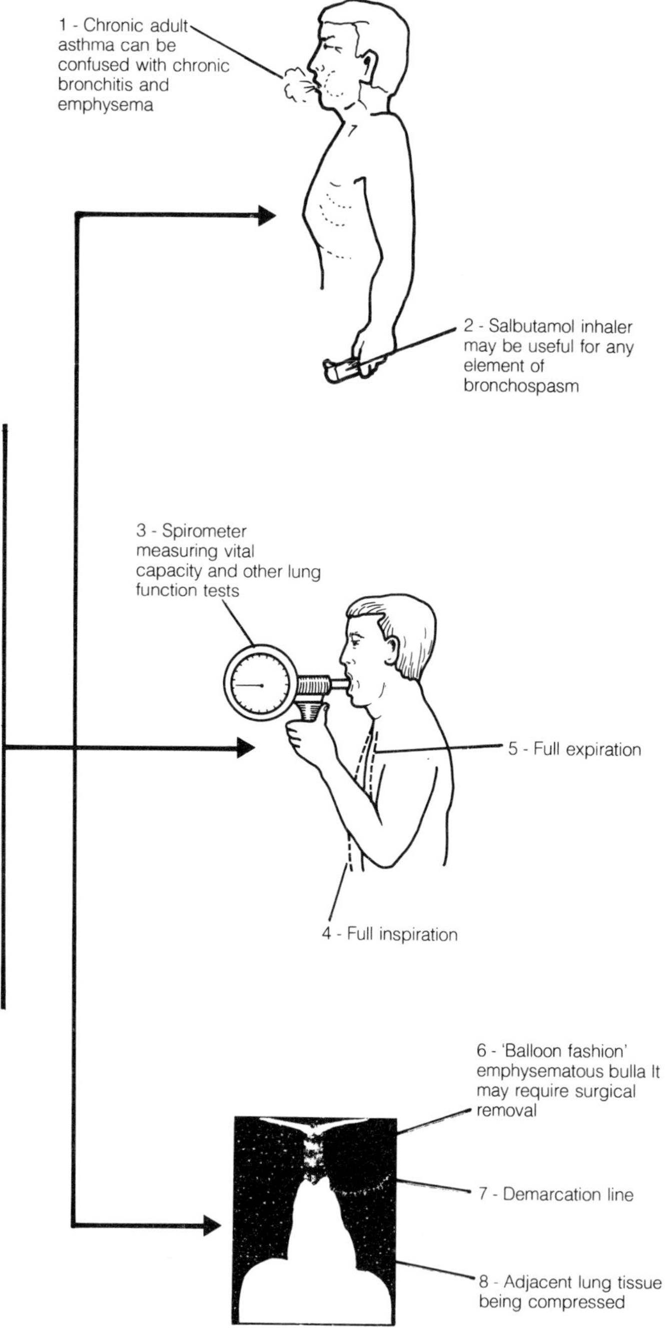

The other cause of sudden breathlessness in COAD is pneumothorax, often through a burst, peripherally-sited emphysematous bulla. This too is diagnosed by chest X-ray, and accentuated in an expiratory film. One further possible cause of a sudden deterioration in respiratory function is pulmonary thromboembolism which is not uncommon in advanced COAD.

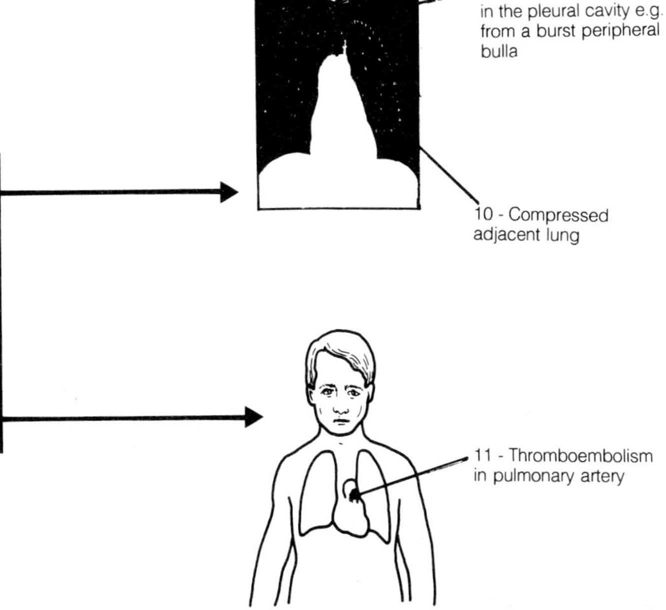

Idiopathic or primary emphysema occurs throughout the acini of all lobes. The cause is often unknown but the familial deficiency of the antiprotease $\propto_1$-antitrypsin, (which neutralises pulmonary macrophage elastase and collagenase) is associated with emphysema: one can envisage unchecked enzymic destruction of acinar anatomy due to this mechanism, but this is unproven. There is

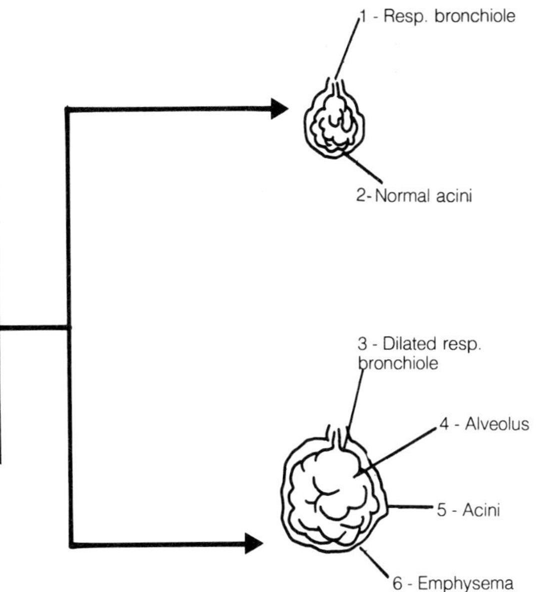

airways obstruction due to premature collapse of weakened airways in expiration. Breathlessness is the main symptom and it progressively worsens: cough is often insignificant. Breathing is laboured and "pursed-lip". On chest examination the over-inflated chest is resonant as described above and on auscultation the expiratory phase is often prolonged, sometimes with rhonchi. The heart sounds may be distant. The low FEV_1/FVC and high RV/TLC ratios are as described above and if the FVC is less than the VC, then air trapping may be deduced to be

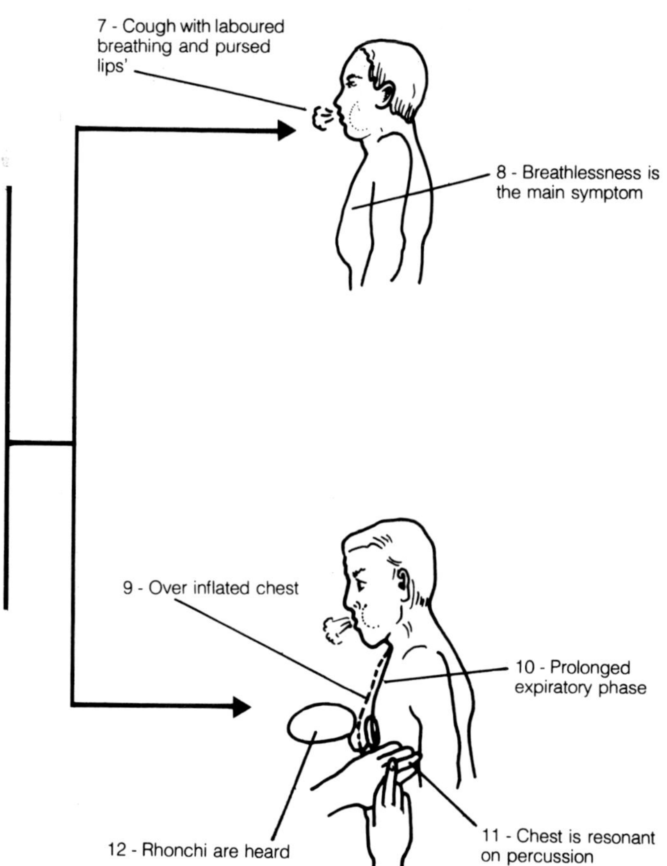

occurring. The DLCO is reduced. Unlike COAD where chronic bronchitis predominates, there is often preservation of respiratory drive and blood gas tensions remain near normal for a long time due to the energetic respiratory efforts, (hence the nickname **"pink puffers"** – i.e. not cyanosed). The chest X-ray is as described above.

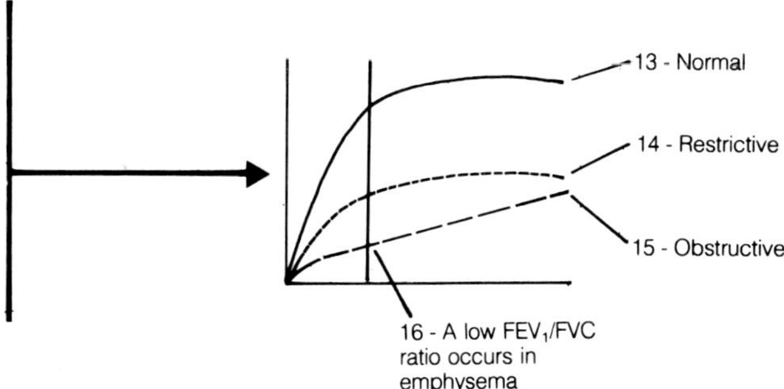

Idiopathic emphysema is irreversible and management involves excluding other treatable conditions (e.g. reversible airways obstruction), active and early treatment of respiratory infections and oxygen administration when necessary (if possible by a light apparatus). Breathing exercises may marginally assist ventilatory efficiency.

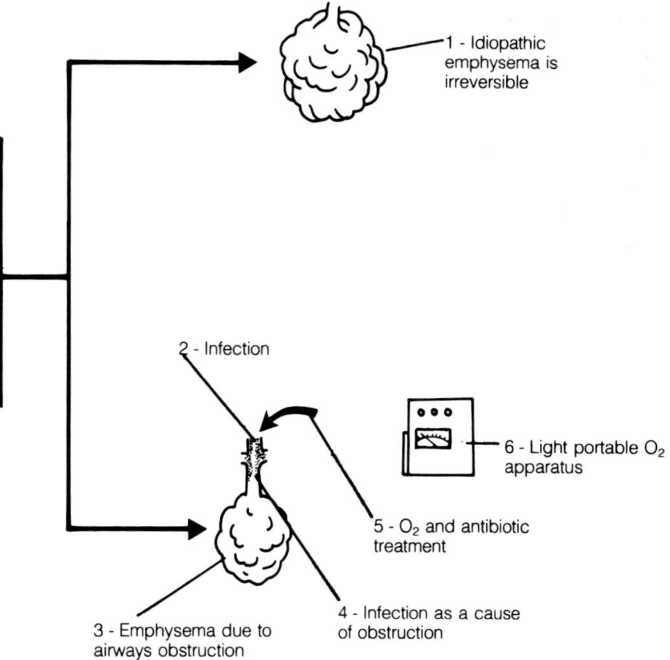

COR PULMONALE

Cor pulmonale refers to hypertrophy (and later heart failure) of the right ventricle resulting from diseases affecting the function and/or structure of the lungs. Causes include COAD, asthma, lung fibrosis from any cause, pulmonary infiltrations or cystic disease of the lungs. Severe kyphoscoliosis may have deformed the lungs sufficiently to cause cor pulmonale in the long term. Pulmonary embolism and idiopathic or drug-induced pulmonary hypertension are further important causes.

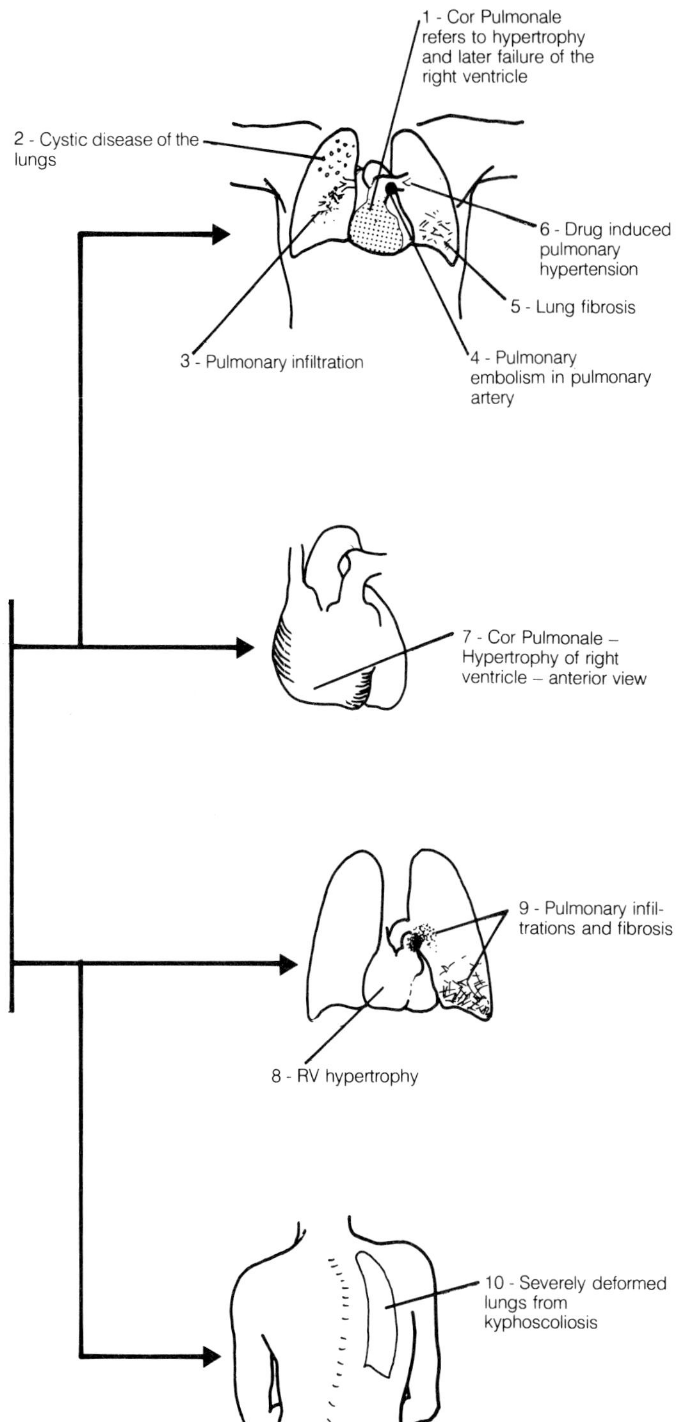

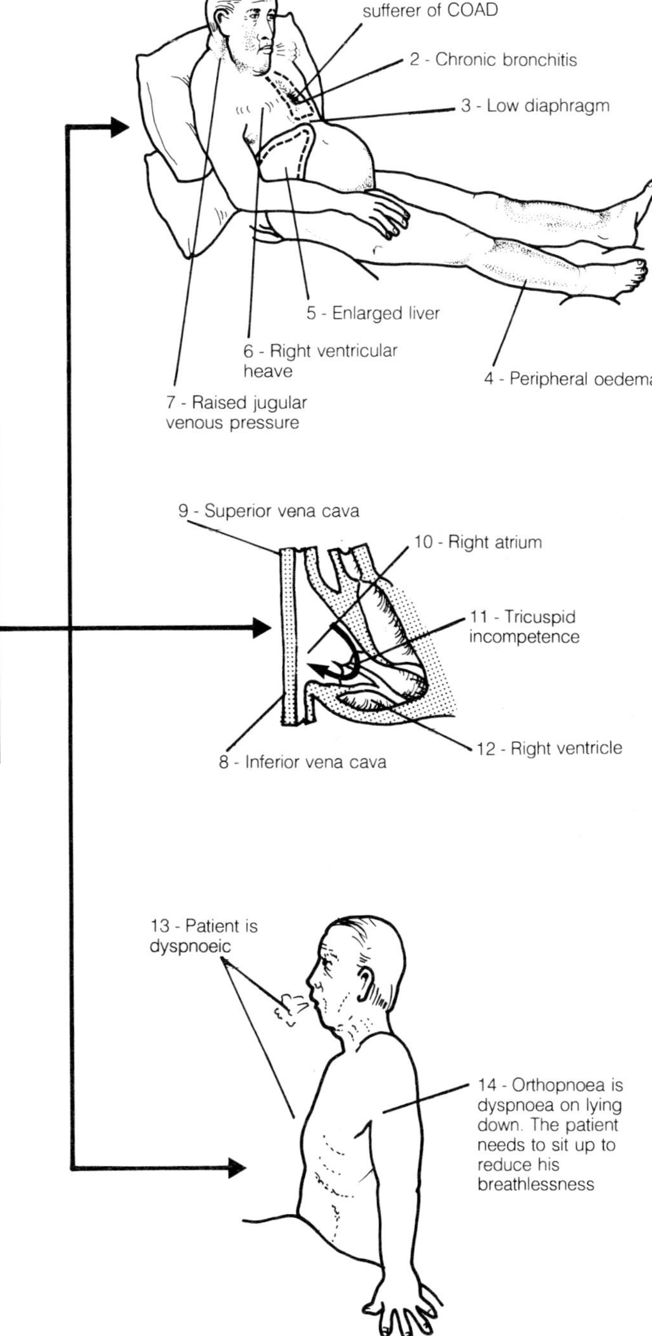

The typical patient is a known sufferer of COAD who is admitted with an infective episode of his chronic bronchitis with all the signs described previously but with peripheral oedema, a raised jugular venous pressure, hepatomegaly (but diaphragm often low due to emphysema), a right ventricular heave occasionally and perhaps even functional tricuspid incompetence if right ventricular dilatation is marked. The dyspnoea and orthopnoea are marked. The ECG shows right atrial and ventricular hypertrophy and the chest X-ray shows cardiomegaly with dilated main pulmonary arteries. Treatment is directed at the infective exacerbation of the COAD with its attendant type II respiratory failure, because the hypoxaemia is a major contributor to the cor pulmonale. Diuretics are the best additional therapy for the cor pulmonale, ensuring that one does not "overdo" the diuresis and that potassium is preserved. Hypnotics and sedatives are to be avoided.

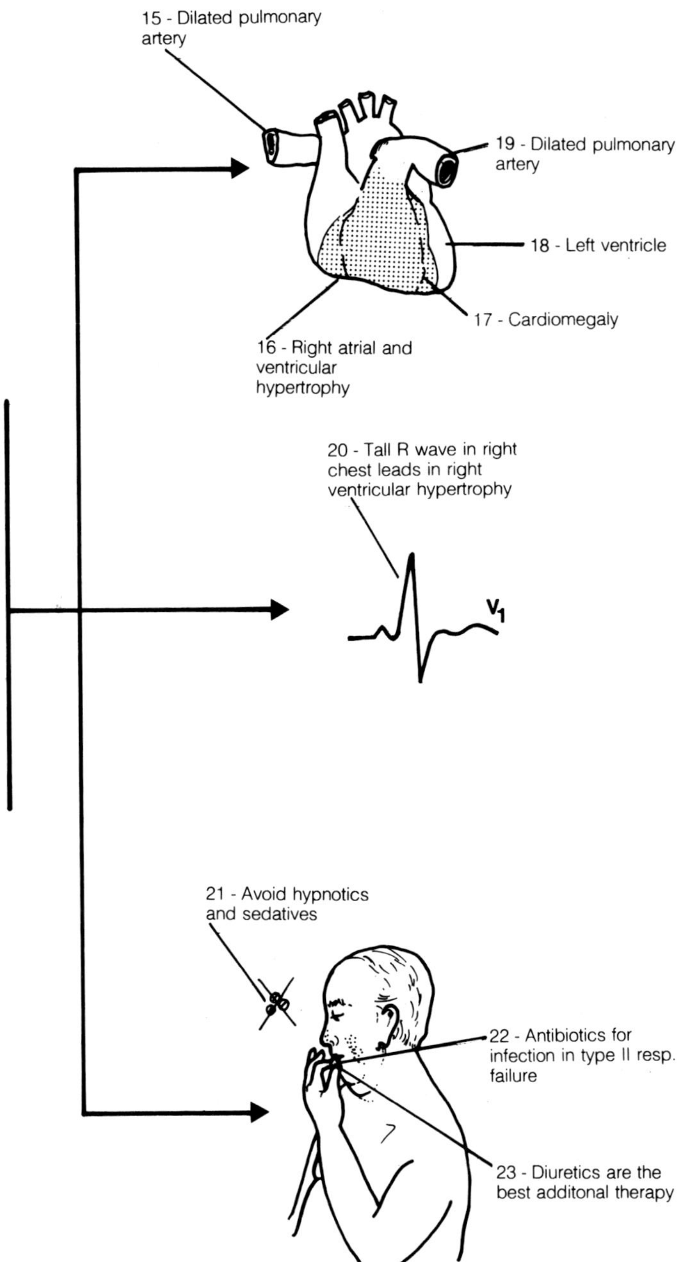

The effect of long term, controlled oxygen therapy, delivered for at least 15 hours each and every day, on the survival of patients with COAD and cor pulmonale is still under clinical research trials.

Patients with cor pulmonale due to e.g. diffuse pulmonary fibrosis or infiltration, tend to develop oedema later in the course of the disease than in COAD. The cor pulmonale of COAD is also remarkable in that for a period, patients have reversible episodes of cor pulmonale with their infective episodes. Eventually, the cardiac output falls and fatal heart failure may supervene.

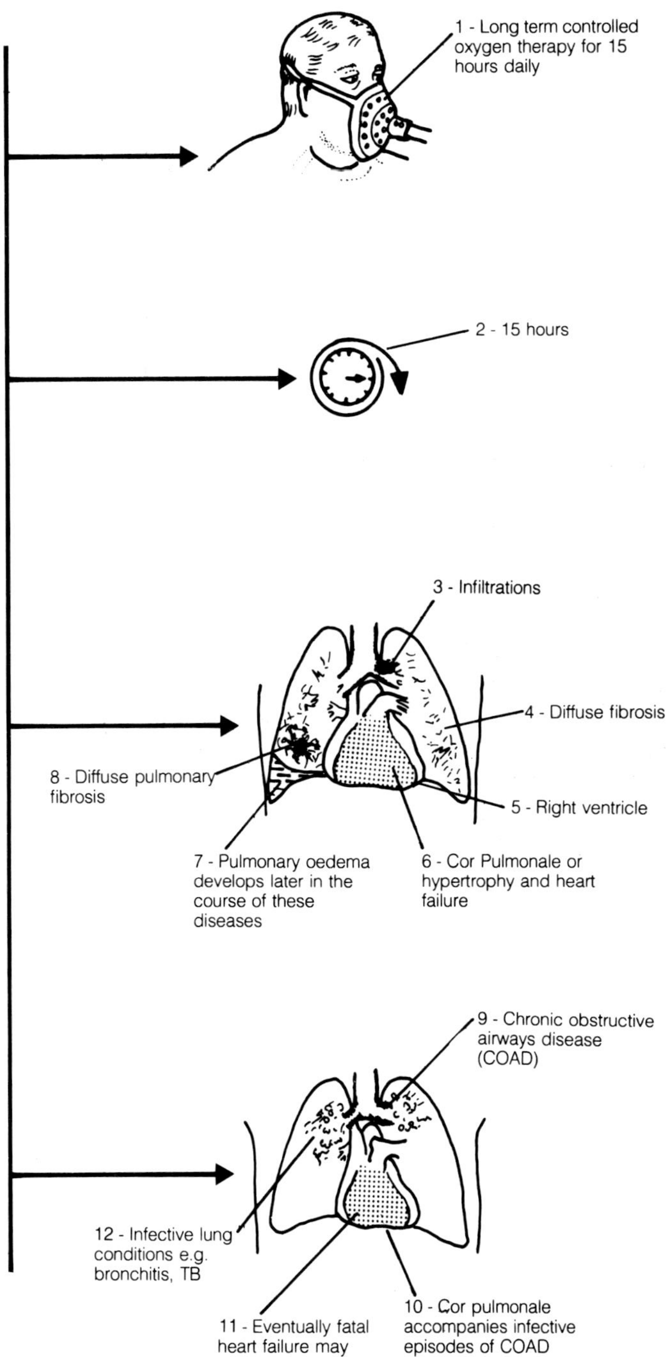

Secondary polycythaemia is a feature of COAD and venesection may improve the exercise tolerance of rare patients, but should not be done unless the haematocrit exceeds 65%: one is balancing increased blood oxygen carrying capacity against the contribution of an elevated blood viscosity to the heart failure. The decision to venesect should be taken by experts.

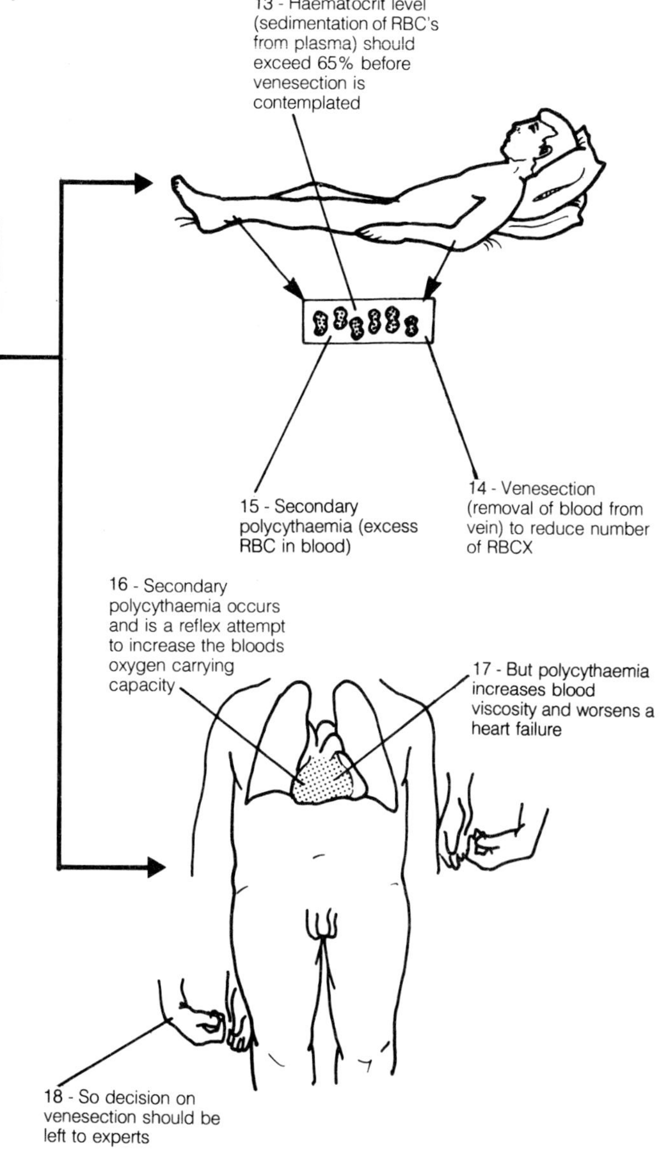

ASTHMA

Bronchial asthma is characterised by paroxysmal attacks of dyspnoea due to the widespread narrowing of airways: between attacks the bronchi return to normal. There are three components to the airways obstruction: firstly, spasm or generalised increased tone of the smooth muscle in the bronchial walls; secondly oedema/swelling of the bronchial mucosa associated with increased local capillary permeability and lastly the endobronchial accumulation of bronchial secretions. All these tend to increase resistance to air flow, especially during expiration.

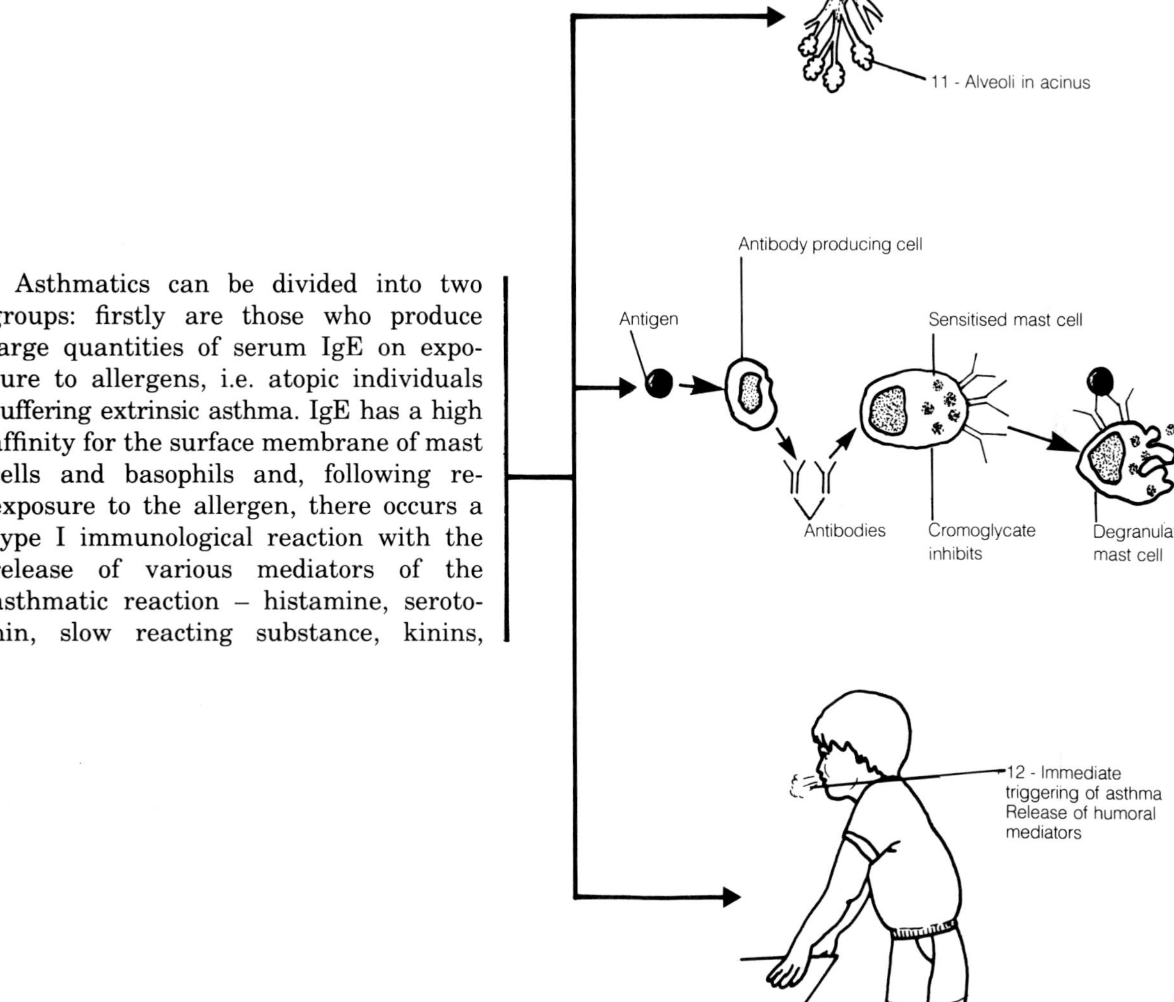

Asthmatics can be divided into two groups: firstly are those who produce large quantities of serum IgE on exposure to allergens, i.e. atopic individuals suffering extrinsic asthma. IgE has a high affinity for the surface membrane of mast cells and basophils and, following re-exposure to the allergen, there occurs a type I immunological reaction with the release of various mediators of the asthmatic reaction – histamine, serotonin, slow reacting substance, kinins,

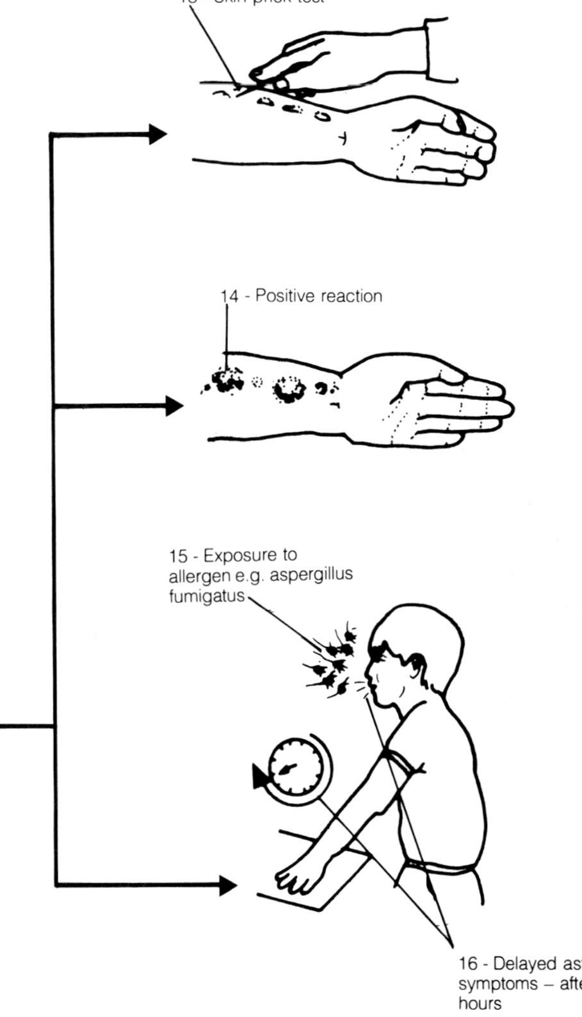

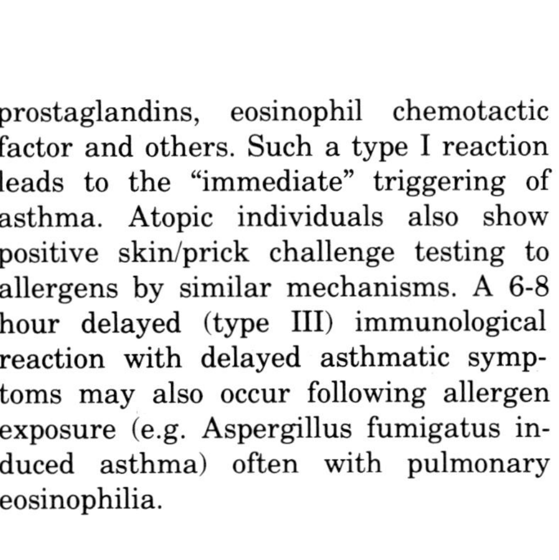

prostaglandins, eosinophil chemotactic factor and others. Such a type I reaction leads to the "immediate" triggering of asthma. Atopic individuals also show positive skin/prick challenge testing to allergens by similar mechanisms. A 6-8 hour delayed (type III) immunological reaction with delayed asthmatic symptoms may also occur following allergen exposure (e.g. Aspergillus fumigatus induced asthma) often with pulmonary eosinophilia.

Non-atopic individuals prone to allergy, possess bronchial hyperreactivity but do not produce excessive amounts of IgE to allergens and the pathophysiological mechanism of asthma production is less understood. Skin-prick testing with allergens is usually negative.

5% of children have asthma to some degree, although half of these will grow out of their symptoms: asthma is commoner and more severe in boys. Most asthmatic children have developed symptoms before the age of seven years – often first masquerading as a chest infection. The vast majority of childhood asthmatic cases are in atopic individuals and between half and three quarters of all cases have a family history of asthma or atopic manifestation. The other atopic features include atopic eczema (more than 50% of infants with atopic eczema subsequently develop asthma) or hay fever.

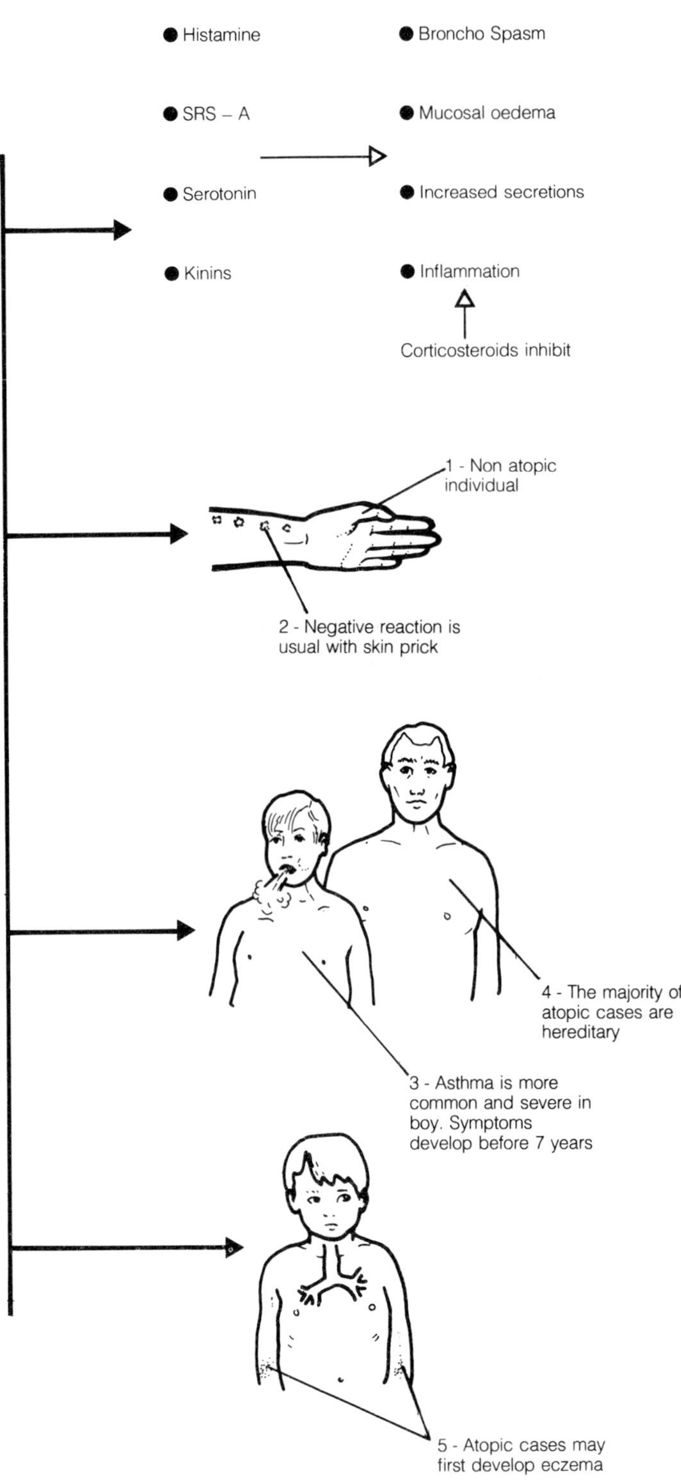

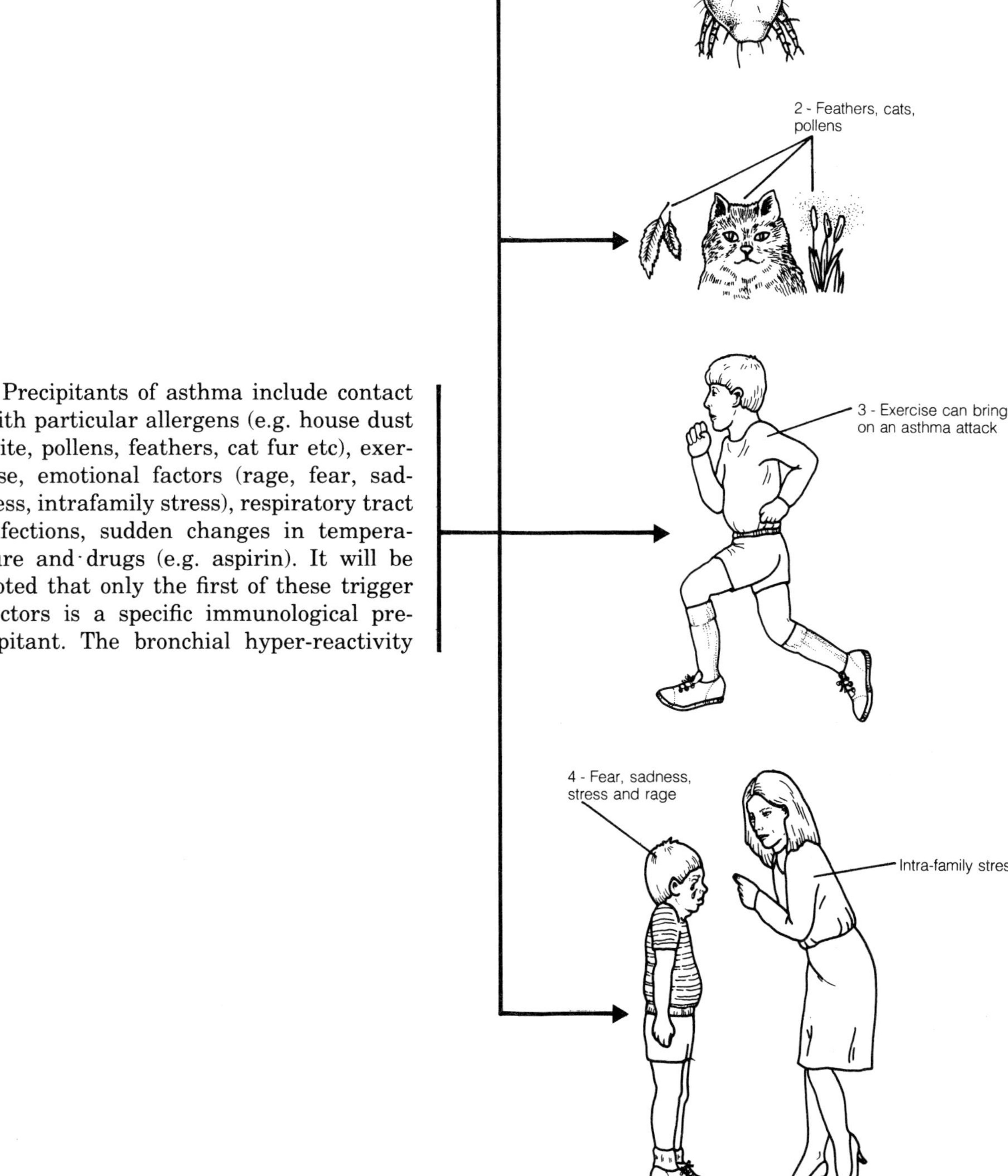

Precipitants of asthma include contact with particular allergens (e.g. house dust mite, pollens, feathers, cat fur etc), exercise, emotional factors (rage, fear, sadness, intrafamily stress), respiratory tract infections, sudden changes in temperature and drugs (e.g. aspirin). It will be noted that only the first of these trigger factors is a specific immunological precipitant. The bronchial hyper-reactivity thus extends to other less specific stimuli and the end result is identical whatever the stimulus – both clinically and with regard to response to treatment.

Adult asthma may be the continuation of childhood asthma or the illness may start in adult life – usually it is then of the intrinsic/non-atopic type. In general, intrinsic asthmatics have less well defined paroxysms of asthma/episodic asthma: the term "chronic asthma" has been used to try to describe the long spells of asthmatic symptoms that they may suffer.

In a typical episodic asthmatic attack, the patient notices a sudden feeling of tightness in the chest and then difficulty in breathing, particularly in expiration which becomes wheezy and laborious. A dry cough is often present or productive of a little viscous sputum sometimes containing mucoid bronchial casts, or the brown, mycelial containing casts of bronchopulmonary aspergillosis. Purulent

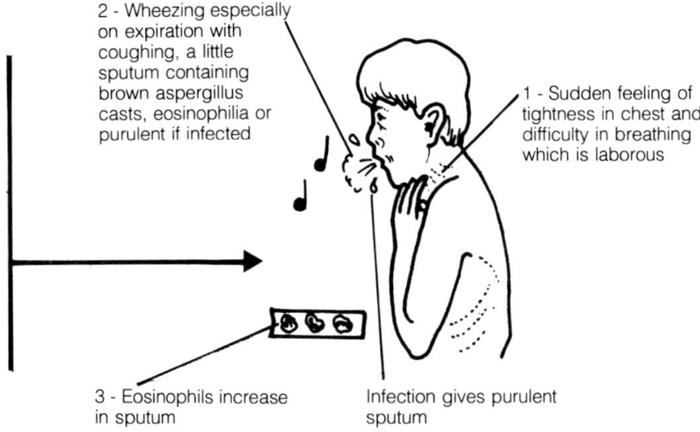

sputum denotes infection or eosinophil excess. The patient usually finds it essential to be upright, fixing the shoulder girdles to bring the accessory muscles of respiration into use. The chest is hyperinflated and there are short inspiratory gasps before the long expiratory wheezes. The auscultatory signs in the chest include quiet respiratory sounds and diffuse added expiratory rhonchi. The term **status asthmaticus** is used to described a prolonged and potentially dangerous attack of very severe asthma.

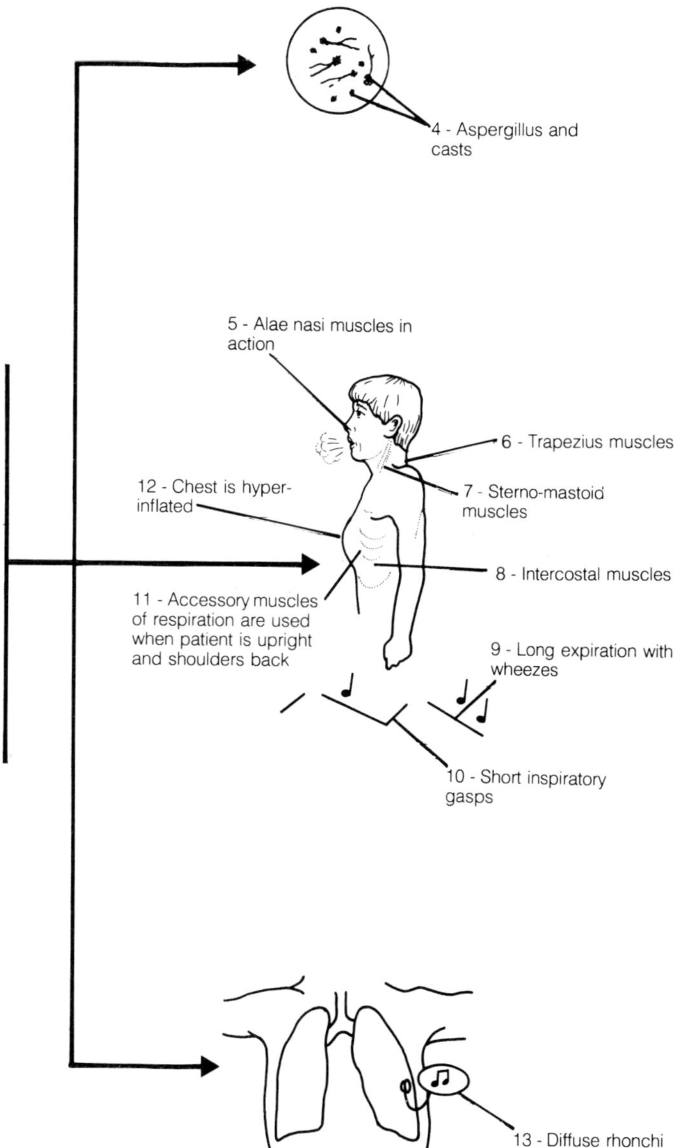

SIGNS OF SERIOUS ASTHMATIC ATTACK

Extra clinical signs denoting serious disease in an asthmatic attack are central cyanosis, a tachycardia of over 130/minute, pulsus paradoxus and a "silent chest" on auscultation (due to hyperinflation and difficulty in producing good-sized tidal volumes).

The PEFR and FEV_1/FVC values and ratio give a reliable indication of the degree of airways obstruction and its response to therapy. Arterial blood gas measurements are only necessary in serious attacks when hypoxaemia is found.

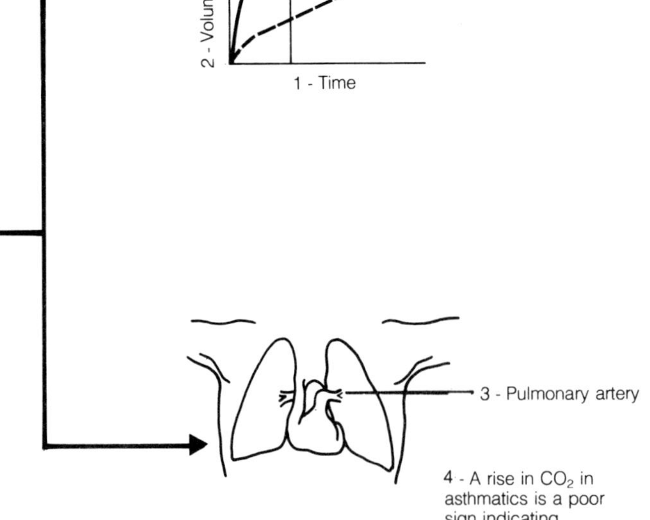

The PaCO$_2$ remains normal or low in most asthmatic attacks; indeed a rise in pCO2 in an asthmatic attack is an ominous sign often denoting exhaustion and weakened ventilatory effort. If maximal therapy has already been implemented, mechanical ventilation may be required.

The chest X-ray is usually normal in asthma although the hyperinflation may be manifest by low diaphragm and horizontal ribs. Patchy parenchymal lung shadowing may occur in cases associated with intense peripheral blood eosinophilia (usually intrinsic asthmatics) or in allergic bronchopulmonary aspergillosis. Mucus impaction in bronchi may cause areas of atelectasis.

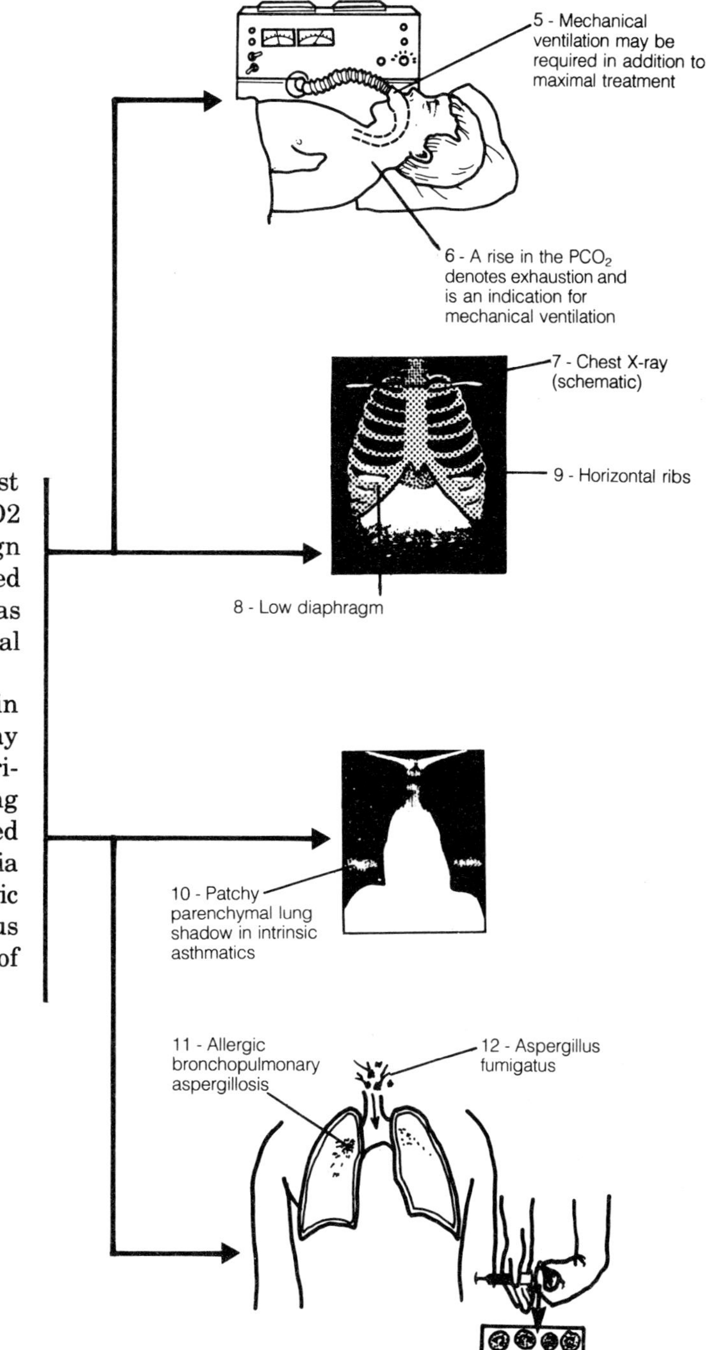

The diagnosis of a typical attack is usually simple, but precipitating and complicating factors (e.g. infection, atelectasis) should not be overlooked. In "chronic asthma", where the episodic nature of the symptoms are less conspicuous and wheezy dyspnoea may persist for weeks along with a productive cough, the diagnosis may well be mistaken for COAD. Clinical features in such a patient that suggest asthma include a recent onset of symptoms (particularly in a non-smoker), or symptoms from childhood, morning chest tightness, nocturnal wheezing attacks, large variations in PEFR on serial measurements and a peripheral blood eosinophilia. Acute left ventricular failure (LVF) causes nocturnal attacks of chest tightness and dyspnoea – even wheezing ("cardiac asthma").

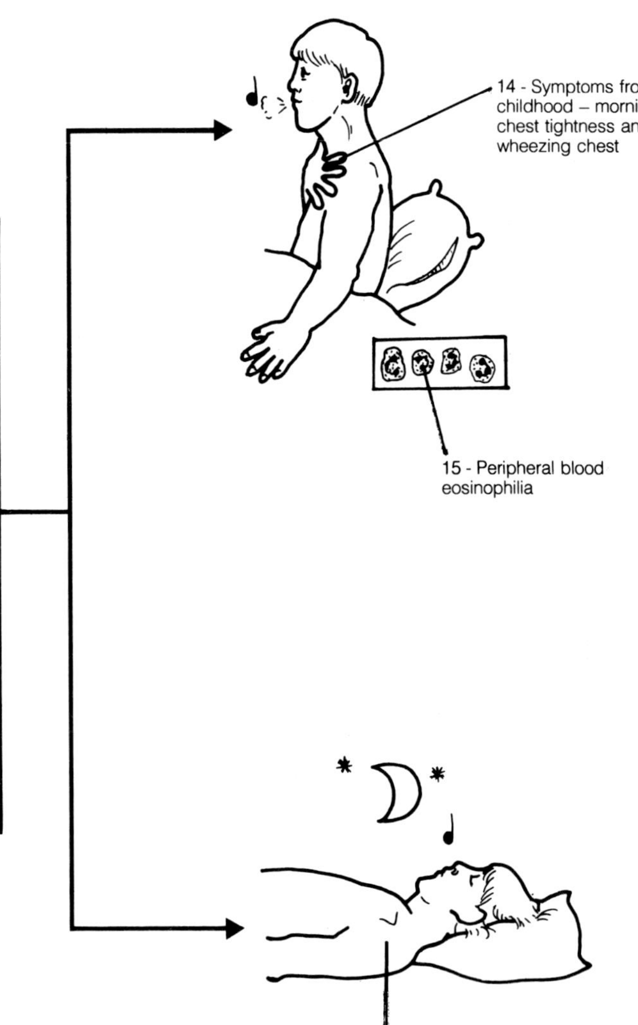

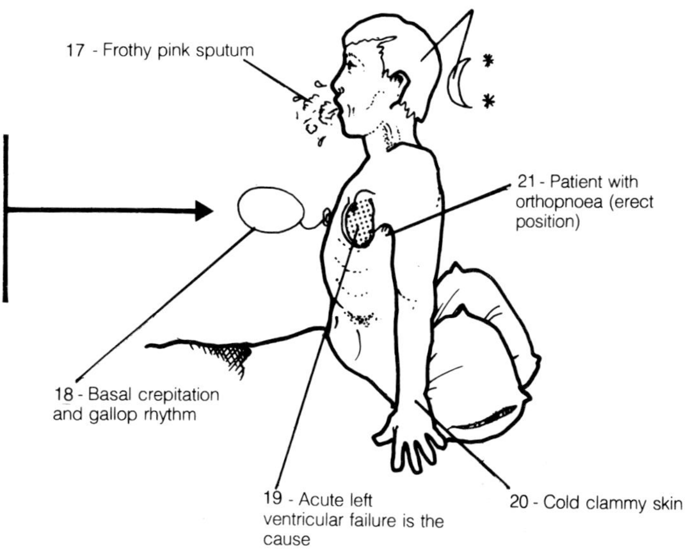

Known heart disease, severe orthopnoea, cold clammy skin, the expectoration of frothy pink sputum, basal crepitations and a perhaps audible gallop rhythm all help to distinguish LVF from asthma but it can be difficult.

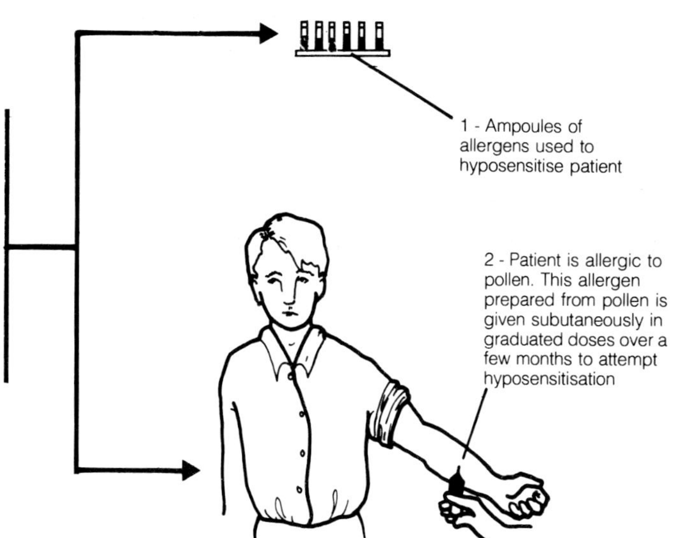

Prevention:– Specific allergens and non-specific bronchial irritants must be avoided. Hyposensitisation by medically supervised, subcutaneous injections of gradually increasing doses of known specific allergens may be worthwhile in selected patients (e.g. with grass pollen allergy). The home environment should be as stable as possible.

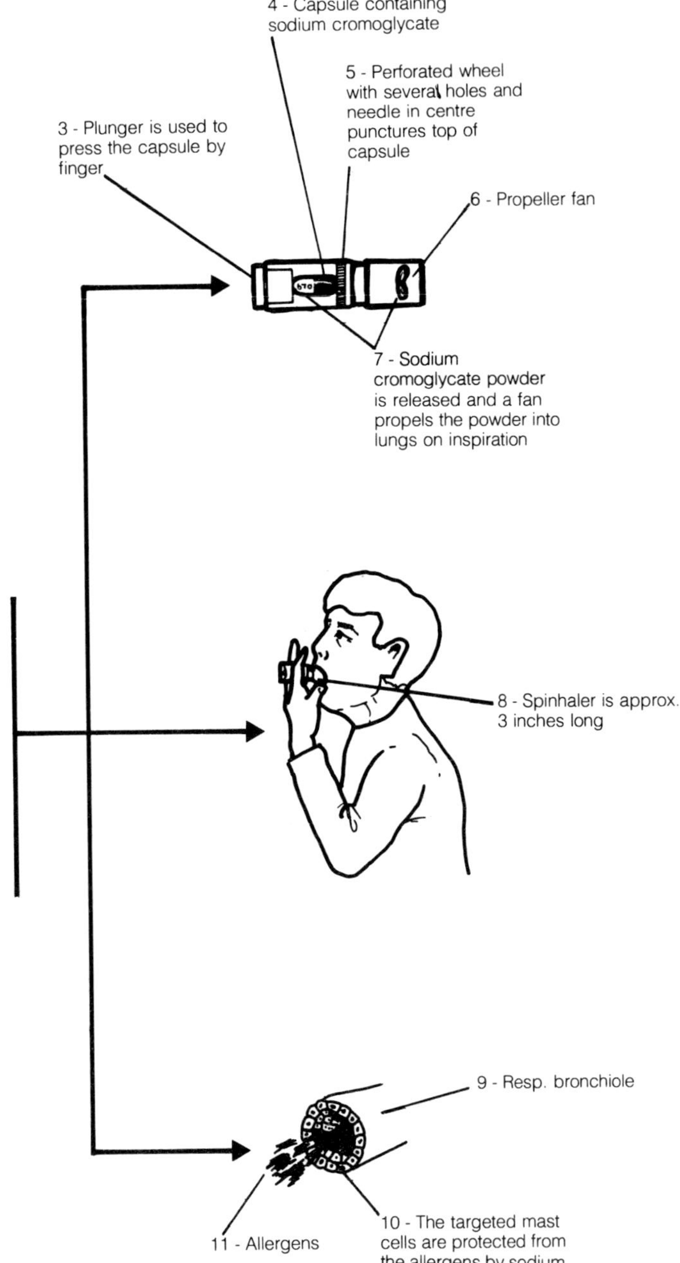

Sodium cromoglycate is a valuable prophylactic drug, particularly in atopic individuals but also some intrinsic asthmatics, and it is administered by inhalation using a "spin-haler" (40-80 mg/day in 4 divided doses). The drug acts by stabilising the mast cell membrane and preventing the release of the humoral mediators of asthma. It is virtually free of side effects.

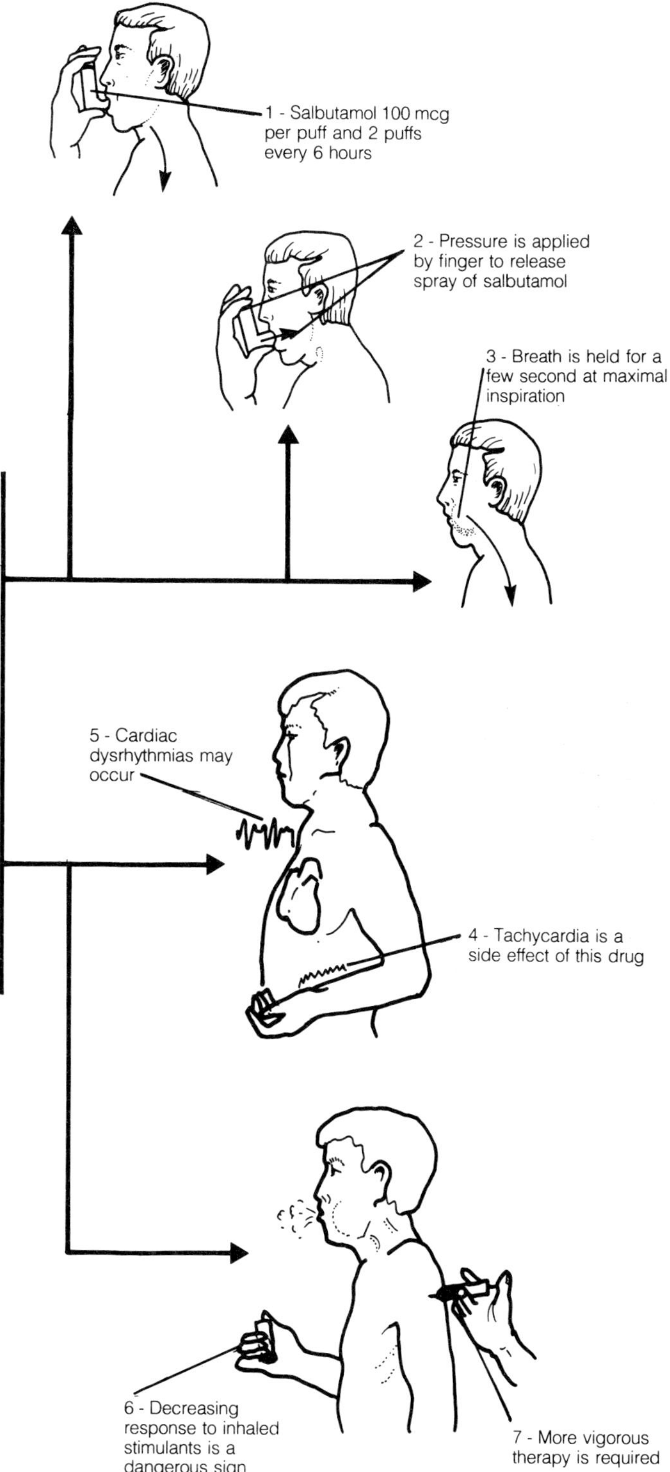

The Asthmatic Attack:– Moderate attacks of asthma are controlled by the patient himself using a pressurised aerosol delivery of a adrenergic stimulant drug (e.g. salbutamol 100 μg per "puff") each patient is given an upper limit of doses that can be administered each time (e.g. 2 puffs 6 hourly). He must learn to synchronise drug delivery with his early inspiratory effort and breathhold for a few seconds at maximal inspiration. Tachycardia (and rarely more severe dysrhythmias) and tremor are side effects of these drugs. A decreasing therapeutic response to inhaled stimulants is a warning of severe asthma requiring more vigorous medical therapy.

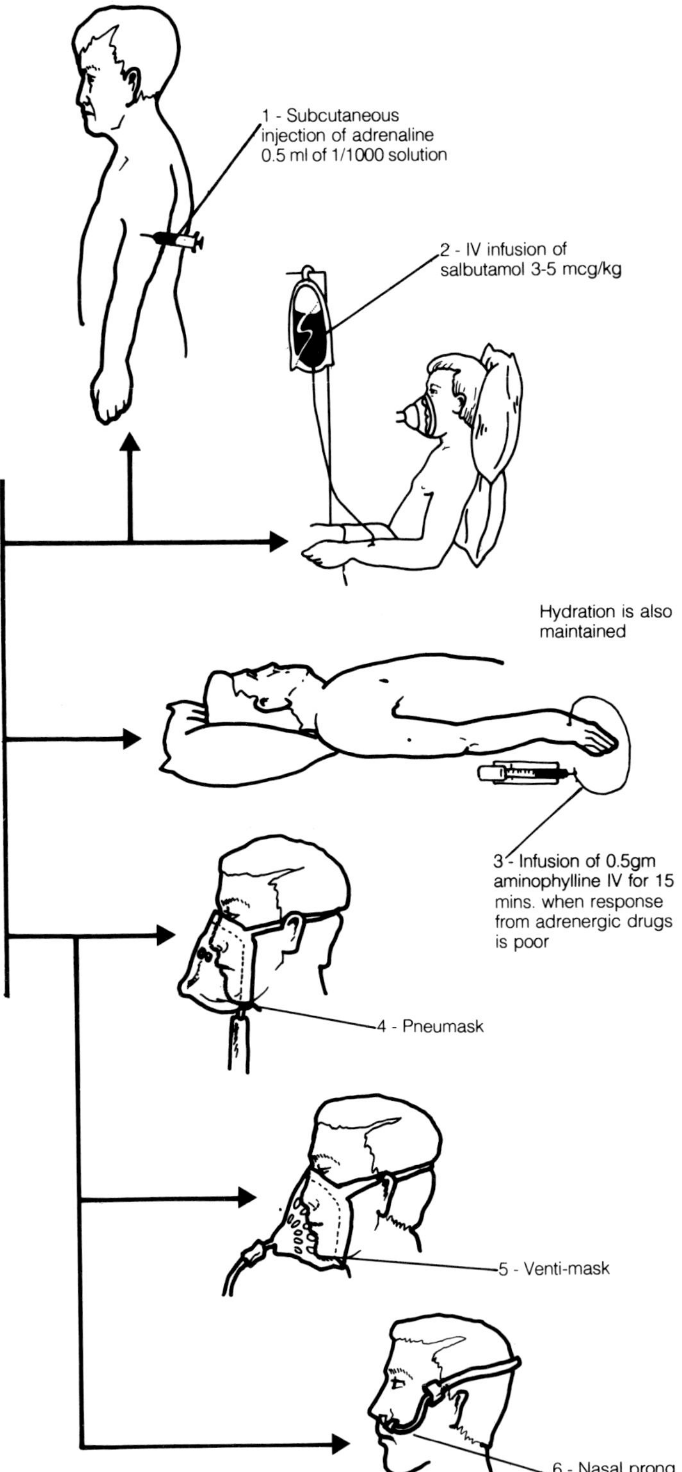

The Severe Asthmatic Attack Systemic administration of adrenergic stimulants is advised: adrenaline 0.5 ml of 1/1000 solution subcutaneously is effective, but an intravenous infusion of salbutamol 3-5 μg/Kg is the modern and more logical alternative. Aminophylline 0.5 g (adults) by slow intravenous injection over 5 minutes (or by infusion) is recommended when there is not a rapid response to adrenergic drugs. An intravenous infusion is advisable to maintain hydration, and hydrocortisone 100-200 mg is administered early and repeated 4 hourly until the attack subsides. Oxygen therapy is delivered to counteract hypoxaemia by mask or nasal prongs, and

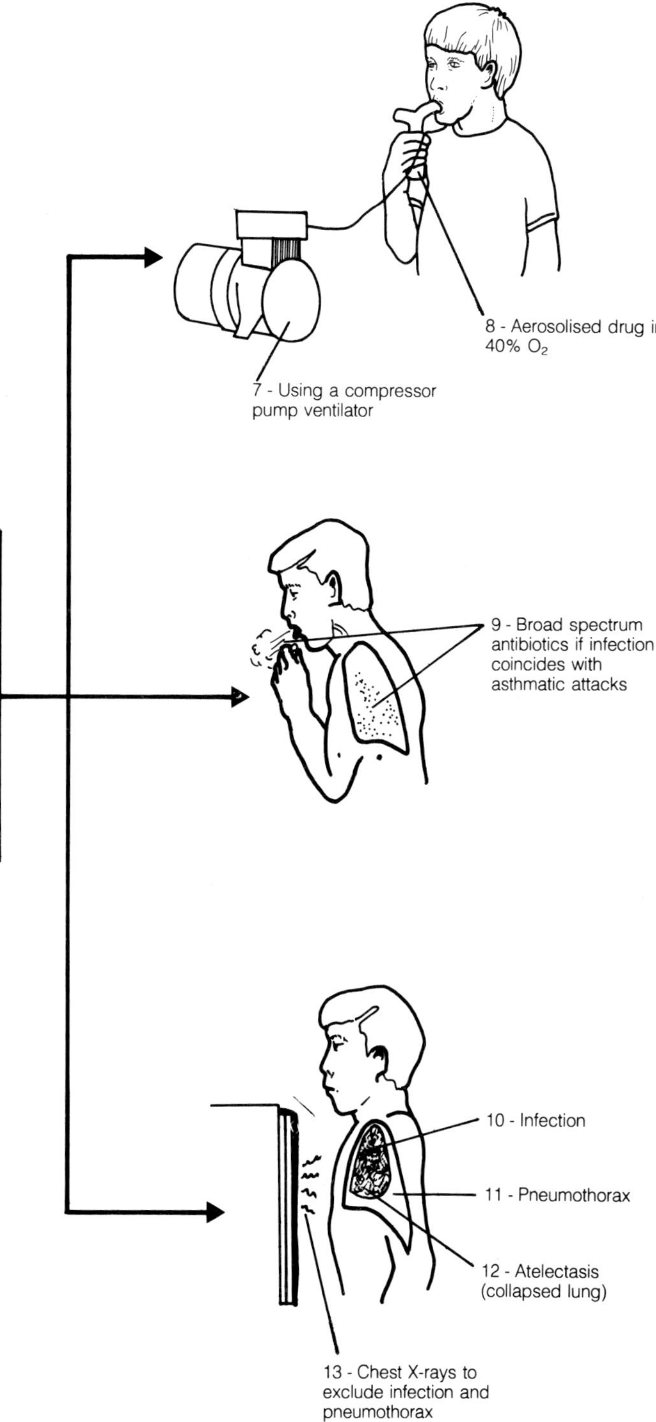

adrenergic stimulants are continued to be administered 2-4 hourly, by inhalation of aerosolised drug in 40% oxygen via a patient triggered ventilator (Bennet or Bird ventilators). Any suggestion of a respiratory infection co-existing with the asthmatic attack is an indication for a broad spectrum antibiotic. A chest X-ray (to exclude infection, atelectasis, pneumothorax etc.) and blood gases are performed. Pulse rate, respiratory rate and

PEF are monitored. Mechanical ventilation is required in exhausted, patients in severe respiratory distress and in addition to worsening hypoxaemia, a rising $PaCO_2$. A powerful volume-cycled ventilator is employed following intubation with a cuffed endotracheal tube. Such patients will be nursed in "intensive care" facilities.

The place of corticosteroid therapy in asthma management needs a further note. Steroids are effective in the control of chronic asthma and very important therapy in the treatment of severe attacks. Oral prednisolone is effective in prophylaxis of asthma but because of the cushingoid side effects, steroid drugs are witheld unless certain indications are present. Steroid aerosols will not terminate a severe attack of asthma but are an important alternative in chronic asthma and in preventing bad asthmatic attacks, as they do not cause such severe cushingoid features, e.g. beclomethasone dipropionate inhaler 400 mcg/day. It is imperative that it is explained to the patient that the corticosteroid inhaler is largely for prophylaxis and so he must take it regularly during periods of bad asthma. In a **"chronic asthma" spell,** when a patient is taking both stimulant and steroid by inhaler, the stimulant should be inhaled 5 minutes before the steroid,

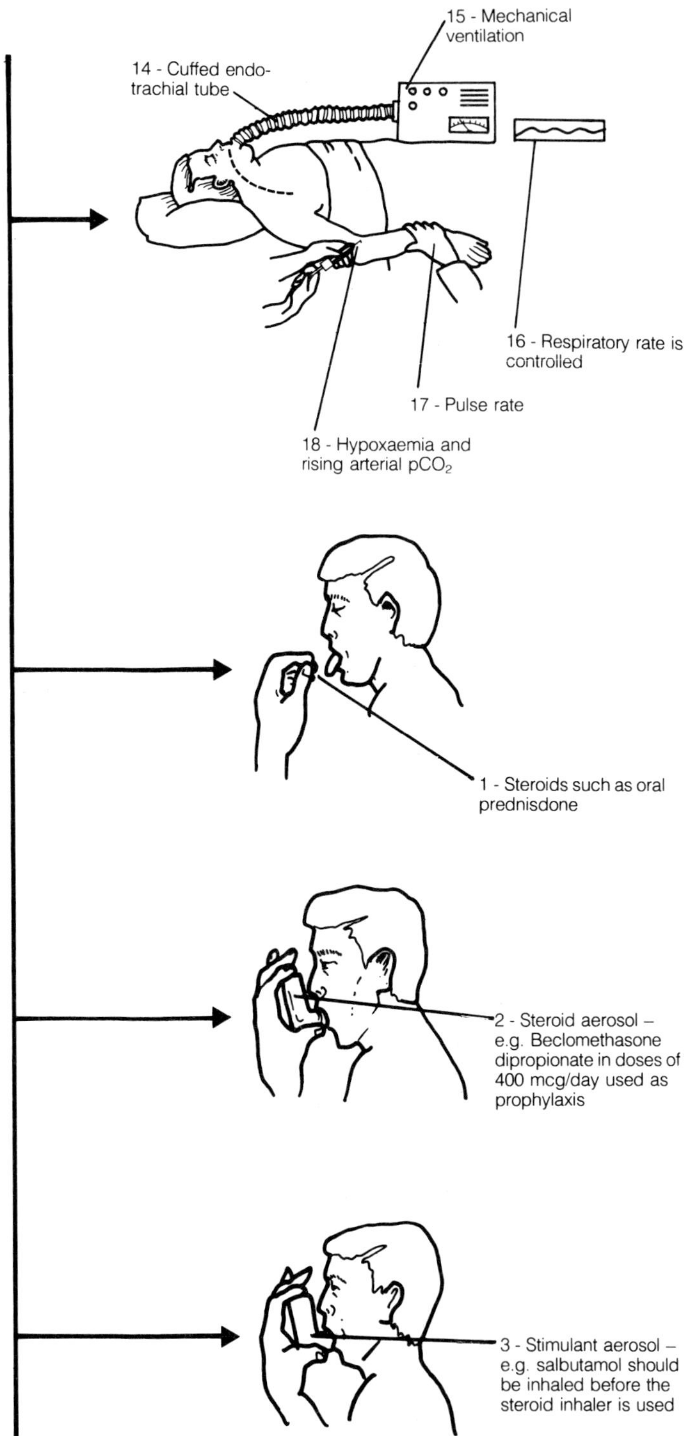

(as it thus allows better inhalation of the steroid). Long term oral steroids (prednisolone tablets e.g. 20 mg/day in divided doses for adults are only prescribed for bad asthmatics not satisfactorily controlled by other measures (including inhalational steroids) and in whom it has been demonstrated by PEFR and FEV_1 measurements that steroids are efficiacious.

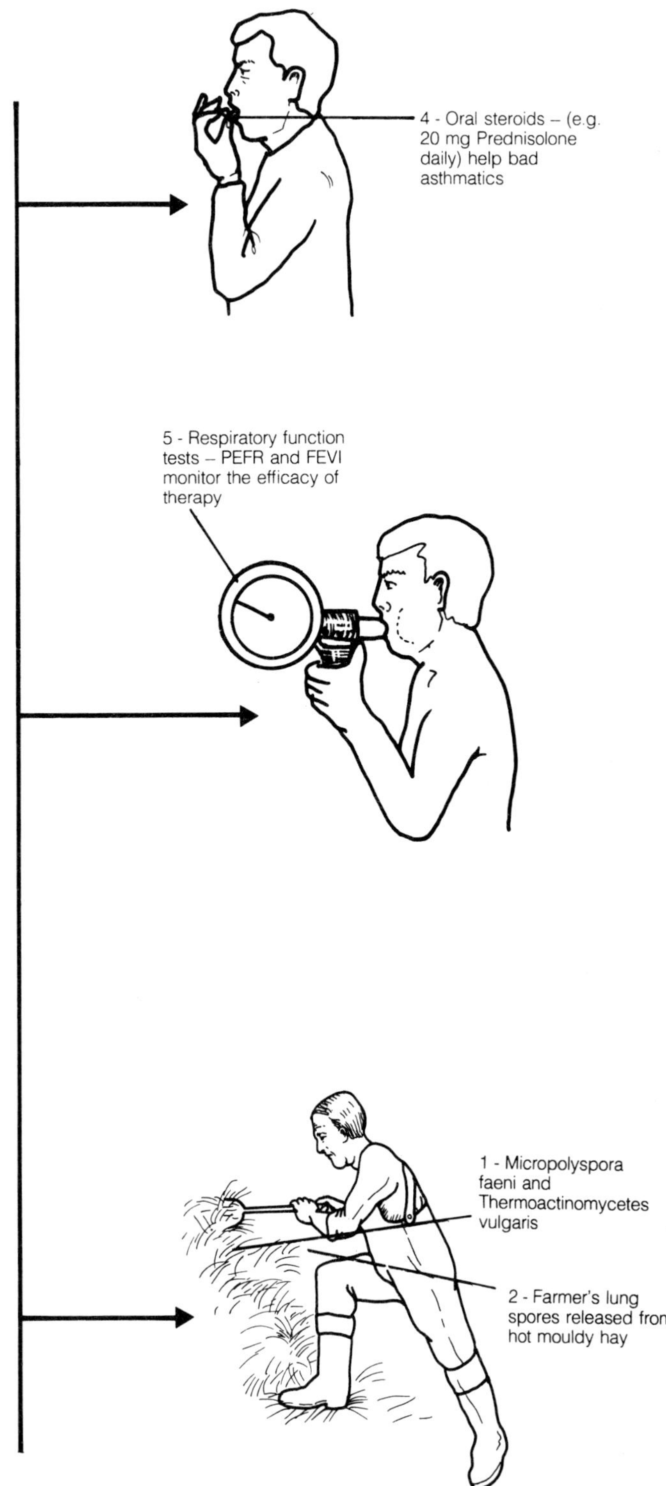

EXTRINSIC ALLERGIC ALVEOLITIS AND EXTRINSIC NON-ATOPIC ASTHMA

This form of allergic lung disease is caused by organic dusts (usually in non-atopic individuals), which generate antibodies that on re-exposure to the allergen react in a type III immunological reaction. This clinically manifests 3-4 hours after exposure, becomes maximal 7-8 hours after exposure and subsides (unless the allergen exposure persists) after 24 hours. An associated rise in the peripheral white cell count (including eosinophils) is not a feature.

Many organic dusts are capable of causing this reaction – "Farmer's lung" due to spores from Micropolyspora faeni, Thermophilic actinomycetes or Thermo-actinomyces vulgaris – all from hot, mouldy hay, "Bagassosis" due to exposure to hot, mouldy sugar cane bagasse – again often T. vulgaris and T. actinomycetes implicated and also in "mushroom picker's lung". Bird fancier's lung, Furrier's lung, Woodworker's lung are due to sensitivity to avian protein, animal hair and sawdust extracts respectively. There are many other recognised allergens.

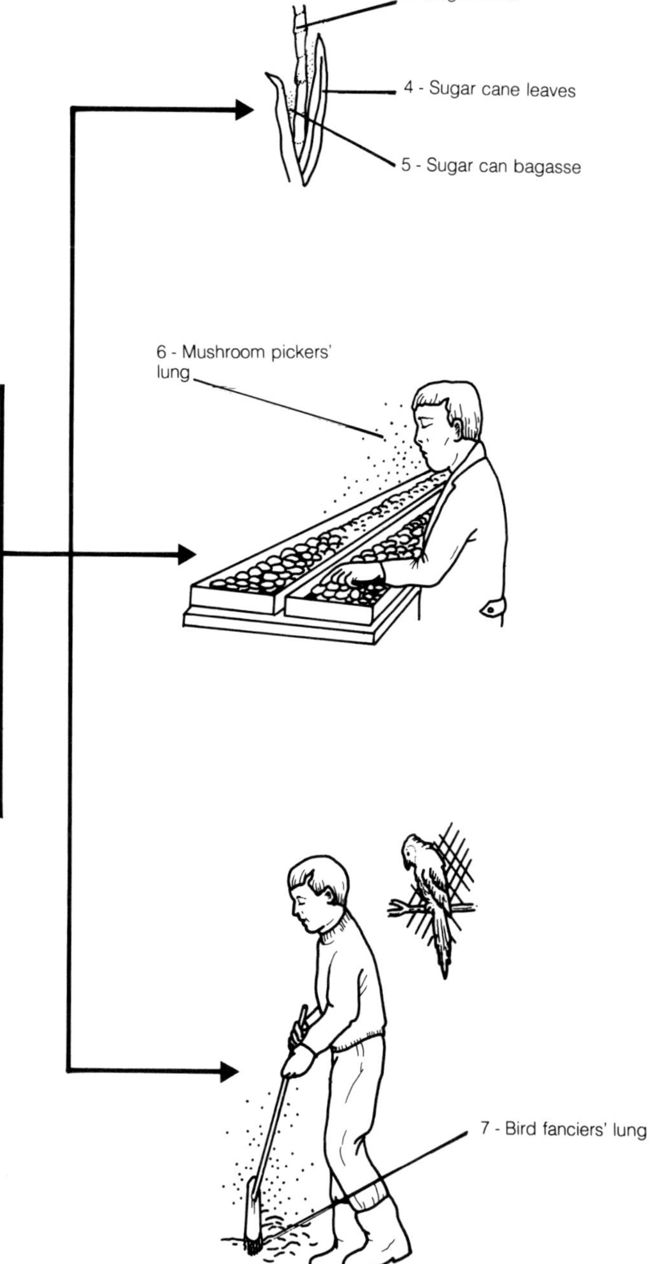

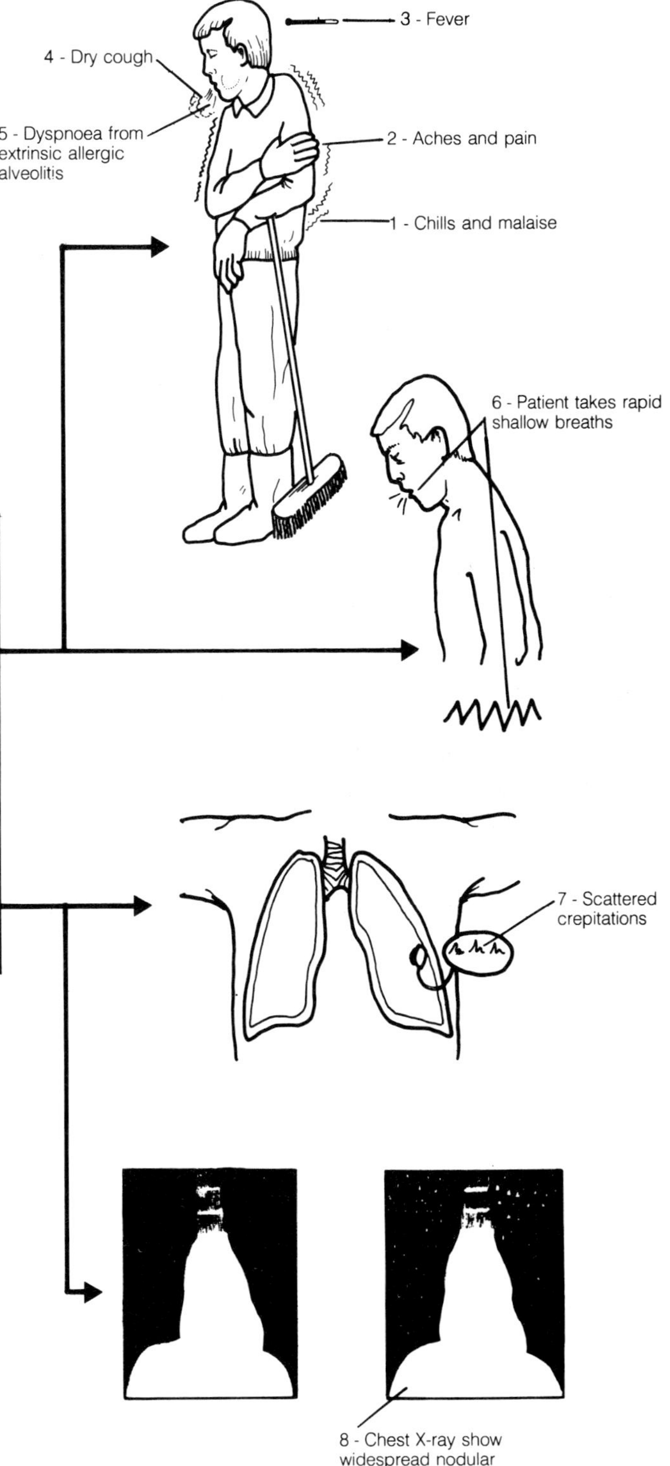

The clinical picture starts 3-4 hours after exposure and constitutional symptoms may be prominent with fever, chills, malaise, aches and pains. The chest symptoms of the alveolar reaction (extrinsic allergic alveolitis) manifest as a severe dyspnoea with a dry cough: wheezing is not present. On examination the patient is taking rapid shallow breaths and on auscultation there are scattered crepitations. The lung function tests show a restrictive ventilatory defect with a decrease in VC, FVC and DLCO. The chest X-ray shows widespread nodular shadowing.

Sometimes a bronchial reaction overrides the alveolar reaction, then called extrinsic, non-atopic asthma. Again, 3-4 hours after allergen exposure a tightness of the chest occurs with wheezing and asthmatic clinical features – often more refractory to immediate therapy (e.g. salbutamol).

Continuing exposure to the allergen leads to more insidious systemic and chest symptoms. The progression of the extrinsic alveolitis reaction is to lung fibrosis and severe lung destruction.

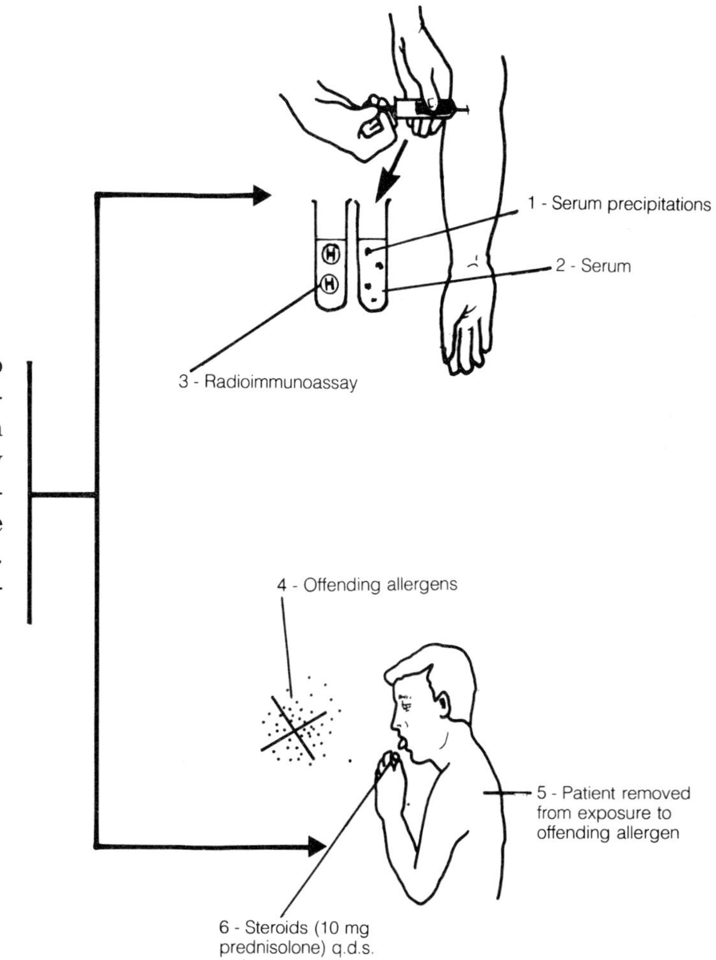

The detection of serum-precipitins to the allergen assist diagnosis, and radio-immunoassays have been important in making monitoring quantitative. The only certain way to ensure cure is to permanently remove the patient from exposure to the offending allergen. Steroids (e.g. prednisolone 10 mg qds) reduce the severity of attacks.

PULMONARY EOSINOPHILIA

This is not one condition but a group of quite different pulmonary conditions but all associated with a peripheral blood and pulmonary eosinophilia.

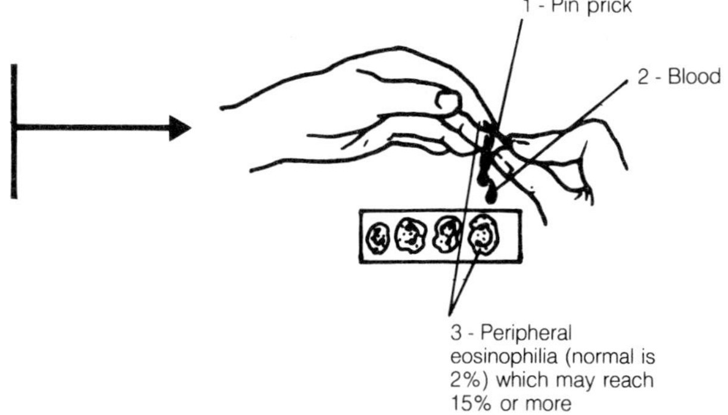

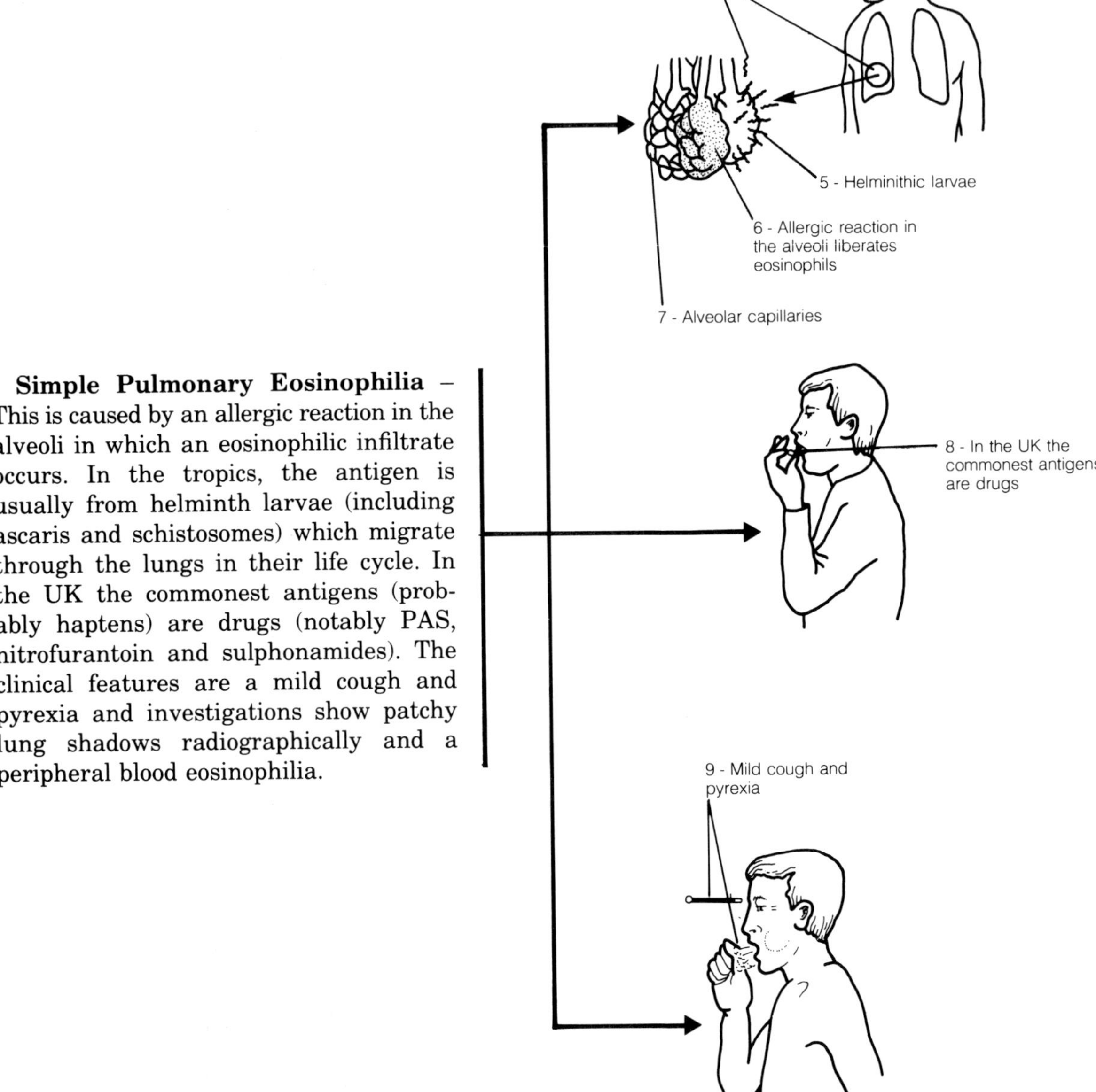

Simple Pulmonary Eosinophilia – This is caused by an allergic reaction in the alveoli in which an eosinophilic infiltrate occurs. In the tropics, the antigen is usually from helminth larvae (including ascaris and schistosomes) which migrate through the lungs in their life cycle. In the UK the commonest antigens (probably haptens) are drugs (notably PAS, nitrofurantoin and sulphonamides). The clinical features are a mild cough and pyrexia and investigations show patchy lung shadows radiographically and a peripheral blood eosinophilia.

Asthma with Pulmonary Eosinophilia
– Although eosinophilia is a frequent accompaniment of asthma, concomitant pulmonary infiltration is not. When it occurs in the UK, it is usually in extrinsic asthmatics and due to combined types I and III immune sensitivity to Aspergillus fumigatus. The asthmatic symptoms of this allergic bronchopulmonary aspergillosis have been described; the pulmonary lesions may take the form of infiltrates of areas of collapse/atelectasis. Bronchiecta-

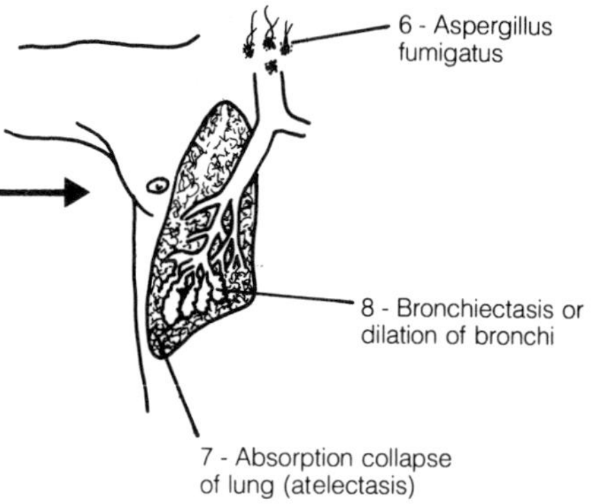

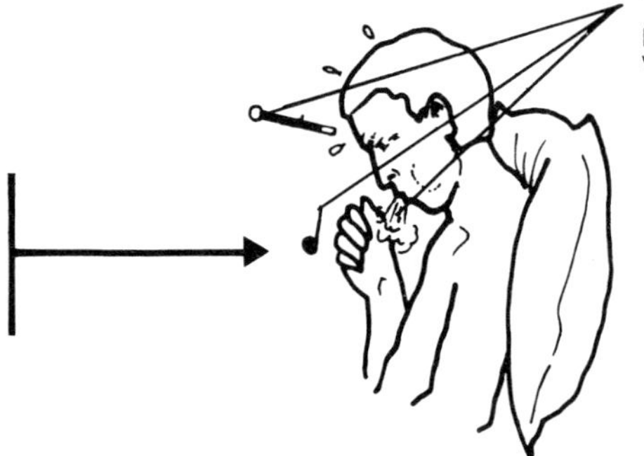

sis not infrequently occurs in collapsed lobes and lung destruction can be serious. Aspergillus is found in the sputum and proves very refractory to antifungal treatment.

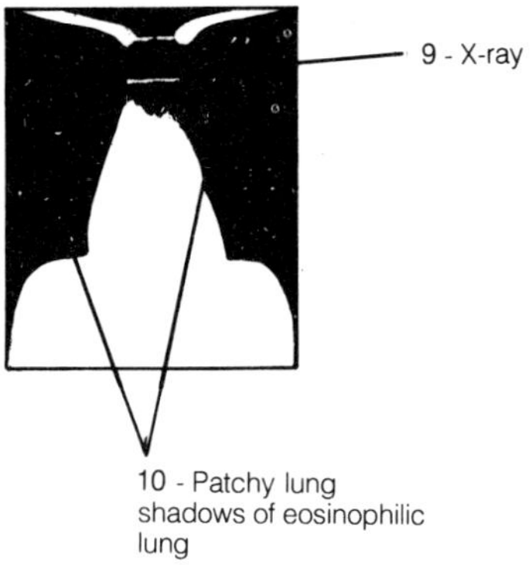

Tropical pulmonary eosinophilia with asthmatic symptoms occurs mainly in India and Ceylon. It is due to an allergy to microfilariae in the lung. There is a

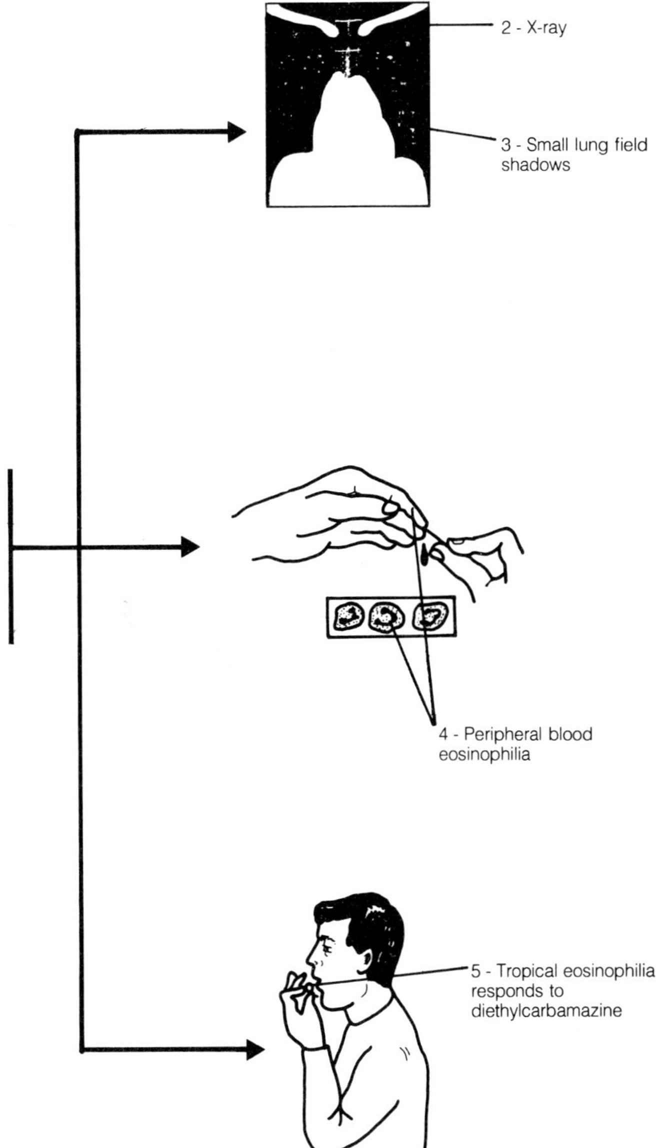

persistent dry cough and wheeze and the patient may be febrile. The chest X-ray shows small nodular lung field shadowing and there is a peripheral blood eosinophilia. The condition responds to antifiliarial chemotherapy e.g. diethylcarbamazine.

Polyarteritis Nodosa (PAN) and Wegener's Disease – PAN is a connective tissue disorder of less certain auto-immune basis than other disorders of this group. Approximately one third of cases have lung involvement and some of these develop asthma associated with eosinophilia, whilst others suffer progressive lung destruction without these features. An allied disorder, Wegener's disease, is often accompanied by necrotising granulomata in the lungs and it is commonly associated with serious renal disease also, (as may indeed occur in PAN). High dose corticosteroids may retard the progress of these serious diseases (e.g. prednisolone tablets 20 mg tds).

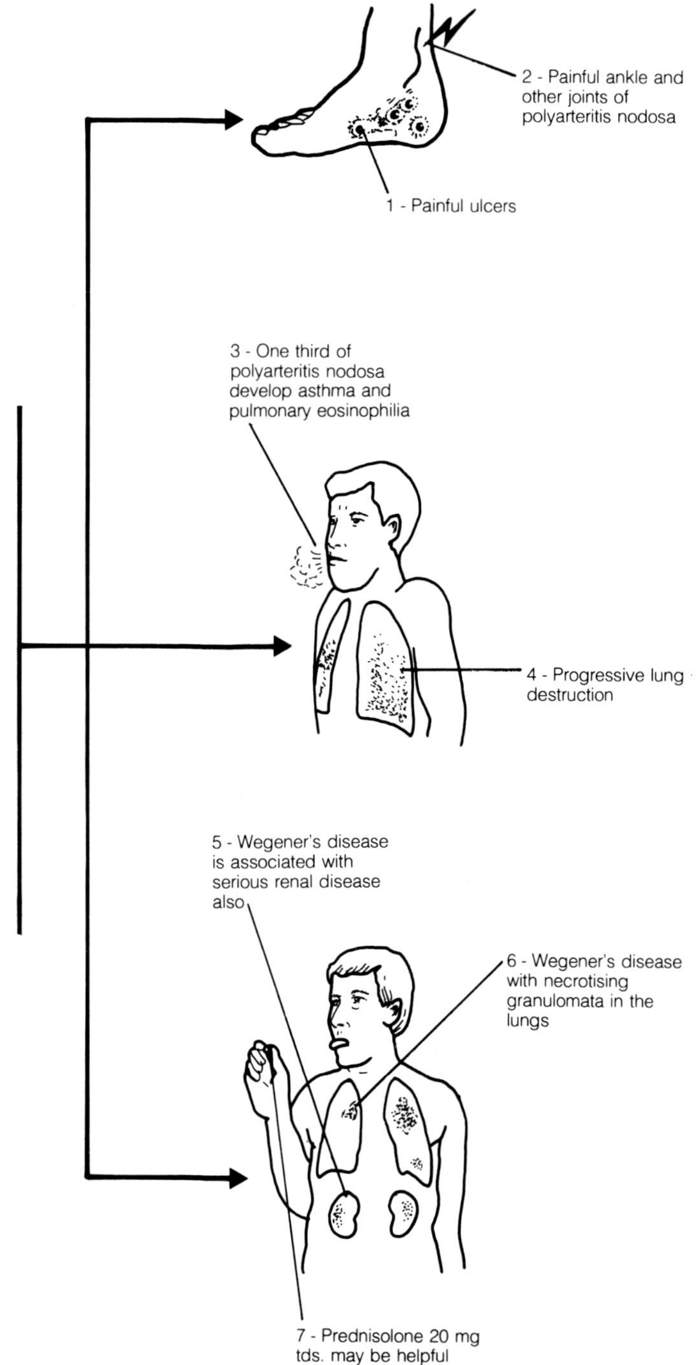

SARCOIDOSIS

Sarcoidosis is a disease of unknown aetiology that most commonly afflicts young adult women, (the F:M ratio is 3:2). Sarcoidosis is most commonly encountered in temperate climates and it is uncommon throughout Africa, India and China. The pathological hallmark of the disease is the **sarcoid granuloma** which may occur in many different organs of the body. The lungs, lymph nodes, liver and spleen are most commonly affected. Each granuloma consists of a focal collection of large pale staining histiocytes (epithelioid cells) among which there may be multinucleate giant cells. Superficially these granulomas resemble T.B. granulomas but caseation does not occur and M.tb is absent. An associated immunological phenomenon is depressed type IV immune reactivity, such that skin reactions to purified protein derivative (PPD) and Candida albicans are reduced and skin sensitisation to dinitrochlorbenzene is difficult to achieve. The **clinical manifestations** are protean, but there are certain commoner presentations.

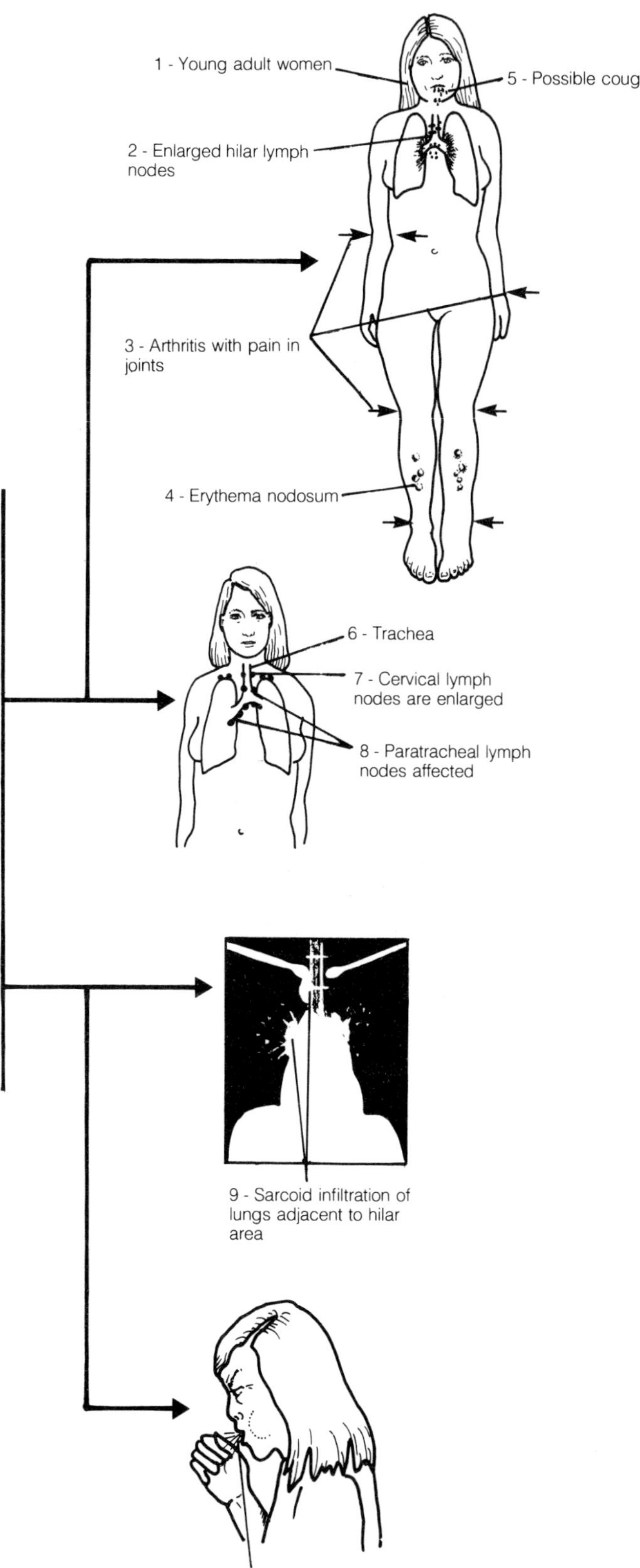

The first is a syndrome of fever, poly-arthralgia (particularly of larger joints), erythema nodosum (on fronts of shins) and bilateral hilar lymphadenopathy. The bilateral hilar lymphadenopathy (BHL) may be symptomatic with cough or may be asymptomatic. On chest X-ray it is usually fairly symmetrical on the two sides and the paratracheal (and cervical) nodes may also be enlarged. There may be radiological evidence of sarcoid infiltration of the lungs adjacent to the hila, showing up as patchy nodular or reticulonodular shadowing usually in both lungs in the middle third of the lung fields. Such patients usually have a dry irritating cough. Sarcoidosis is occasionally diagnosed in an asymptomatic individual who has BHL perhaps with lung shadowing on a routine chest X-ray.

The vast majority of patients with BHL and associated symptoms do not progress to chronic sarcoidosis but resolve. Indeed one estimate shows that 9 of 10 individuals with BHL have normal chest X-rays 2 years later. The early infiltrative lung lesions may also resolve. Nevertheless, an unfortunate minority of patients do progress and may develop progressive pulmonary fibrosis or sarcoidosis of the nervous system (presenting in many possible ways from focal signs to menigoencephalitis or transverse myelitis) or eye, bone or heart lesions. Patients with sarcoidosis have an abnormal sensitivity to vitamin D and persistent hypercalcaemia may occur with all its problems.

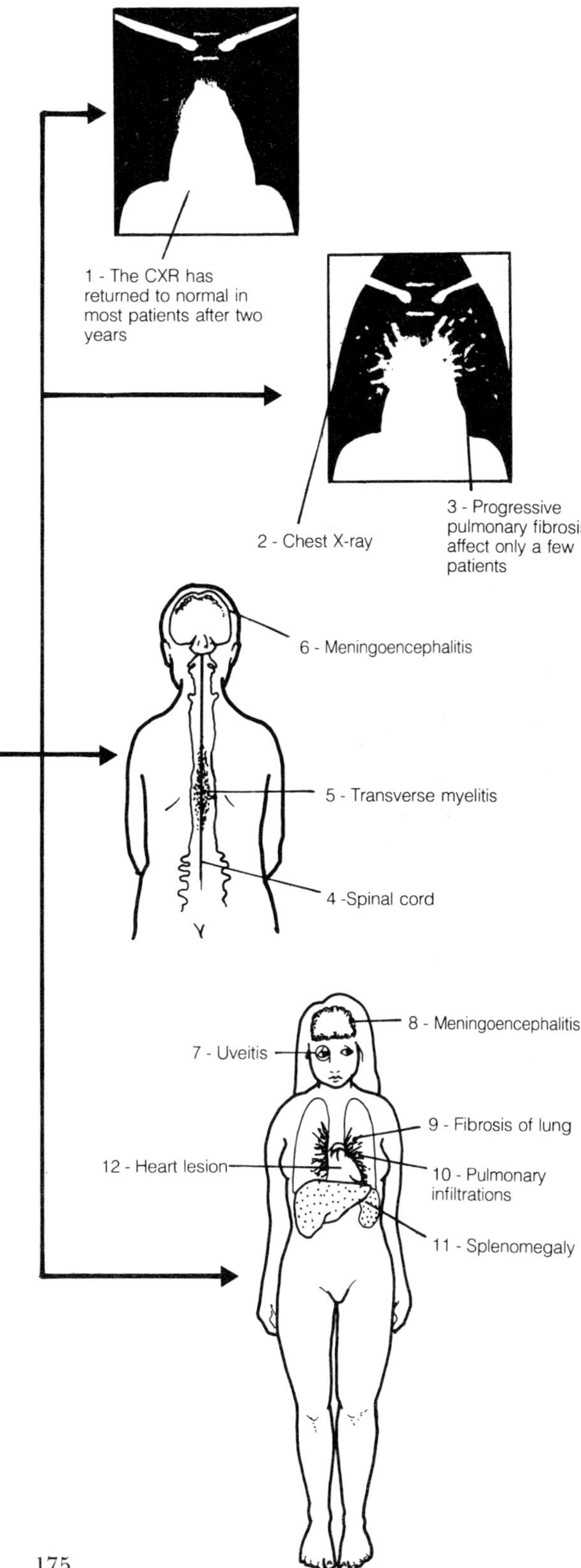

Ocular sarcoidosis may be a presenting complaint when it presents as an acute uveitis or iridocyclitis. A more chronic form of uveitis may not give rise to the pain and photophobia (the acute eye complaints), and this may lead to serious eye damage before diagnosis. Rarely it is associated with swelling of the parotid and sometimes lacrimal glands.

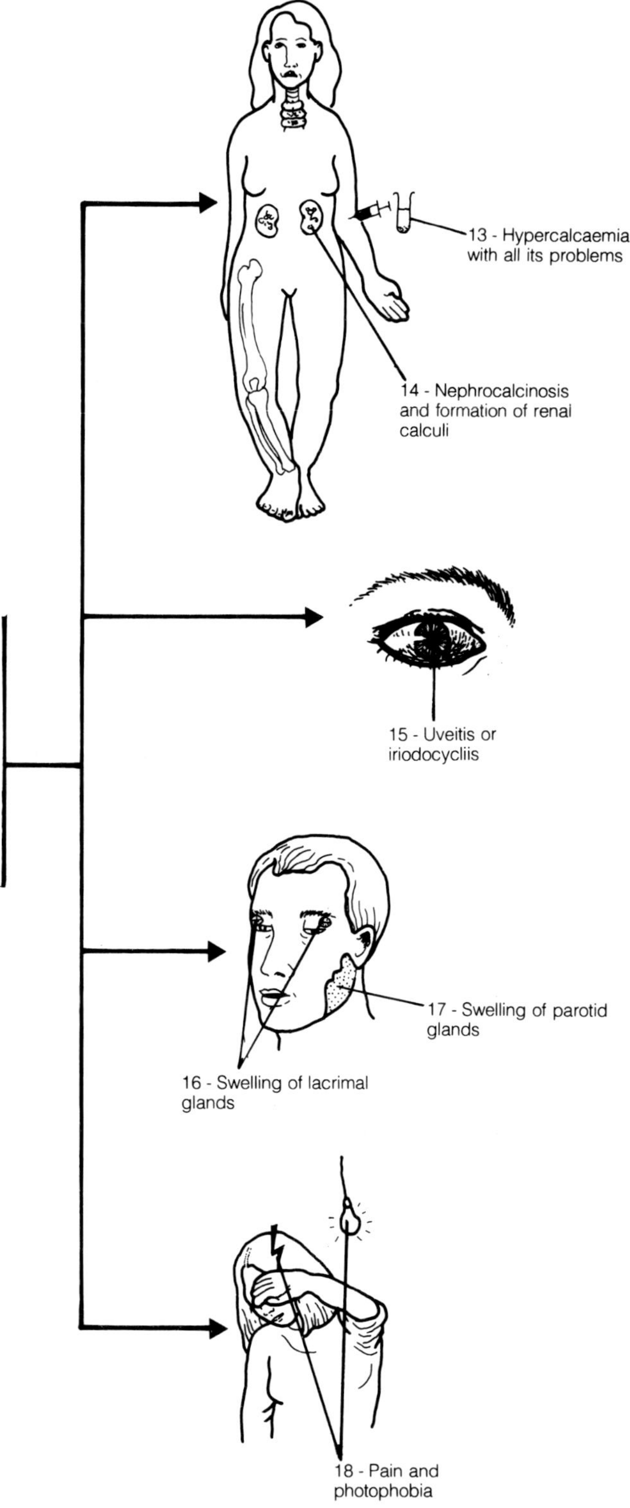

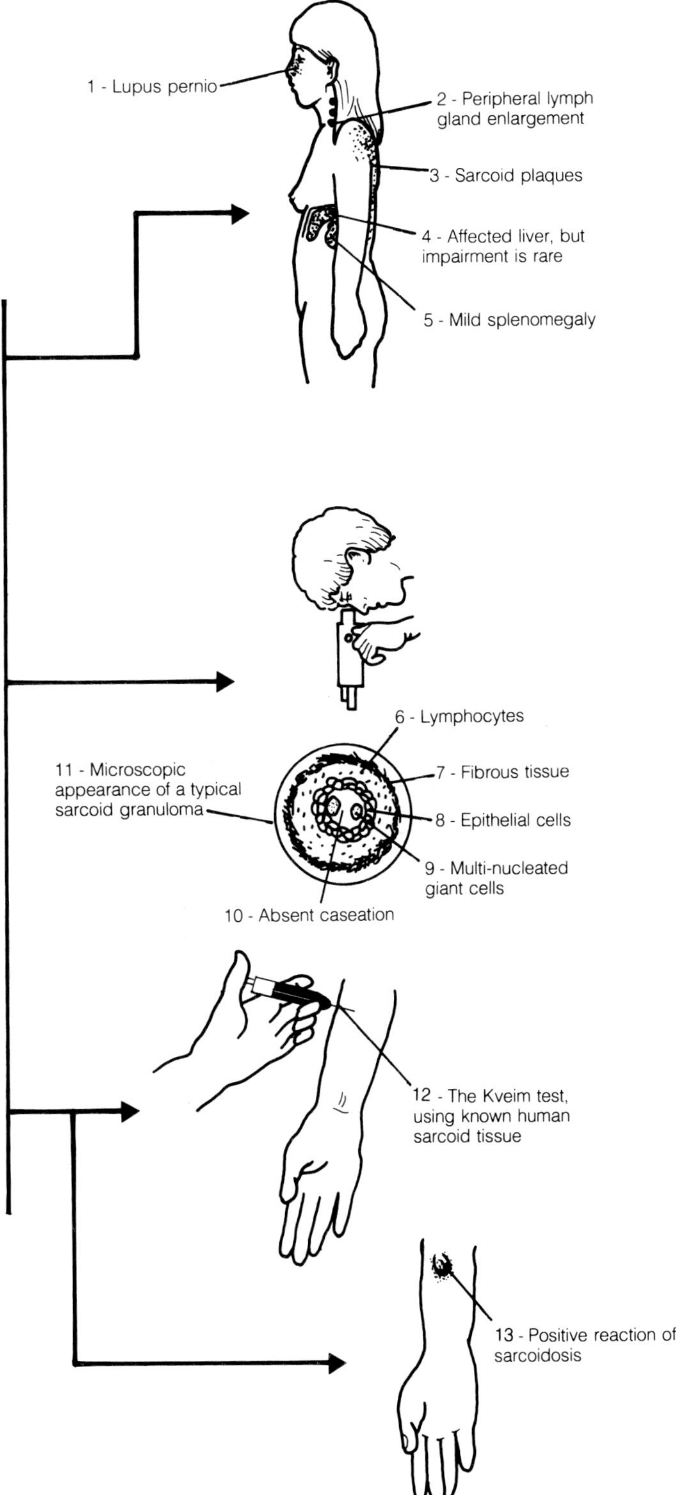

Skin sarcoidosis may comprise lupus pernio, sarcoid plaques or nodular infiltration in progressive sarcoidosis. Peripheral lymph gland enlargement is not uncommon in active sarcoidosis, particularly in the neck. The liver is very commonly affected in active sarcoidosis but severe impairment of liver function is rare. Modest splenomegaly due to involvement is also common.

The **diagnosis** of sarcoidosis is a tissue diagnosis (i.e. made by a histologist on biopsy material) demonstrating widespread non-caseating epithelioid cell granulomatosis. The Kveim test comprises an intradermal injection of a suspension

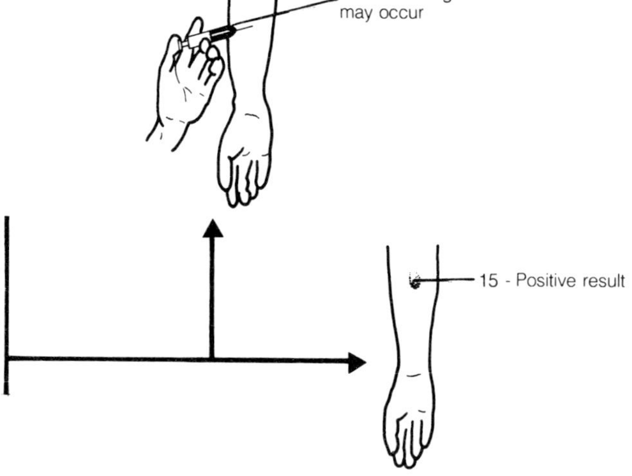

of known human sarcoid tissue. A positive result, which comprises the development of a sarcoid granuloma at the site of injection by 6 weeks, supports the diagnosis of sarcoidosis, but false negatives occur.

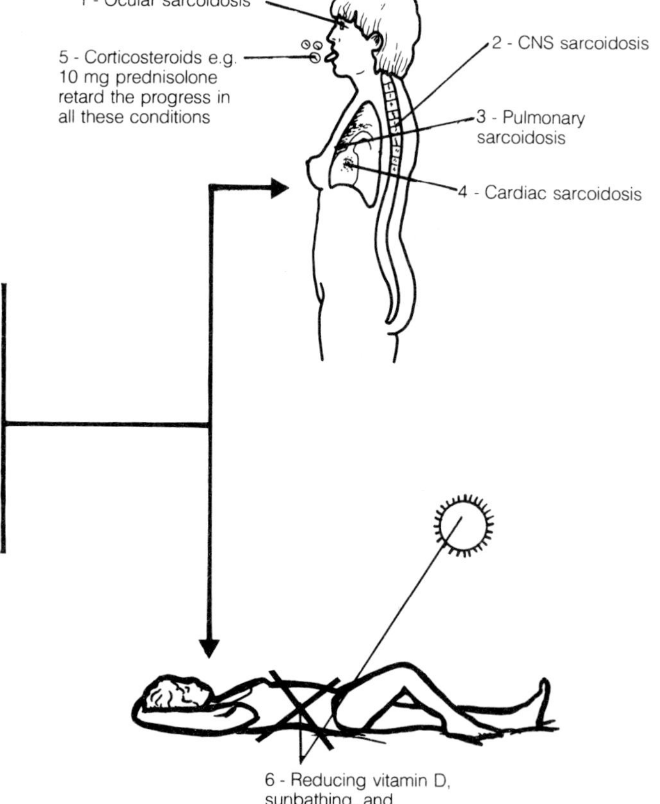

Treatment: Most patients recover spontaneously and completely and require no treatment. Corticosteroids are the most effective agents at retarding the progress of sarcoidosis and are indicated in ocular, central nervous system and cardiac sarcoidosis. They may be also indicated in more severe cases of pulmonary sarcoidosis (e.g. prednisolone tablets

10 mg b.d.). Hypercalcaemia is managed by reducing vitamin D intake, sunbathing and excessive calsium intake along with oral phosphate, corticosteroids and a high fluid intake.

FIBROSING ALVEOLITIS

Diffuse **pulmonary fibrosis** and **alveolitis** occurs in a number of conditions. It may be the sequel to chronic extrinsic alveolitis (e.g. farmer's lung), sarcoidosis or the pneumoconioses. It may follow pulmonary radiation or follow some drugs used in therapeutics (e.g. busulphan, chlorambucil, bleomycin). There remain two similar types of fibrosing alveolitis which may have a common immunological aetiology: the first is cryptogenic fibrosing alveolitis and the second is the fibrosing alveolitis associated with connective tissue disease, notably systemic sclerosis, systemic lupus erythematosus and rheumatoid arthritis.

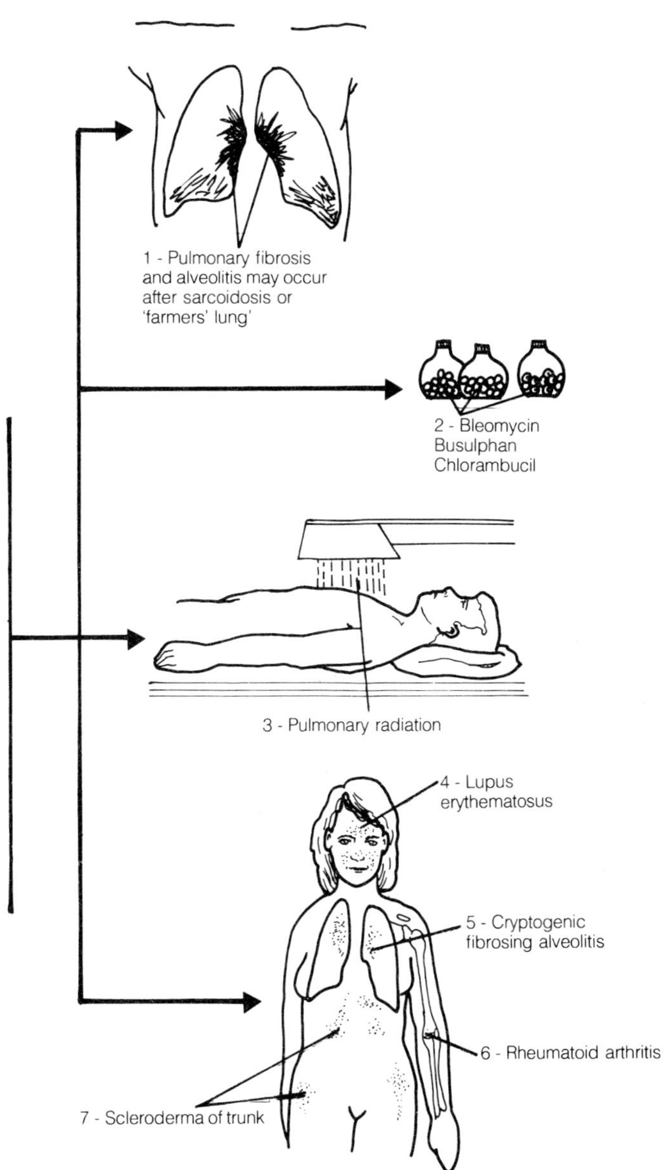

Cryptogenic fibrosing alveolitis (CFA) – A rare disease with world-wide distribution that tends to affect middle aged men slightly more commonly than other adults. The aetiology is unknown but an immunological basis seems likely. The typical histological features of the lungs are cellular thickening of the alveolar wall with (later) fibrosis and a mononuclear cell infiltrate within the alveoli. If the first feature dominates the histological pattern is termed "mural CFA" (cryptogenic fibrosing alveolitis), if the latter feature is most conspicuous the pattern is "desquamative CFA". Approximately one third of patients with CFA have a positive serum antinuclear factor and many of these have a positive serum rheumatoid factor; circulating immune complexes and IgG with complement deposition in alveolar capillaries, have also been demonstrated in CFA.

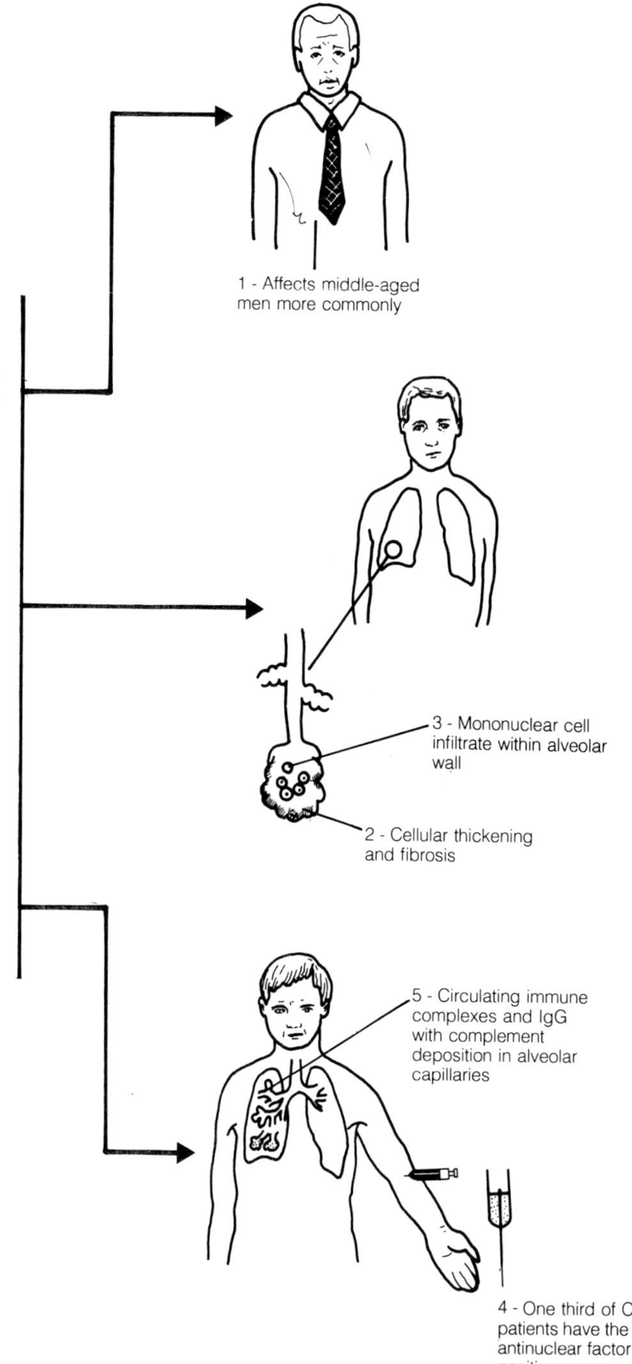

The presenting **clinical symptom** in CFA is progressive dyspnoea on effort, but the pace of onset and progression is enormously variable. A dry cough is a later feature and, like many restrictive lung conditions, is precipitated by deep inspiration. A rheumatoid-like polyarthralgia may occur and the patient may suffer modest general malaise. **Examination** reveals finger clubbing in two-thirds of patients, variable dyspnoea, diminished chest expansion and end-inspiratory, bilateral, basal crepitations, (to be distinguished from the basal crepitations of acute left ventricular failure).

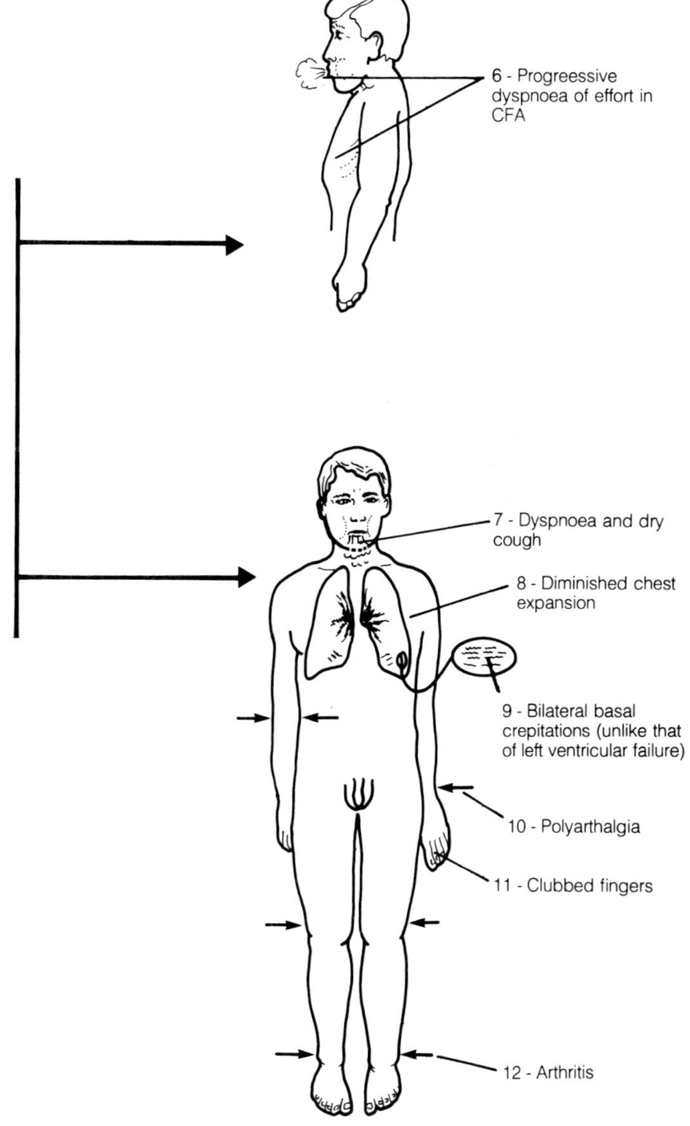

The pulmonary function tests show a restrictive ventilatory defect with a reduced DLCO, and the V/Q mismatch leads to hypoxaemia without hypercapnia. Radiologically, the lung fields are small with bilateral, reticular basal shadowing, even a honeycomb appearance. The diagnosis is made by a lung biopsy. The disease may spread to other lung areas to cause widespread fibrosis.

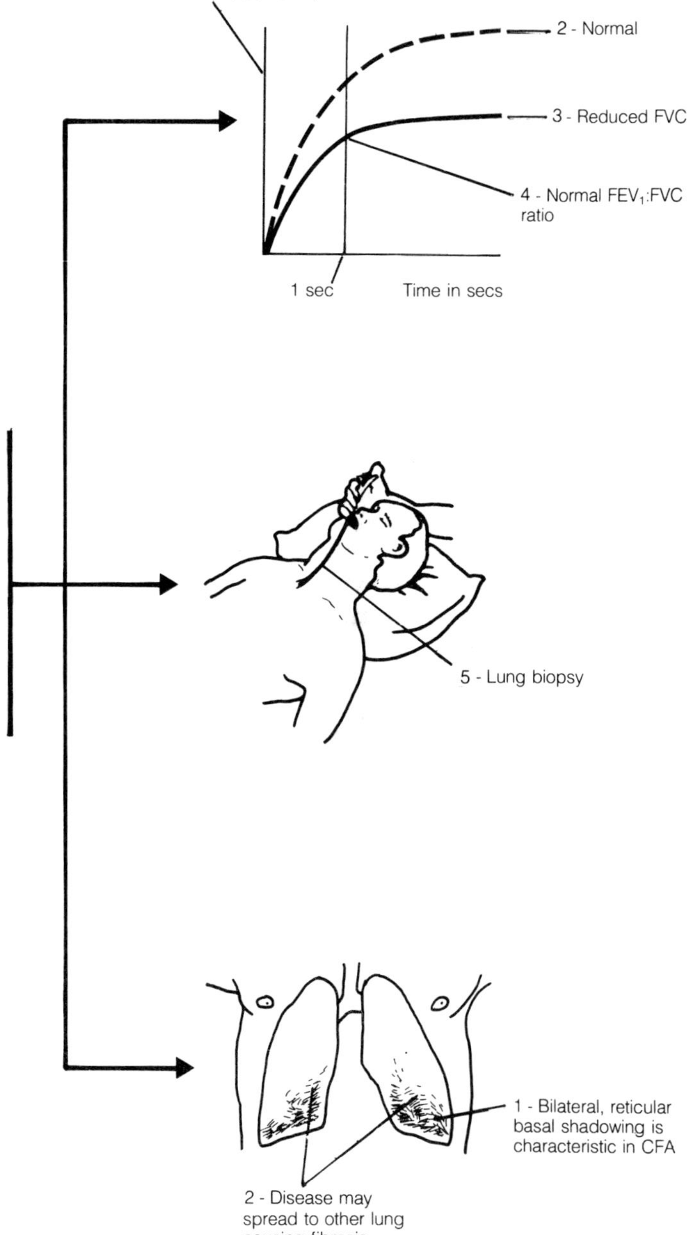

The **natural history** of the disease varies — some patients progressing to respiratory failure within months, others have indolent disease changing little over the years. Prednisolone tablets (40 mg/day) influences the course of the disease in some patients but is not a cure. In patients who are progressing rapidly, corticosteroids should be given a trial.

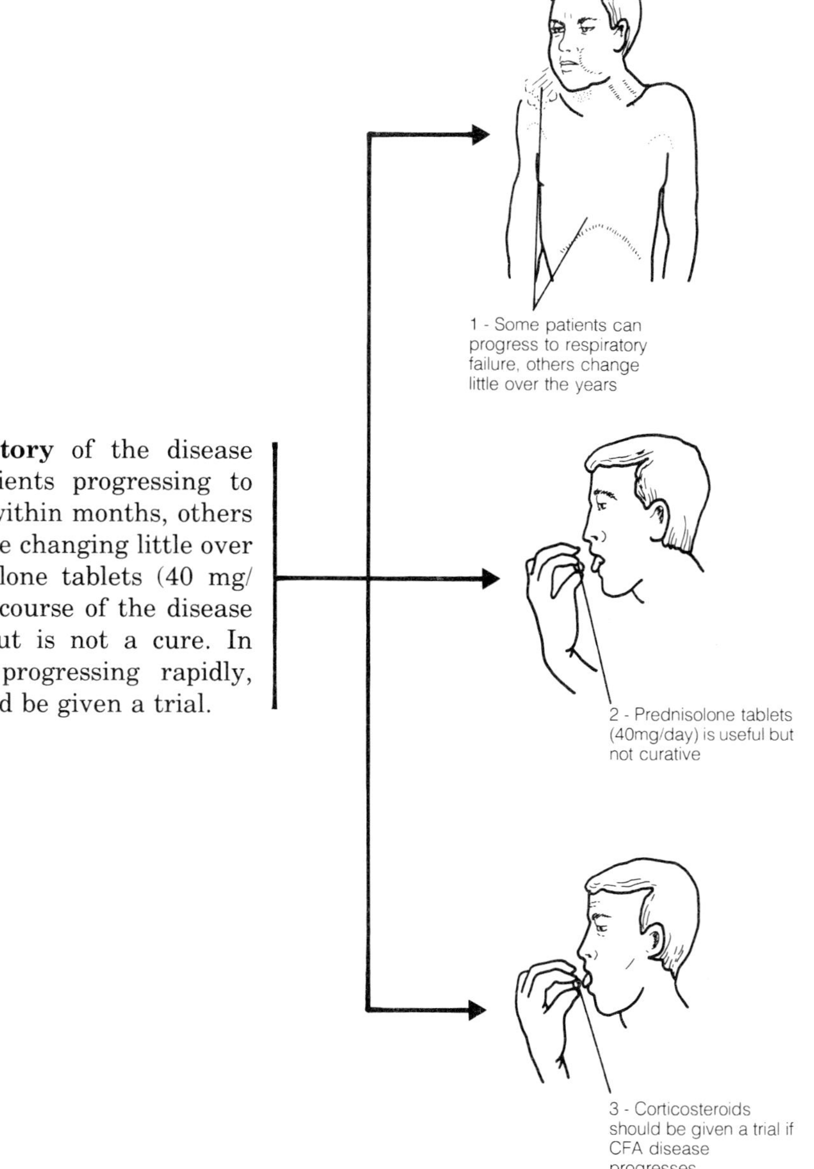

PNEUMOCONIOSES

The **pneumoconioses** are a group of occupational lung diseases acquired from the inhalation of inorganic dusts – the dust particles being small enough to reach the alveolar level. If the lung clearance mechanisms (e.g. pulmonary macrophages and ciliated transport) are unable to excrete the dust particles they remain there and may engender a fibrotic and destructive lung disease.

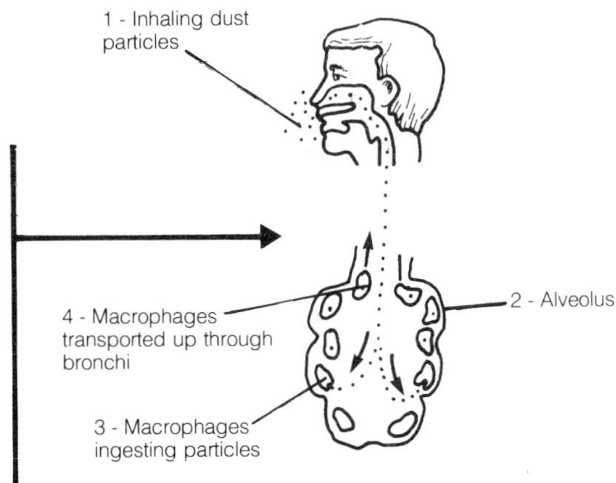

Fibrotic Pneumoconioses – Coal worker's pneumoconiosis (anthracosis) is due to dust accumulation in the lungs and in "simple" cases gives rise to small nodular lung shadowing on chest X-ray with minimal symptomatology. However, lung fibrosis may occur, sometimes where the mined coal has a high silica content, sometimes where there has been high

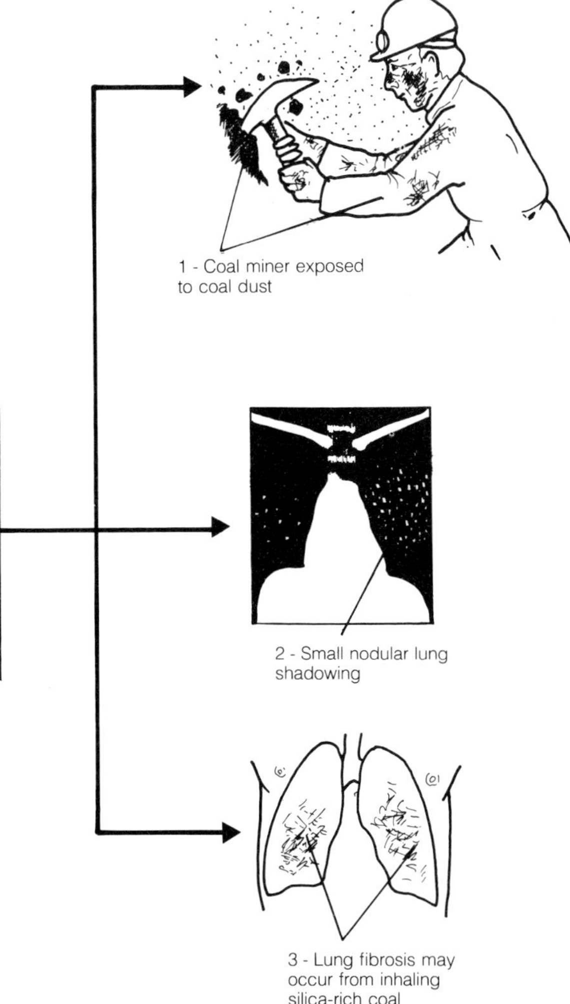

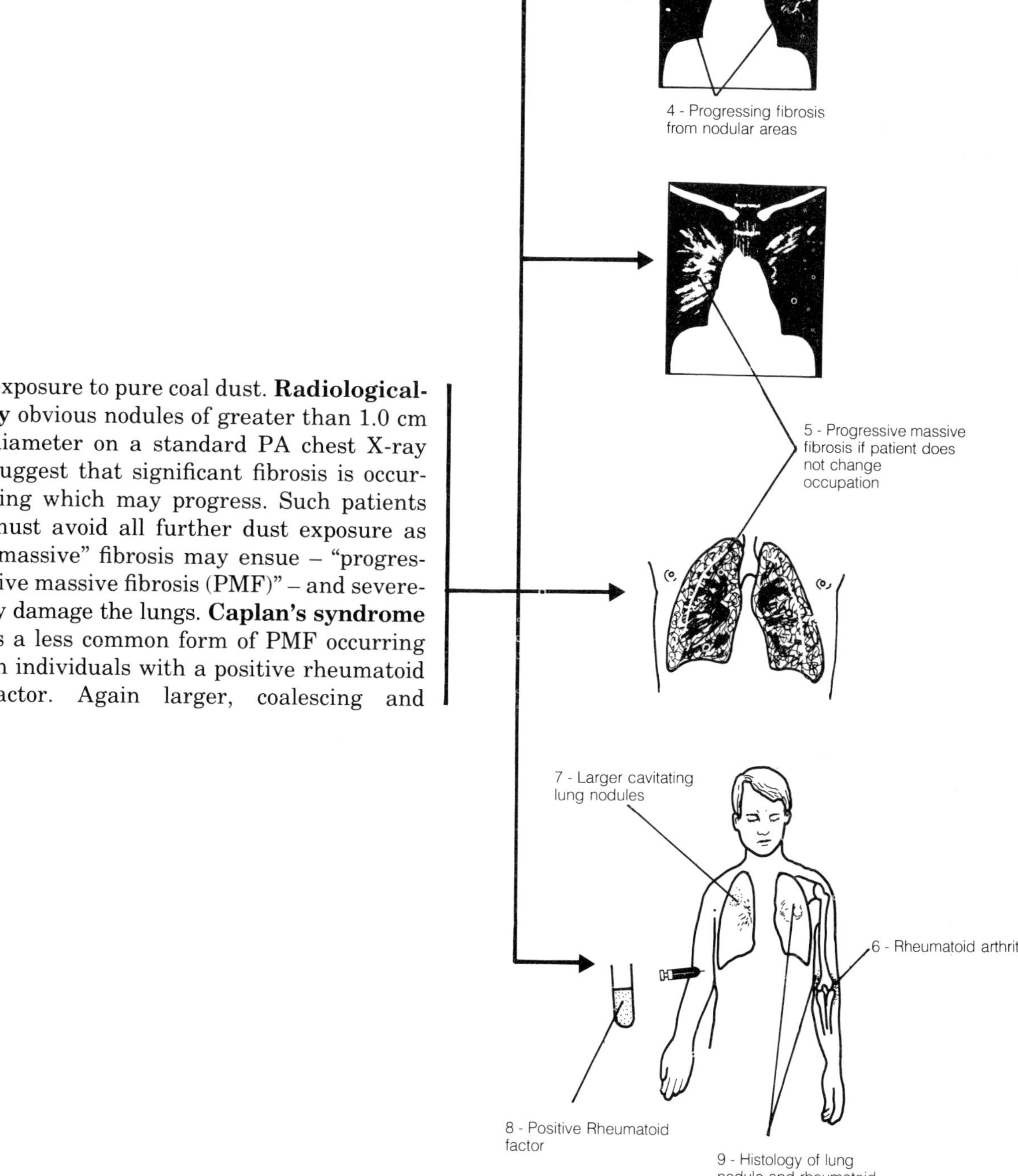

exposure to pure coal dust. **Radiologically** obvious nodules of greater than 1.0 cm diameter on a standard PA chest X-ray suggest that significant fibrosis is occurring which may progress. Such patients must avoid all further dust exposure as "massive" fibrosis may ensue – "progressive massive fibrosis (PMF)" – and severely damage the lungs. **Caplan's syndrome** is a less common form of PMF occurring in individuals with a positive rheumatoid factor. Again larger, coalescing and

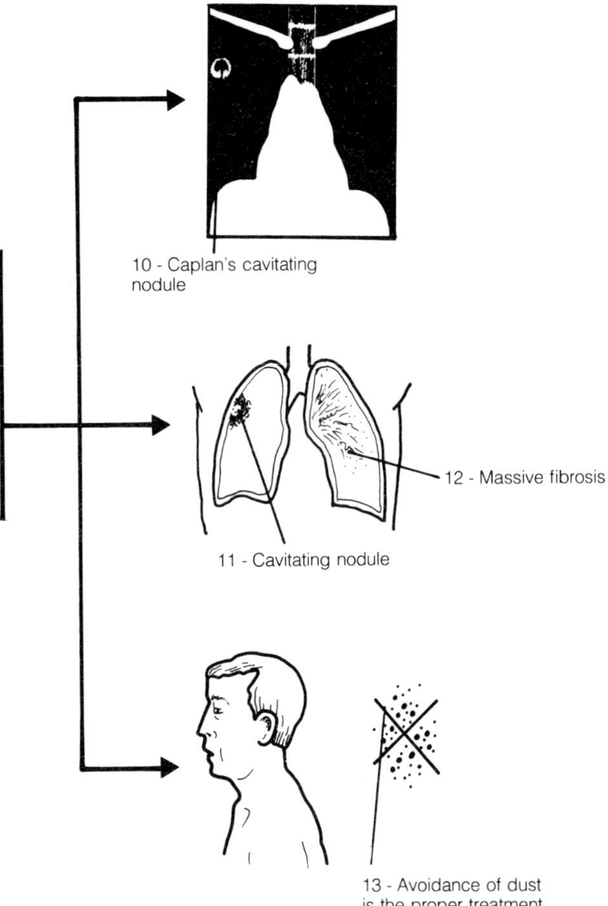

10 - Caplan's cavitating nodule

11 - Cavitating nodule

12 - Massive fibrosis

13 - Avoidance of dust is the proper treatment

perhaps cavitating nodular lung lesions are present and these may progress to PMF. Interestingly, the histology of the nodules resembles that of rheumatoid nodules and this adds credence to the notion that there is an immunological component to PMF. **Management** is dust avoidance from the time of diagnosis of simple pneumoconiosis on chest X-ray.

Silicosis is caused by inhalation of free silica dust mainly from mining or working with silica containing rock (flint, quartz, etc). The typical lesion tends to

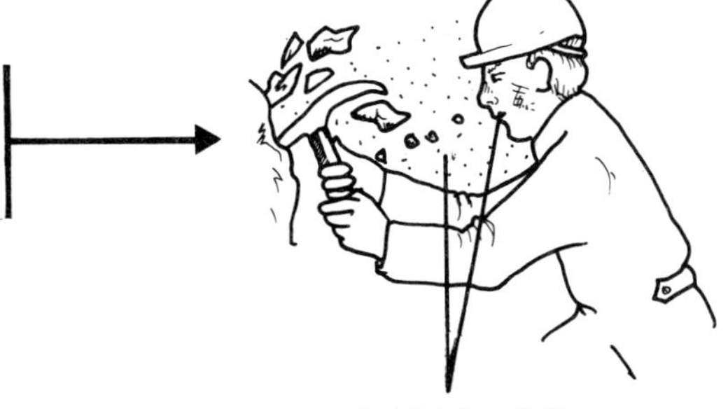

1 - Inhalation of silica dust from working with flint, quartz etc.

occur in the upper lobes and is a grey nodule, 2-5 mm diameter with a whorled pattern due to concentric collagenous fibrosis around the silica: once again, there may be an immune reaction that contributes to this host response. The nodules may enlarge, coalesce and cause fibrotic lung disease, even PMF. Other cases do not progress. Silicosis predisposes to infection by M.tb.

Mixed dust fibrosis results from inhalation of silica dust with another dust e.g. iron oxide in *haematite* miners. The siliceous element is probably the promotor of the fibrosing pneumoconiosis.

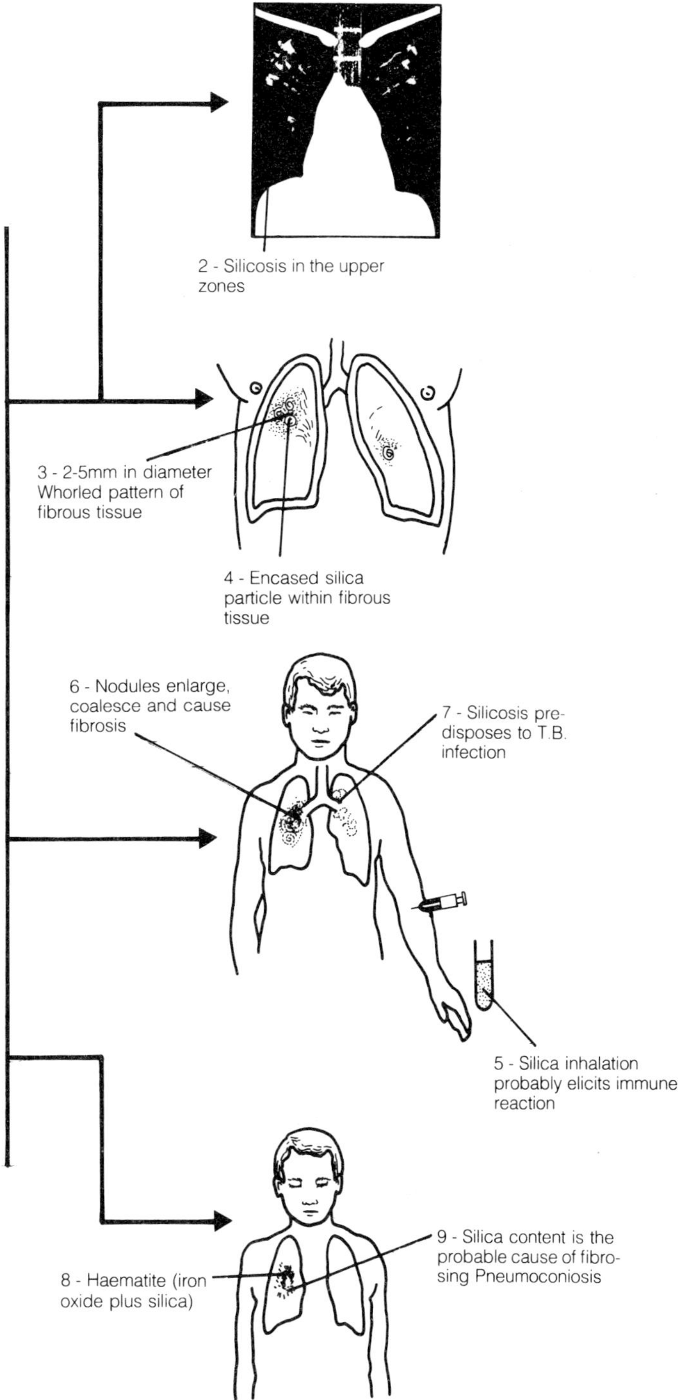

Chronic exposure to beryllium dust may lead to a chest disorder resembling sarcoid including BHL and reticuloendothelial involvement. A fibrotic pneumoconiosis is part of the syndrome.

The **pulmonary dysfunction** from the fibrotic pneumoconioses depends on the degree of fibrosis, but PMF leads to severe breathlessness, grossly disturbed respiratory function tests (perhaps an early restrictive defect with uneven ventilation and reduced DLCO) progressing to respiratory failure perhaps with cor pulmonale.

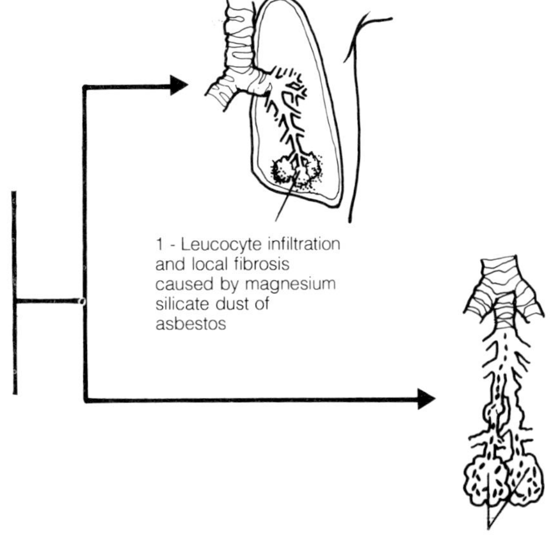

Asbestosis is due to the inhalation of asbestos dust (a magnesium silicate). The asbestos fibres impact in the distal bronchial tree where they engender a leucocyte infiltration and local fibrosis. Part of the host reaction is to coat the asbestos fibres with a protein covering – asbestos body.

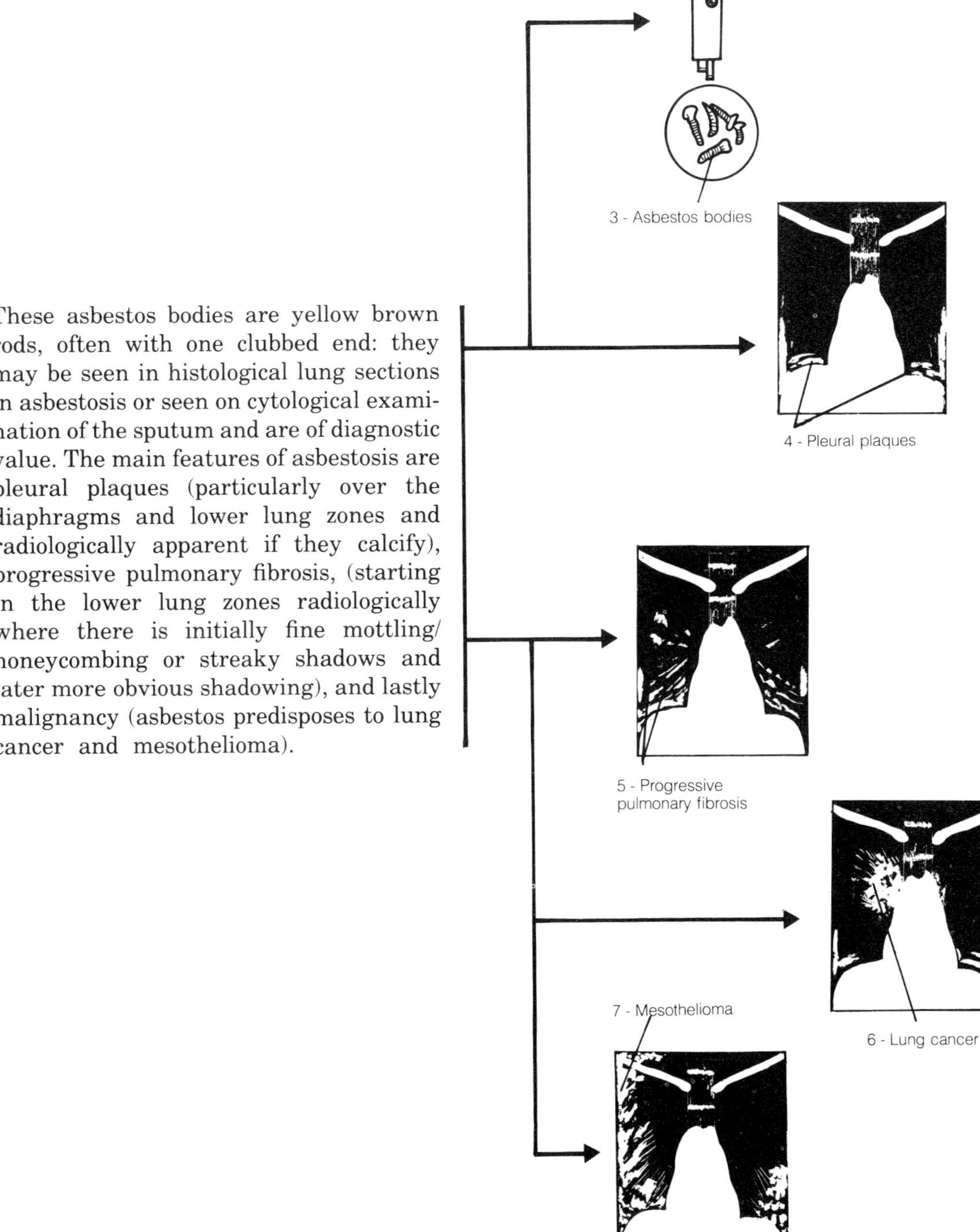

These asbestos bodies are yellow brown rods, often with one clubbed end: they may be seen in histological lung sections in asbestosis or seen on cytological examination of the sputum and are of diagnostic value. The main features of asbestosis are pleural plaques (particularly over the diaphragms and lower lung zones and radiologically apparent if they calcify), progressive pulmonary fibrosis, (starting in the lower lung zones radiologically where there is initially fine mottling/ honeycombing or streaky shadows and later more obvious shadowing), and lastly malignancy (asbestos predisposes to lung cancer and mesothelioma).

The patient presents with progressive dyspnoea and two useful physical signs in asbestosis are the common occurrence of finger clubbing and bilateral basal crepitations. Lung function tests show restrictive ventilatory function. **Diagnosis** is by history of occupational exposure, clinical and investigational findings and perhaps lung biopsy. Treatment is symptomatic. Cigarette smoking is to be deplored as it augments the risk of lung cancer.

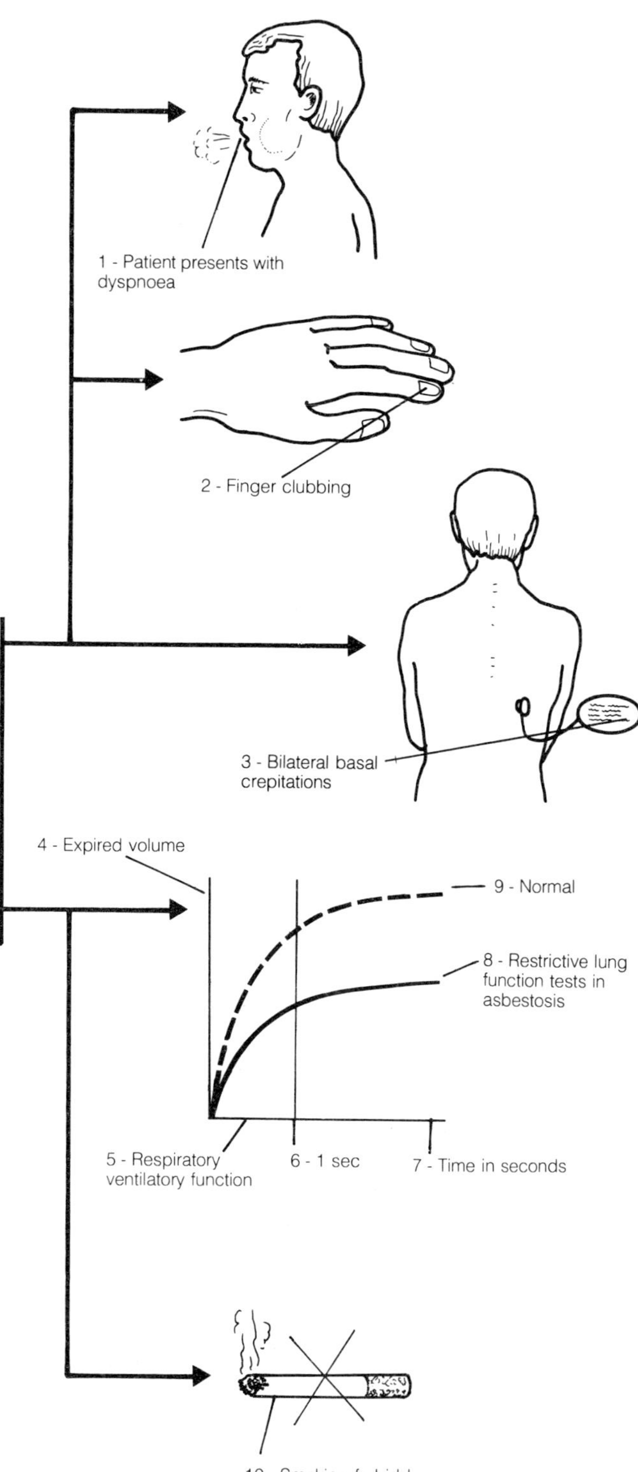

Non-fibrotic pneumoconioses – Radiologically, non-progressing small nodular lung shadowing occurs in workers with iron oxides (siderosis), tin oxide (stannosis), barium sulphate, antimony or chromite dusts.

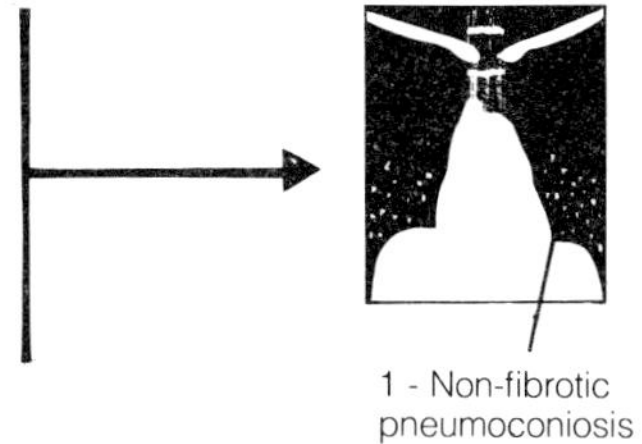

DISORDERS OF THE PLEURA

The pleura is a serous membrane covering the lungs (visceral pleura) and chest wall (parietal pleura). Inflamed pleura may evoke an exudative response (pleurisy with effusion) or not (dry pleurisy).

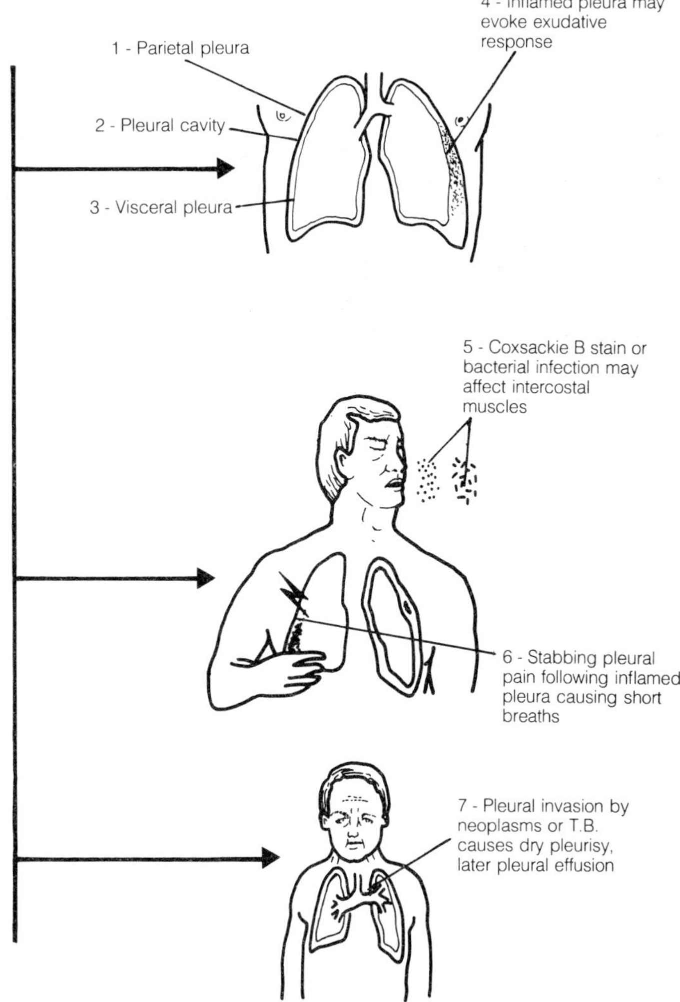

Dry Pleurisy – Inflamed pleura usually occurs over an infected area of lung (e.g. pneumonia either bacterial or viral, or a lung abscess) or over a pulmonary infarct. A particular Coxsackie B strain may infect the intercostal muscles (epidemic myalgia) and cause dry pleurisy. Pleural invasion by neoplasms or T.B. can also give rise to dry pleurisy, usually followed by an effusion.

Particularly in the infectious types of dry pleurisy, the onset of clinical symptoms may be sudden with stabbing pleural pain limiting inspiration to short breaths.

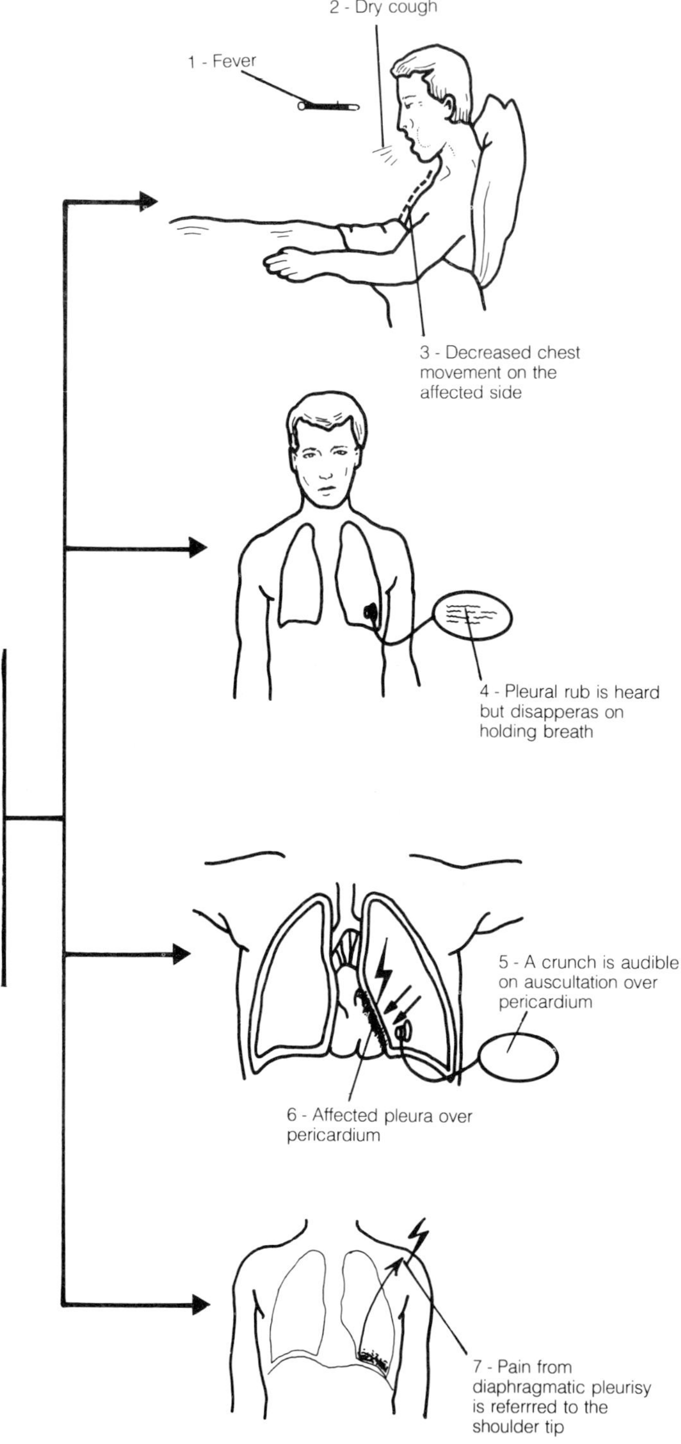

There is usually a fever and a dry cough. On examination, there is decreased chest movement on the affected side and a pleural rub is heard on auscultation. The pleural rub disappears on breath holding except when the pleura over the pericardium is involved; a "crunch" or rub is then audible in time with the cardiac cycle. The pain from diaphragmatic pleurisy is referred to the shoulder tip.

The **differential diagnosis** of dry pleurisy includes the prodromal pain of thoracic herpes zoster, epidemic myalgia, fractured rib, pneumothorax or even upper abdominal disease (particularly in children). A chest X-ray is mandatory but shows nothing specific in dry pleurisy. However, an early effusion manifesting as a bluntened costophrenic angle, should be sought on the PA chest X-ray. Treatment is of the underlying cause, but the pleuritic pain may require a strong analgesic, even an opiate temporarily.

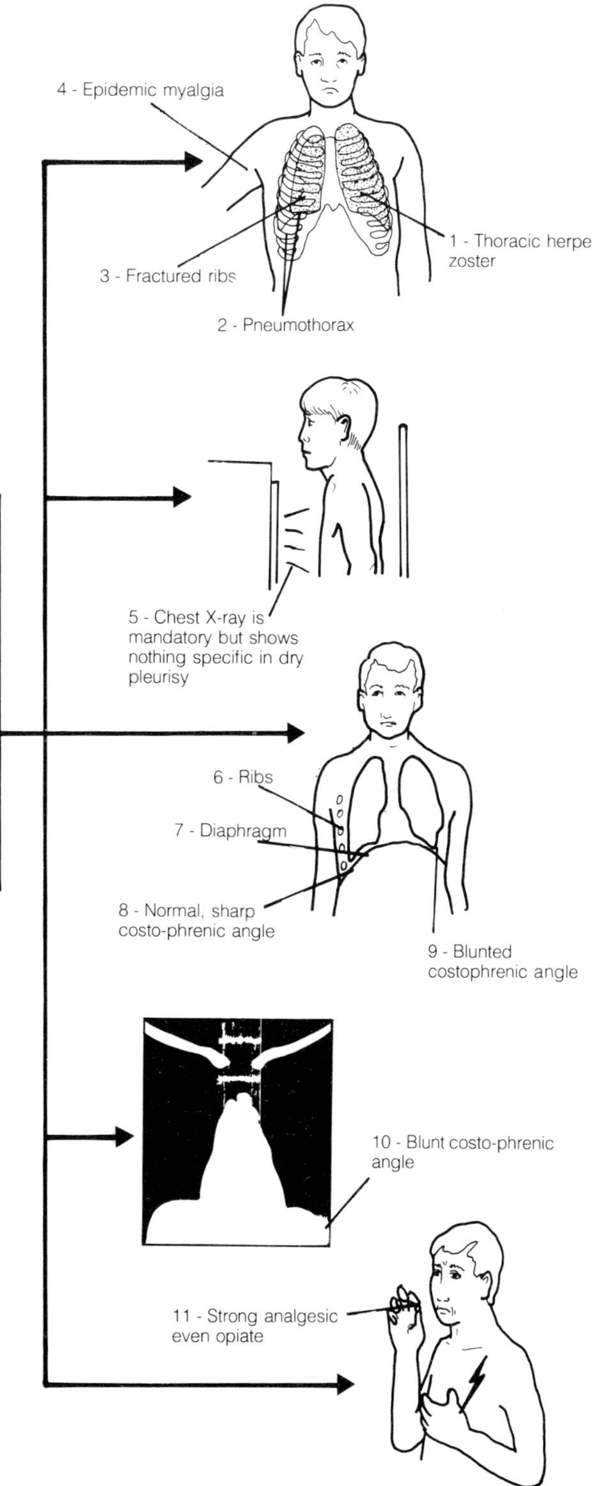

Pleural Effusion – Passive transudation of fluid (a serous effusion with a protein content of less than 30 g/l) into the pleural cavity occurs in heart failure and constrictive pericarditis due to venous back pressure and in hypoproteinaemic anasarca (e.g. nephrotic syndrome, cirrhosis). Inflammatory or neoplastic effusions are more proteinaceous and may be cloudy or even purulent (empyema) or haemorrhagic. These are exudates and occur over a bacterial (including tuberculous) pneumonia, lung abscess, pulmonary infarct or with neoplastic invasion of the pleura. Pleural exudates also occur in the collagenoses.

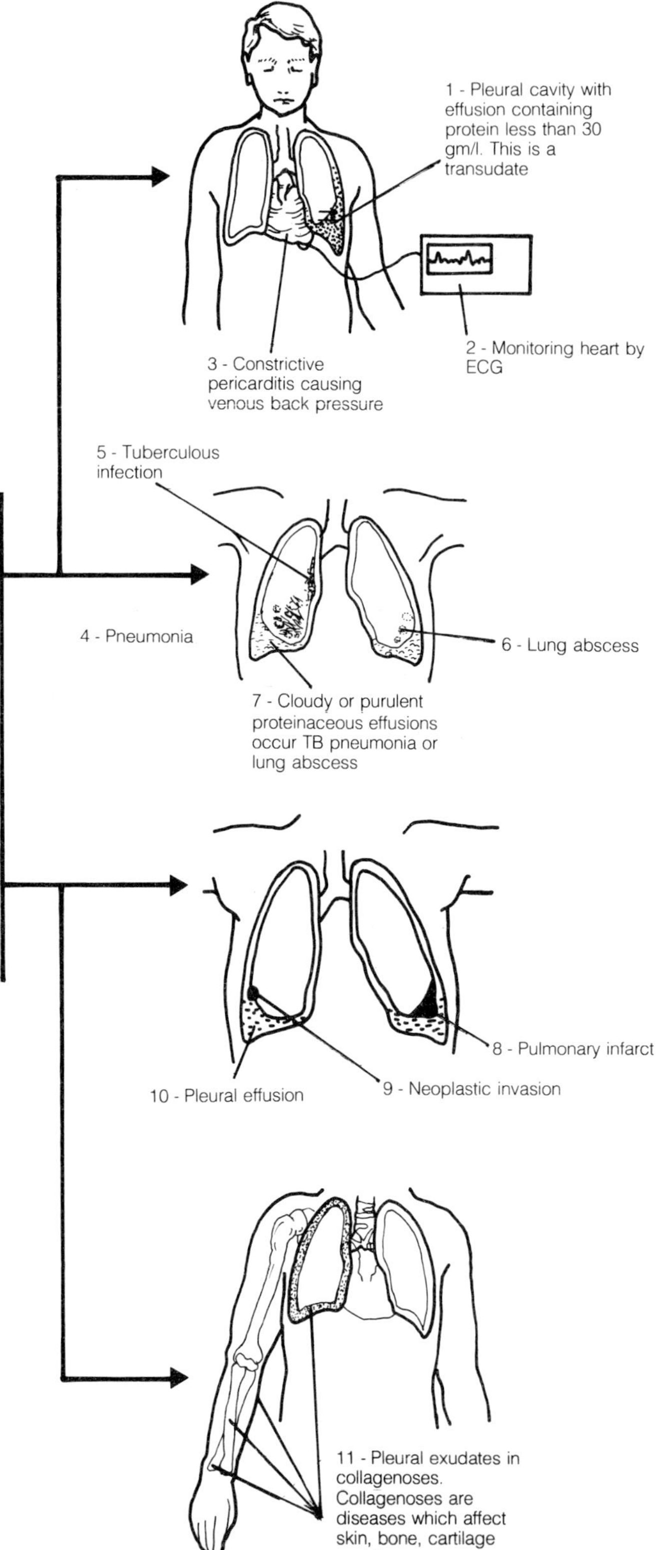

The **clinical symptoms** of "dry" pleurisy often precede the effusion, but in some patients the accumulation of the pleural effusion is clinically silent until the size of the effusion(s) is large enough to cause dyspnoea. The **physical signs** in the chest are those of a fluid collection and the chest X-ray is usually diagnostic. A lateral decubitus chest X-ray demonstrates the gravity dependence of a pleural effusion that is not loculated.

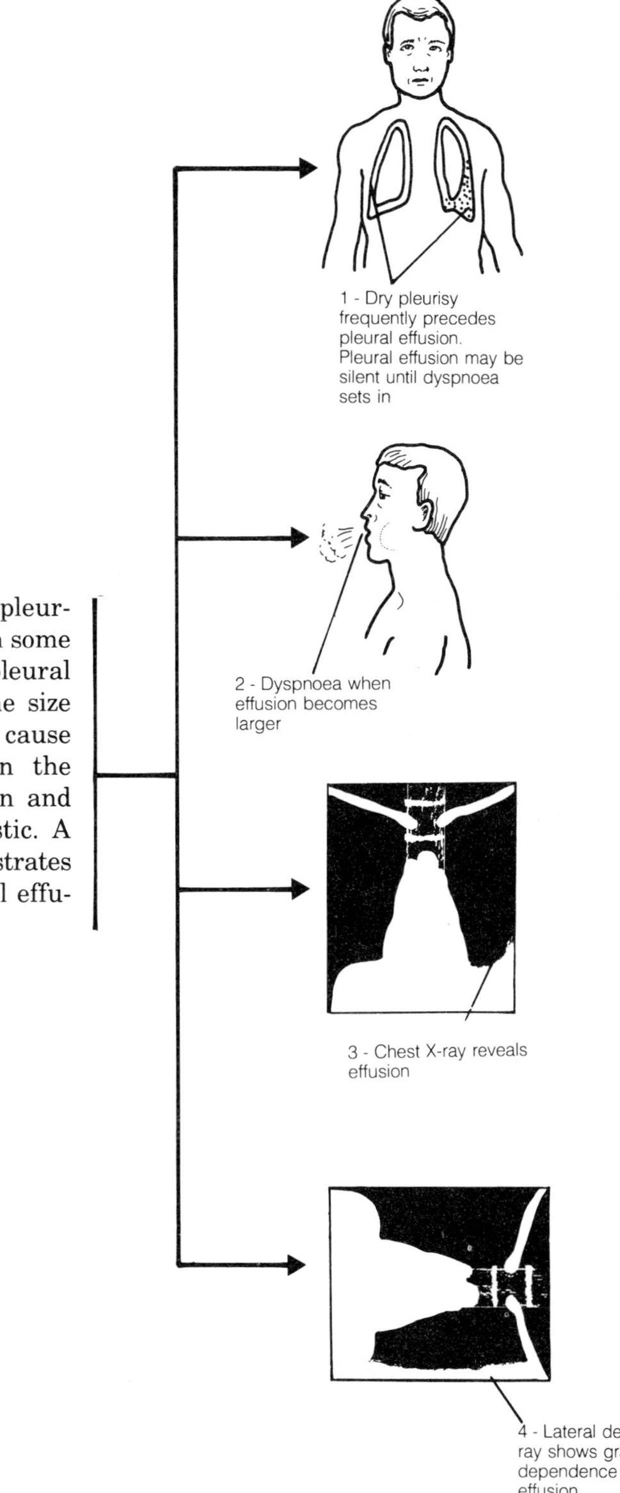

The **diagnosis** of a pleural effusion and its cause is made by fluid sampling — simply performed under local anaesthetic with a Number 1 venepuncture needle inserted through the lower half of the intercostal space that overlies the region of maximal dullness, (remembering the areas of cardiac and liver dullness and the position of the diaphragm and great vessels posteriorly). A more elaborate method (using an Abram's punch) also allows sampling of the pleura for histological examination. The fluid is examined for cells, protein and culture. In suspected infective cases, a Gram stain or Ziehl-Neelsen stain might be requested as an immediate procedure.

The commonest causes of a blood stained pleural effusion are malignancy and pulmonary infarction. In malignancy the effusion progesses and cytology is usually positive whereas in infarction the effusion tends to be smaller and often the fluid contains many eosinophils.

Large unilateral pleural effusions, which tend to reaccumulate, are encountered commonly in carcinoma of bronchus and carcinoma of breast. Repeating needle aspirations through a trocar with cannula, (attached to a three way tap and syringe), allow daily drainage of 1.0 litre volumes of fluid to dryness: the drainage of a large effusion is not performed at one sitting as the mediastinal shift towards the created new space may cause respiratory distress. Where the fluid has tended to recur, a chemical pleurodesis is attempted: following drainage, 500 mg of tetracycline in 50 ml of 0.9% saline is injected into the pleural space and the patient changes his position in bed quarter hourly for an hour. A chest drain connected to an underwater seal is an alternative method (see pneumothorax section). Where the effusion is loculated, drainage is difficult and attempted pleurodesis not indicated.

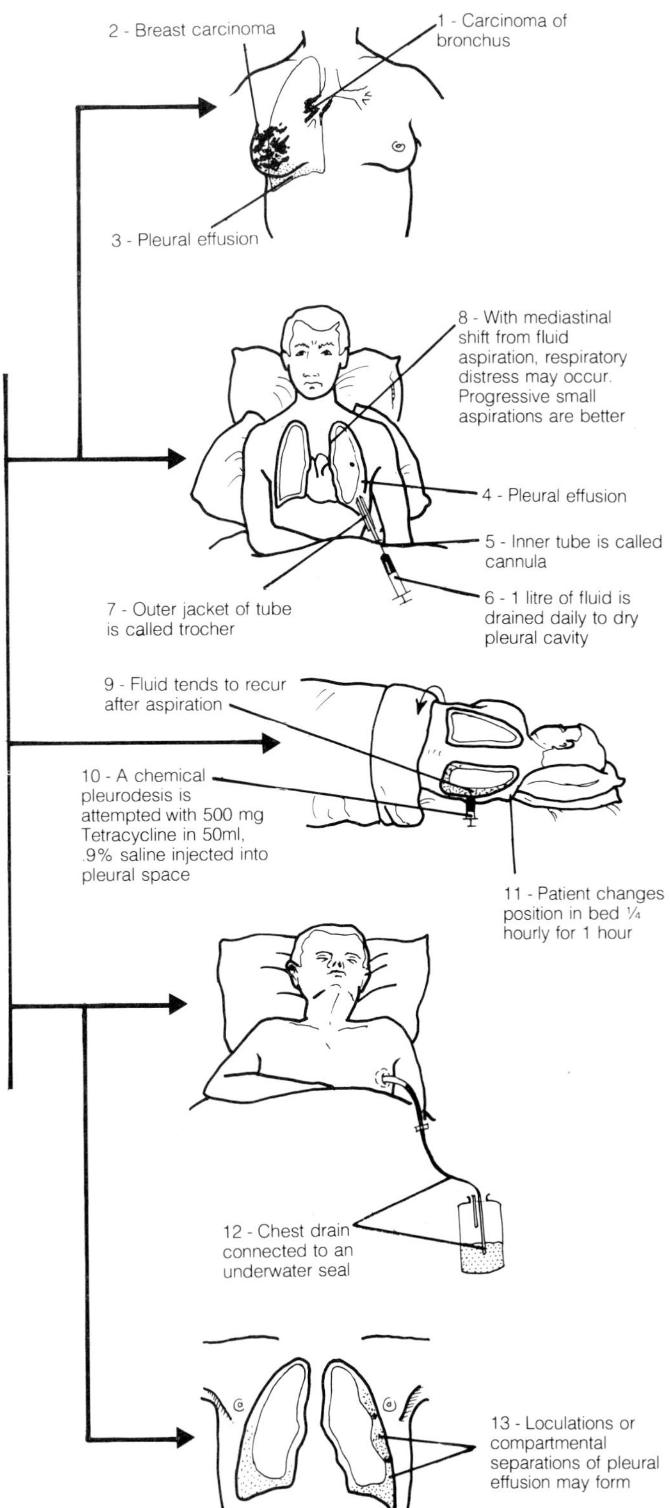

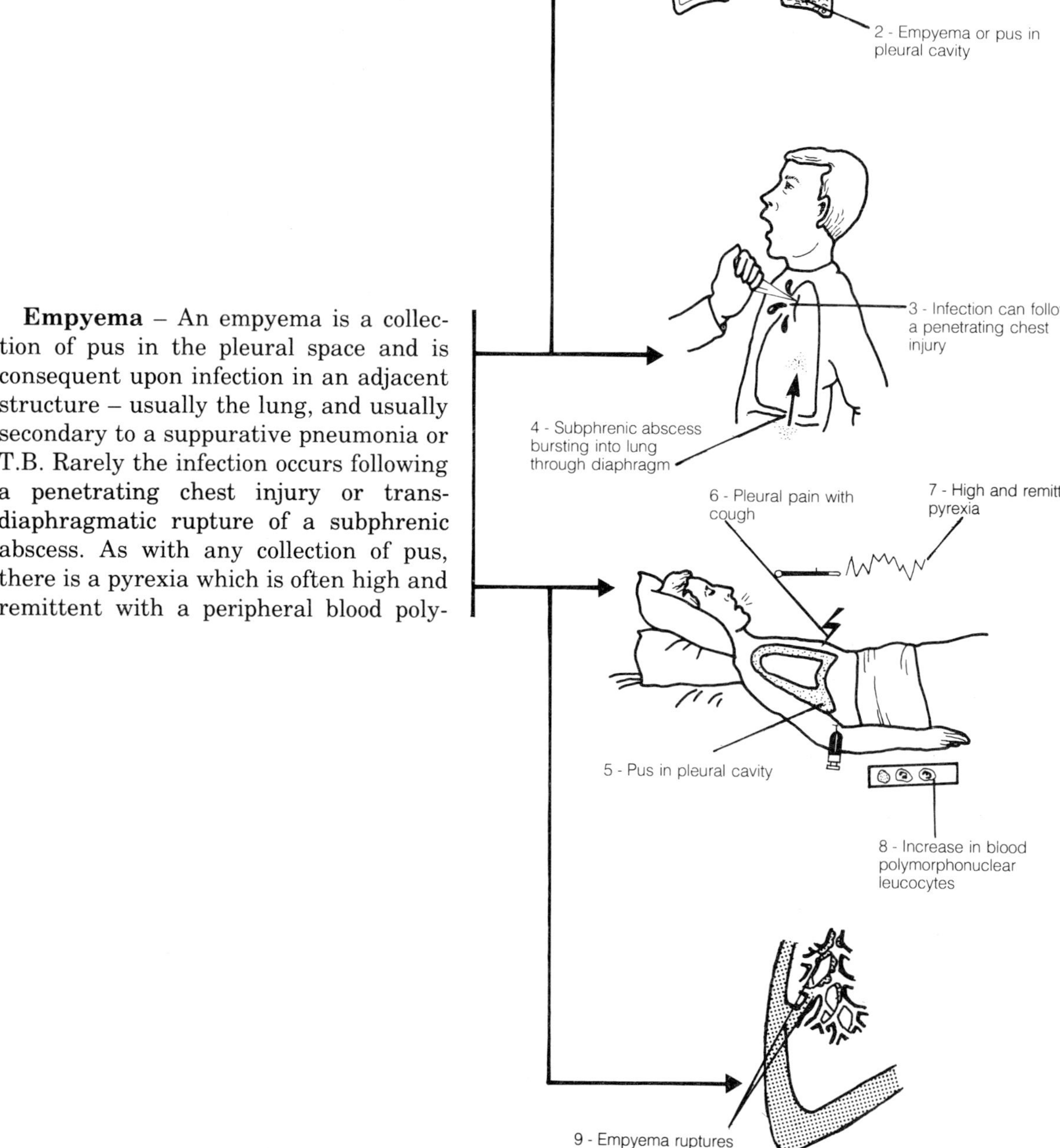

Empyema – An empyema is a collection of pus in the pleural space and is consequent upon infection in an adjacent structure – usually the lung, and usually secondary to a suppurative pneumonia or T.B. Rarely the infection occurs following a penetrating chest injury or trans-diaphragmatic rupture of a subphrenic abscess. As with any collection of pus, there is a pyrexia which is often high and remittent with a peripheral blood polymorphonuclear leucocytosis. There may be pleural pain, with cough and if the empyema ruptures into a bronchus purulent sputum may occur. Another important consequence of such a rupture is the creating of a bronchopleural fistula (see below). The physical and radiological chest signs are those of a pleural effusion.

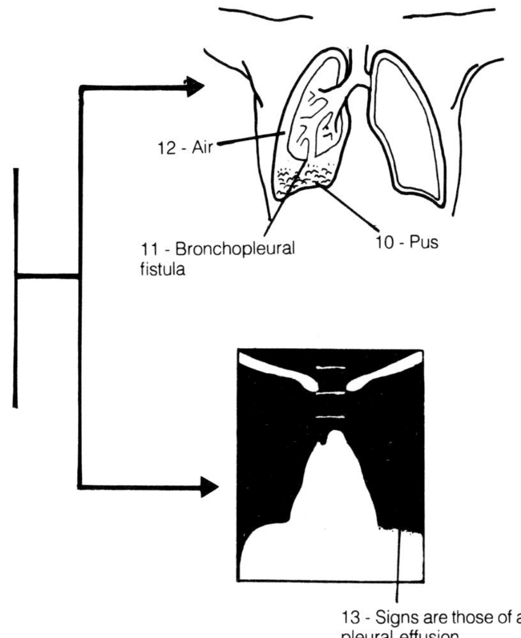

The diagnosis is made by needle aspiration (usually by a wide bore needle because of the high viscosity of pus). Treatment is by drainage and prompt institution of effective systemic antibiotics. If an intercostal tube, placed in the most dependent part of the empyema, provides an inadequate drainage system, (as may happen with thick, loculated pus), a formal surgical resection of a rib portion with insertion of a wide bore drain is required.

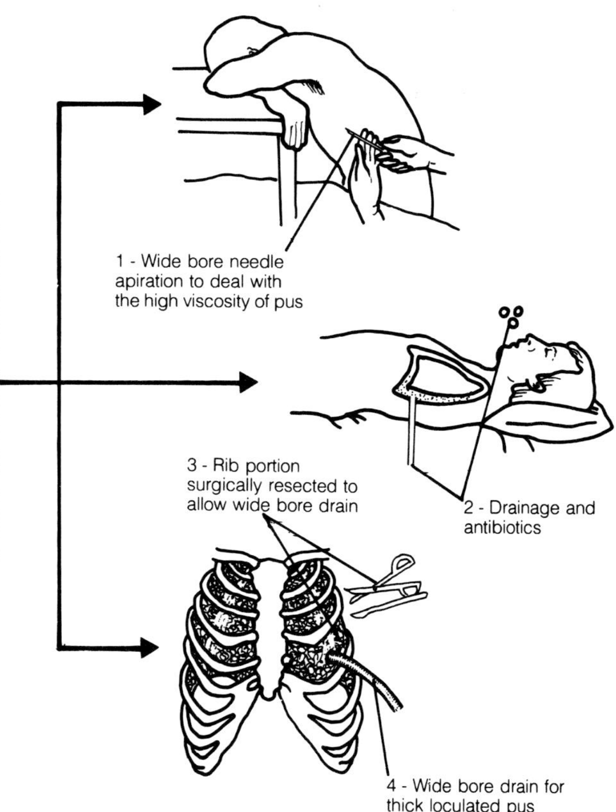

Spontaneous Pneumothorax – A breach in the visceral pleura allows air to escape from the lung into the pleural space – a pneumothorax. When this occurs without apparent reason, it is termed a spontaneous pneumothorax to distinguish this variety from a traumatic cause of air in the pleural space from a penetrating chest injury. If the hole in the visceral pleura closes over, there is no further air leak and this is called a closed spontaneous pneumothorax. If the air continues to leak "in and out" through the hole, a **bronchopleural fistula** is said to have formed (open spontaneous pneumothorax). Occasionally (and dangerously), a valve-like closing of the visceral pleura over the tear allows inspired air into the pleural space, but will not allow air to exit from the pleural space (tension or valvular pneumothorax). The trapped air increases in volume and pressure, and this causes the lung to collapse. As the pressure builds up further, the mediastinal structures may be pushed into the other side of the chest with cardiopulmonary embarrassment and perhaps death. It is possible for this state of affairs to happen startlingly rapidly.

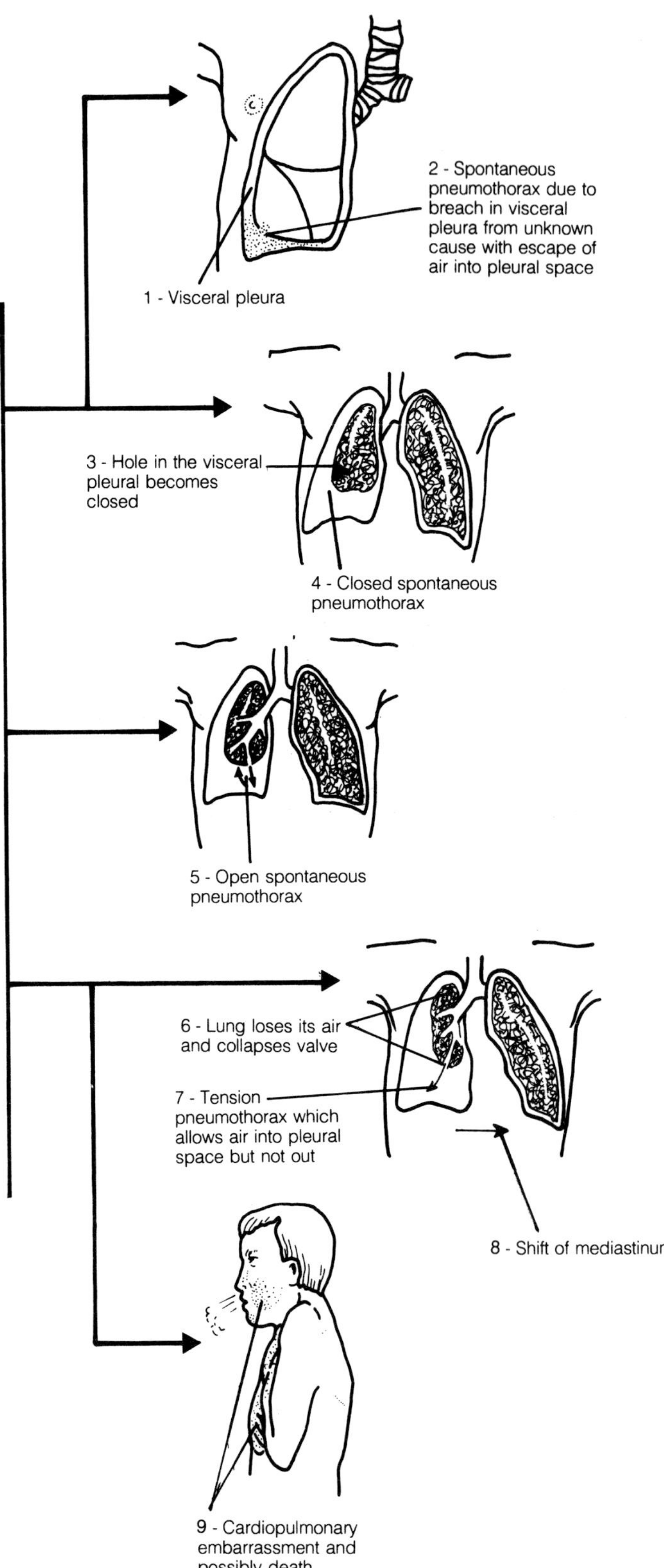

Young thin and tall adult males seem at a higher risk of a spontaneous pneumothorax than others. Patients with COAD, particularly those with emphysematous bullae are perhaps the highest risk group – due to rupture of a bulla into the pleural space, and asthmatics are also at risk during an attack. Other patients at risk of

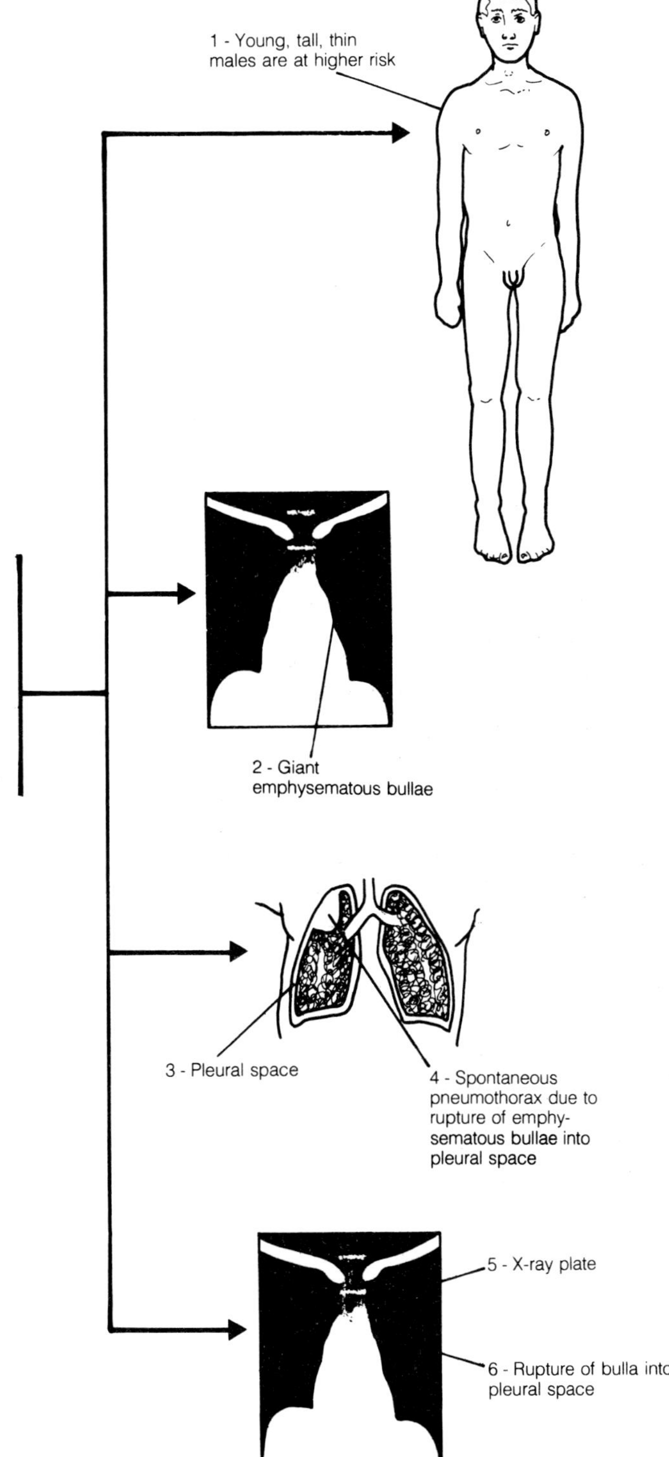

a pneumothorax are premature infants with respiratory distress, patients on ventilators, patients with collagen defects (e.g. **Ehlers-Danlos** and **Marfan's Syndrome**) and patients with cavitating peripheral lung lesions (e.g. carcinoma) or cystic (e.g. staphylococcal pneumonic) lesions.

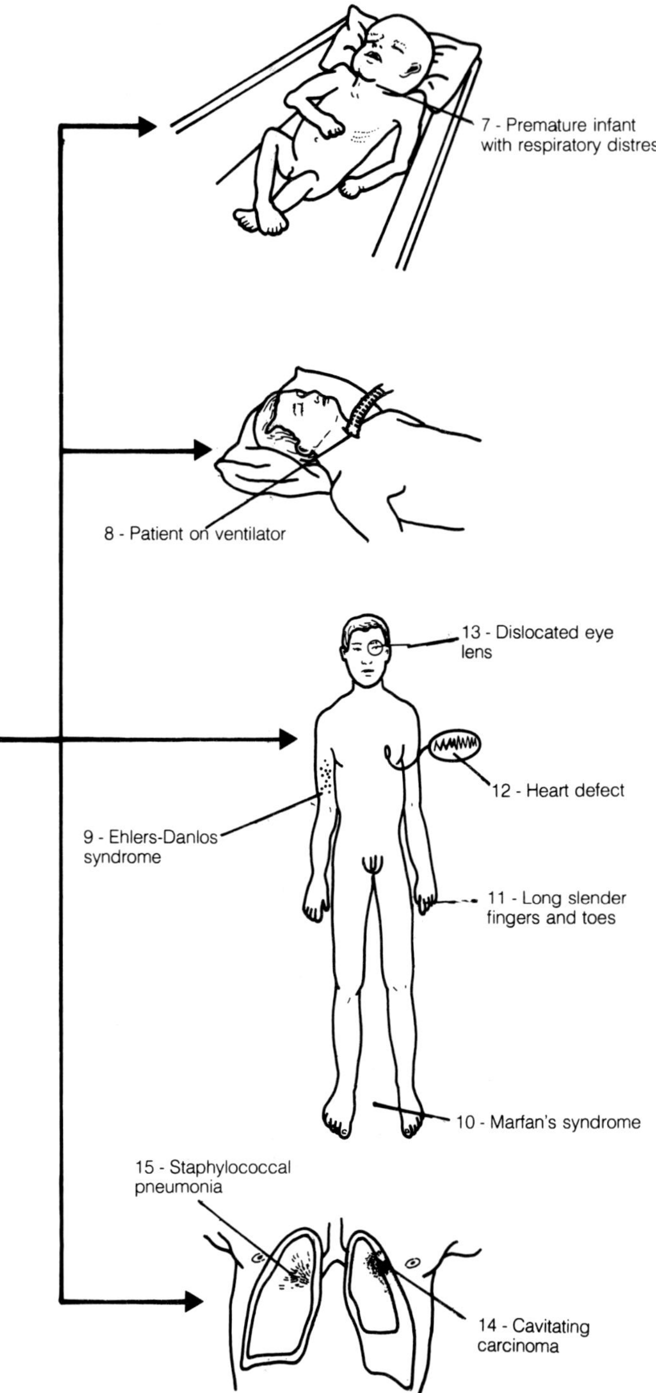

The **clinical onset** is usually sudden with sharp or "dragging" pain or "tightness" on one side of the chest – usually made worse by a deep inspiration or effort. Breathlessness depends on the size of the pneumothorax and the prior respiratory status of the patient: even a small closed pneumothorax can be life-threatening in an emphysematous respiratory cripple. In a tension pneumothorax, the dyspnoea worsens rapidly to asphyxia, if untreated.

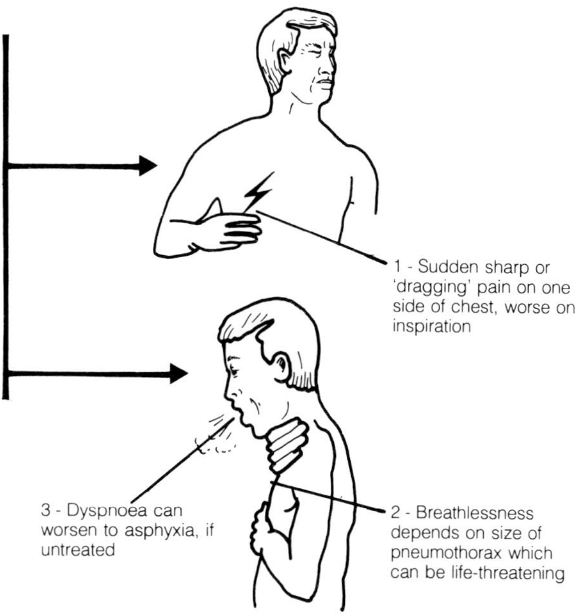

The **physical signs** depend on the size of the pneumothorax and the intrapleural pressure. If the pneumothorax is of some size, there is diminished chest movement on the affected side, hyper-resonance on percussion and diminished or absent breath sounds. If there is tension, respiratory distress, shifted mediastinal structures, central cyanosis and in severe cases a rapid pulse with hypotension, coexist with more accentuated chest signs. The

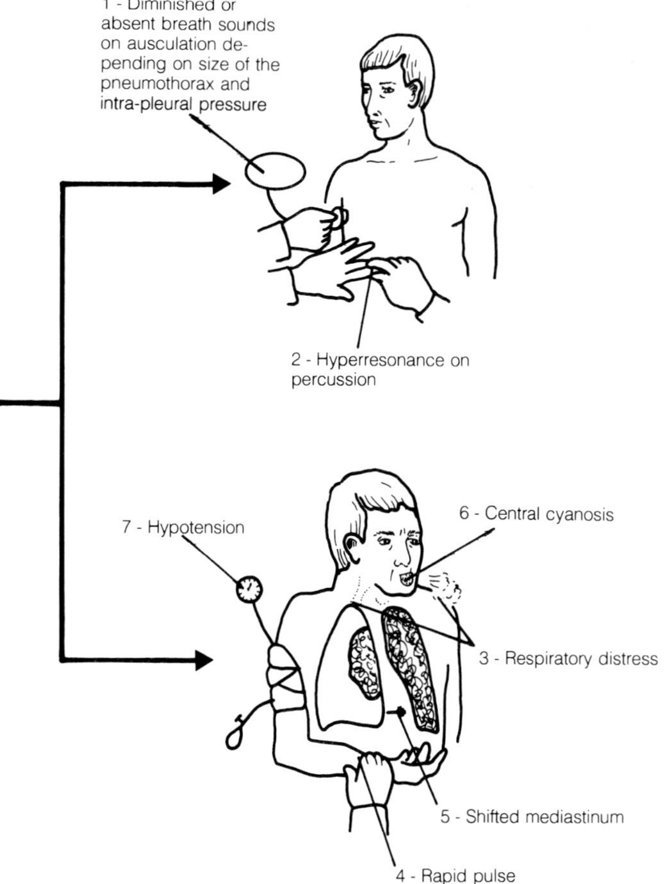

chest X-ray is diagnostic as the visceral pleura is seen as a curved hairline lateral to which there are no lung markings. A pneumothorax is accentuated on an expiratory film, which is thus the requested investigation to define a small pneumothorax.

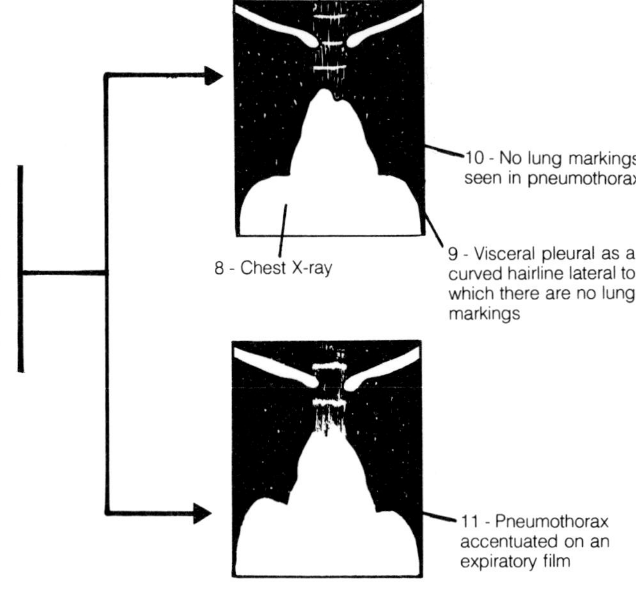

A small pneumothorax (less than one third lung collapse) will usually absorb in a few days and in a fit young man the management involves daily chest X-rays as an outpatient (provided there are rapid hospital admitting facilities should problems arise), and no active intervention is given. A larger pneumothorax with dyspnoea requires the insertion of catheter, preferably draining upwards towards the

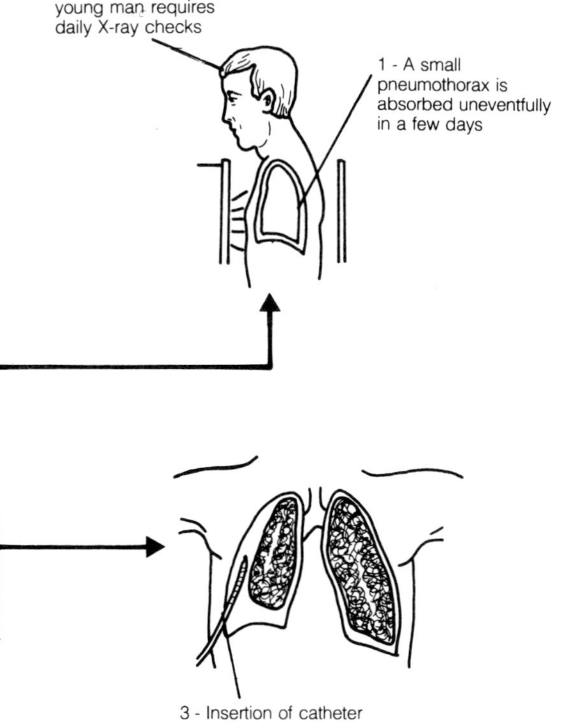

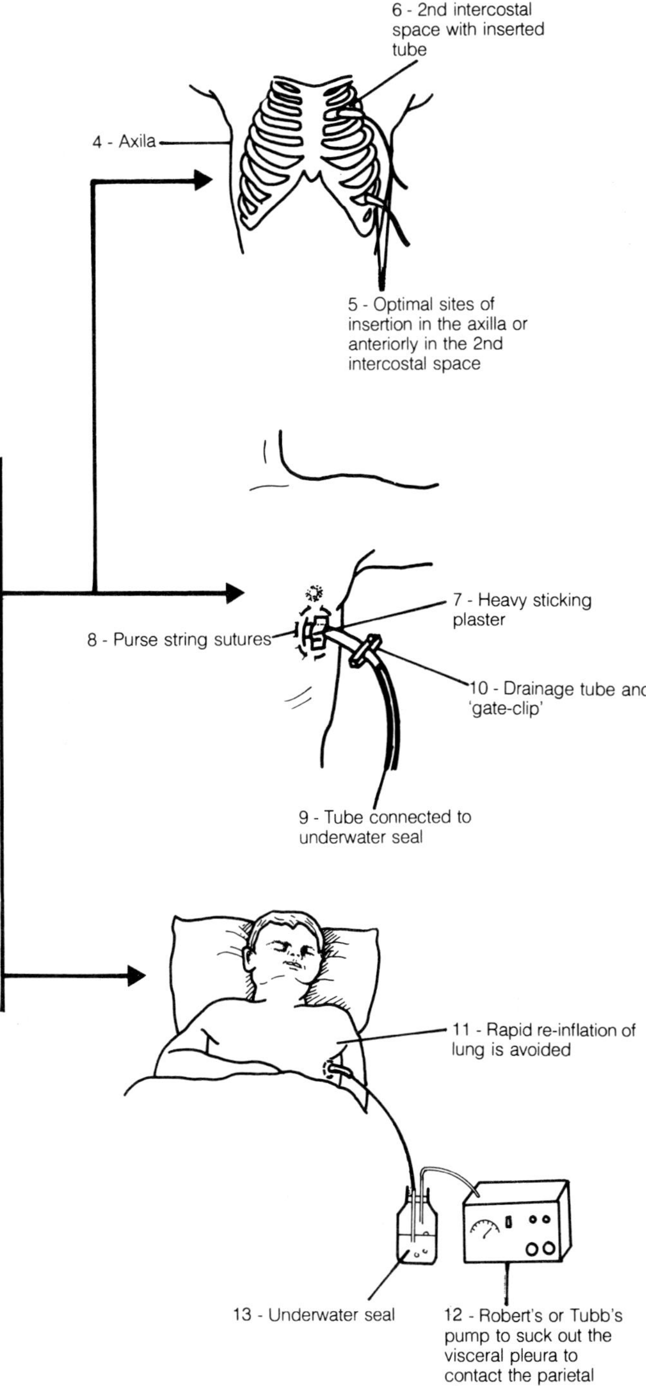

lung apex. The optimal insertion site is in the axilla as the chest wall here is thin and the tube causes least discomfort. However, the second intercostal space anteriorly is an alternative site of insertion. The tube is retained *in situ* by lattice tying it to a skin stitch and by heavy 'elastoplast' overlying it. A purse string suture down to muscle surrounds the tube such that should it "fall out", the hole can be immediately sealed. After insertion of the tube, it is connected to an underwater seal drainage bottle. Air escape is controlled initially as too rapid reinflation of the lung can (paradoxically) lead to respiratory embarrassment, due to pulmonary oedema. This is achieved by a clip on the tubing.

If the pneumothorax is open, air continues to drain and suction on the chest catheter is performed by a Robert's or the more powerful Tubb's pump, connected to the underwater seal. The object is to "suck out" the visceral pleura to contact the parietal pleura for a time and so seal the breach with its bronchopleural fistula. When the lung has re-expanded on the repeated chest X-ray, the tubing to the underwater drainage bottle should be clamped for at least 24 hours and a further repeat chest X-ray should confirm that the pneumothorax is absent before the chest drain is removed. A tension pneumothorax requires immediate action, even a number one venepuncture needle plunged through an intercostal space – but preferably, if time permits, urgent introduction of an intercostal catheter to an underwater seal. Supplementary oxygen is also required.

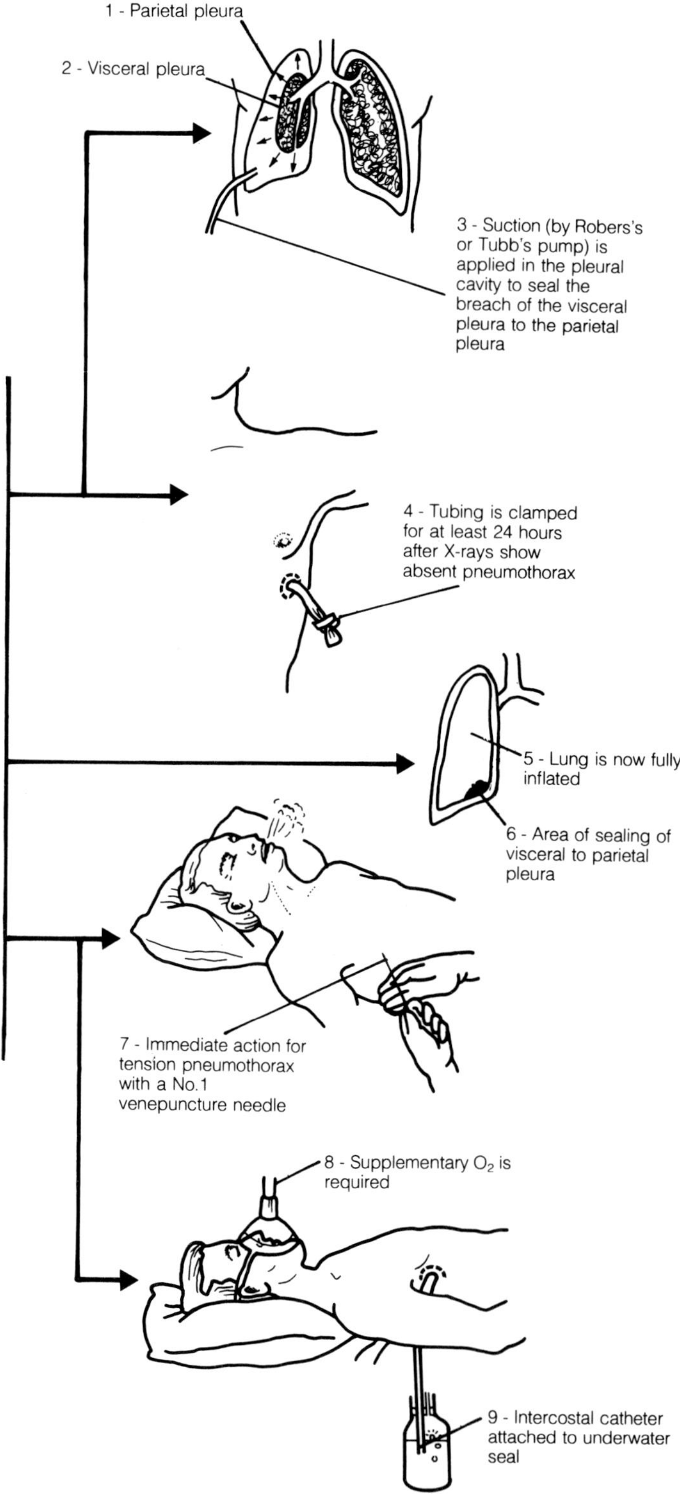

Patients with COAD have a greater than 50% risk of a second subsequent pneumothorax due to the nature of their disease, and after two episodes of pneumothorax, the risk of a third one is very high indeed. Such patients must be considered for surgical pleurectomy – stripping of the parietal pleura, which leads to obliteration of the pleural space. **Surgical intervention** is also required where a bronchopleural fistula persists in causing an open pneumothorax despite suction attempts. Occasionally, the surgeon can oversew a burst bulla. Attempts at **chemical pleurodesis** are now only recommended in those not suitable for surgery.

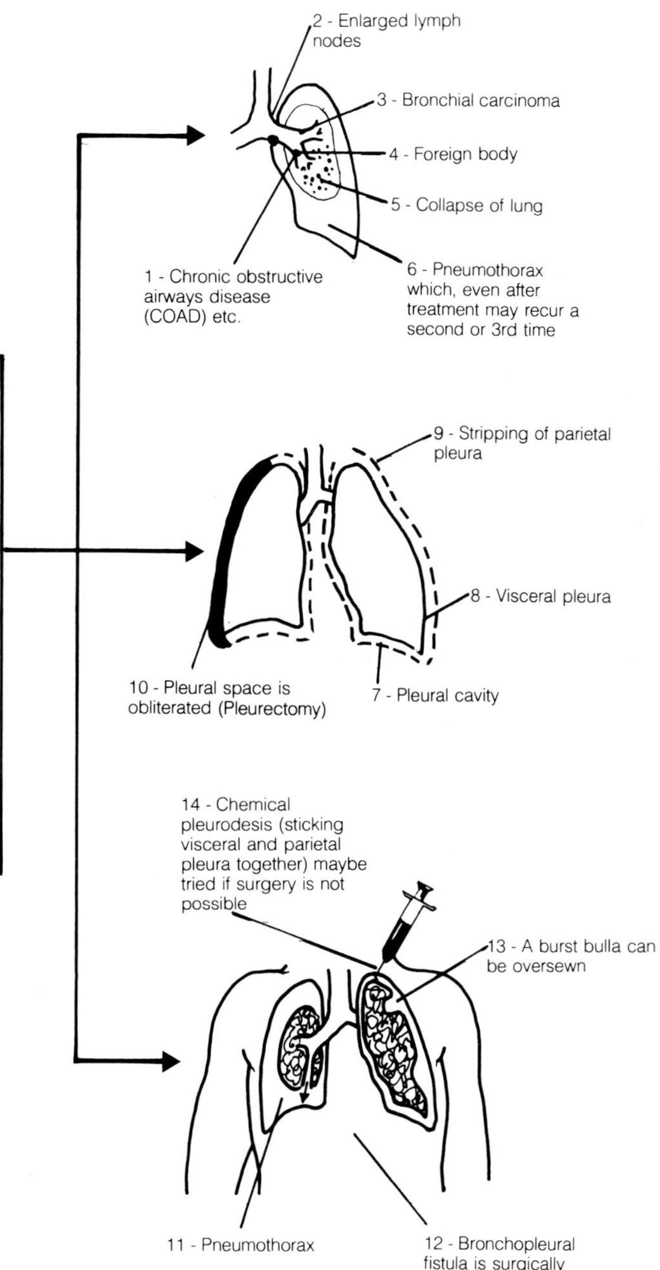

Bleeding may occur at the time of the pneumothorax, and a haemopneumothorax occurs, usually diagnosed by chest X-ray. Occasionally, the bleeding is severe and attended by the clinical features of internal haemorrhage: this is an urgent surgical problem requiring thoracotomy. Other causes of blood in the pleural space (haemothorax) are usually following chest trauma or leaking aortic aneurysm – both serious surgical conditions. If the chest trauma causes rupture of a major lymphatic vessel (notably the thoracic duct), chyle or lymph leaks into the pleural space (chylothorax).

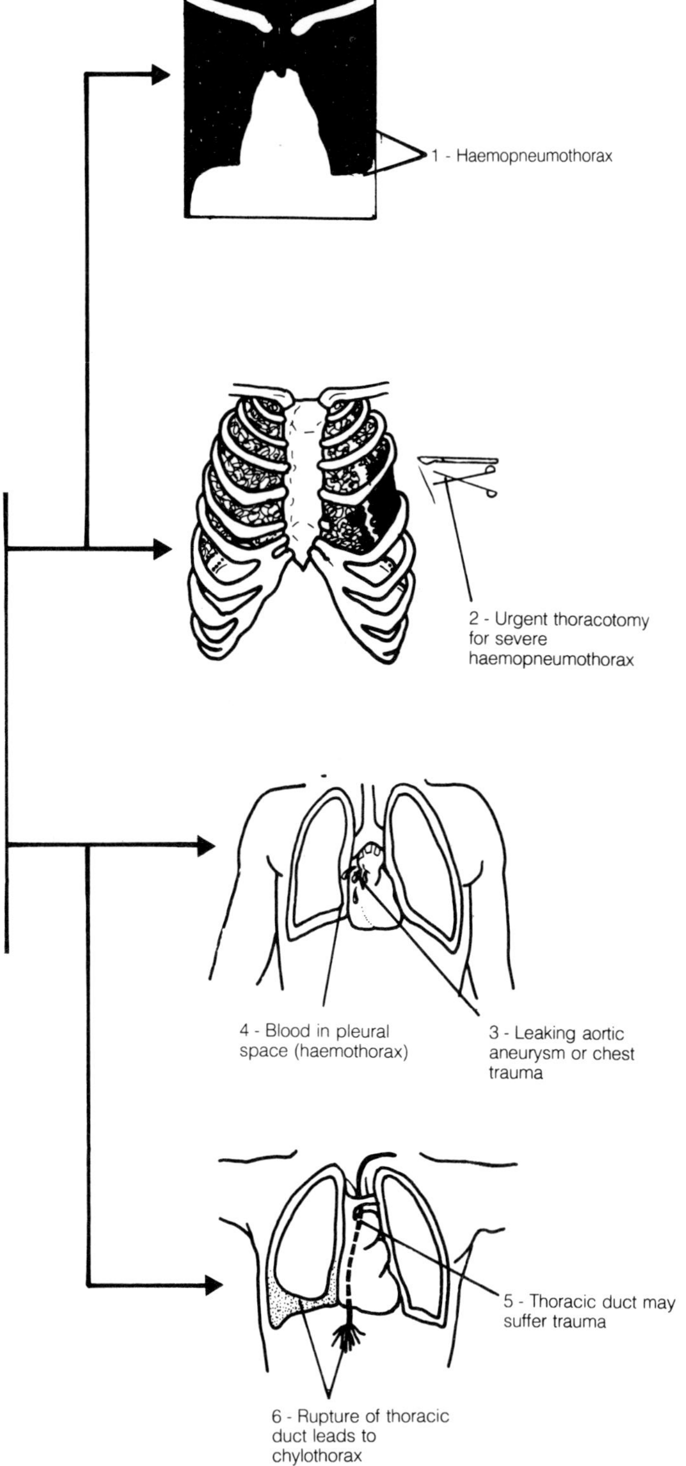

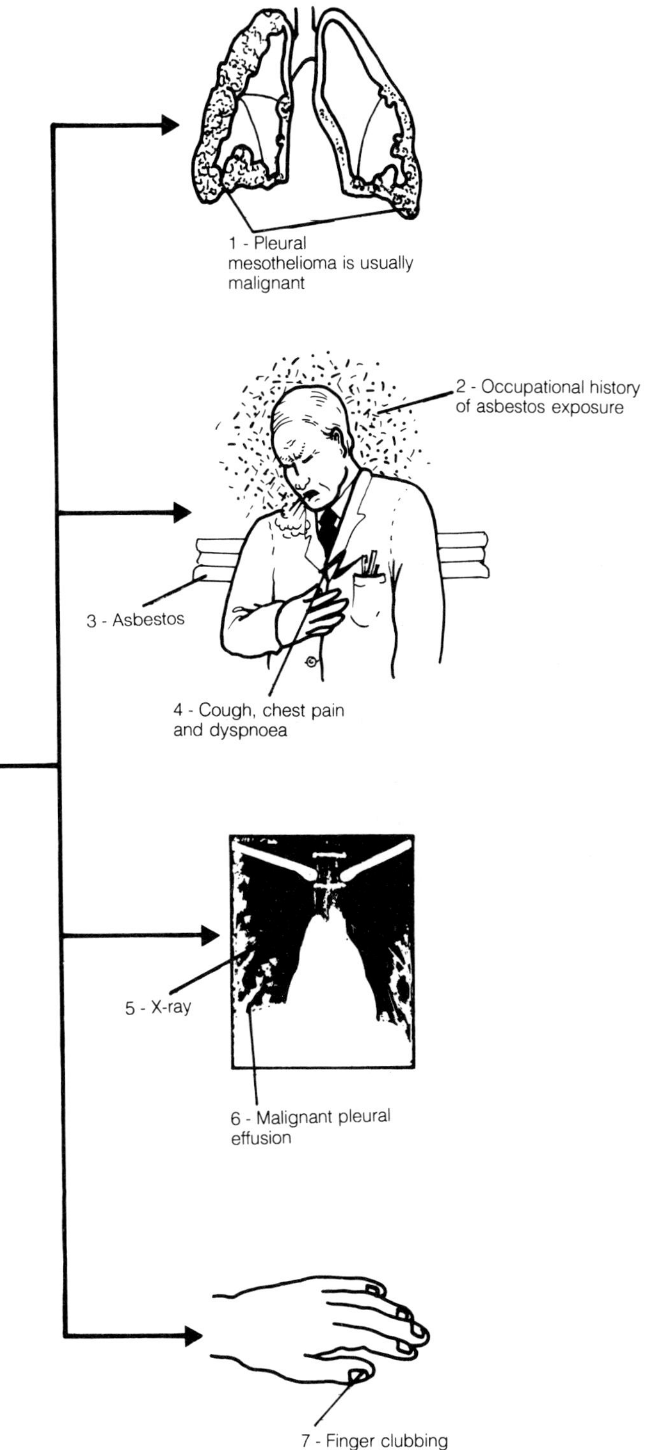

PLEURAL MESOTHELIOMA – This primary pleural tumour is **usually malignant** and the majority of patients have an occupational history of asbestos exposure. The clinical features are usually dyspnoea, cough and chest pain and a malignant pleural effusion is frequently found at presentation. The patients often exhibit finger clubbing. Surgical resec-

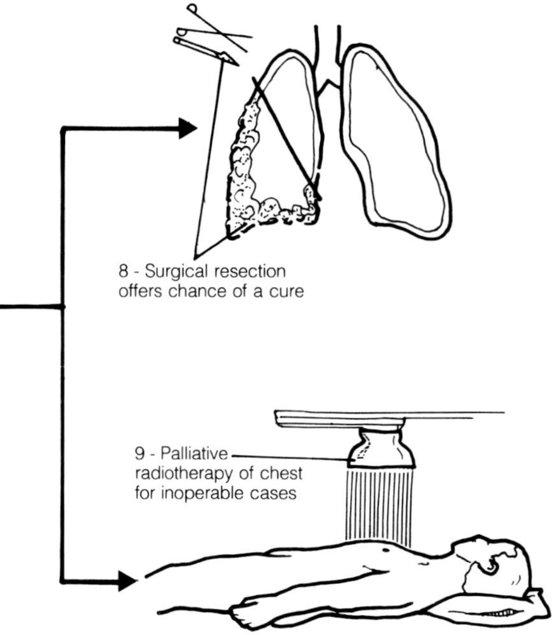

tion is the only modality of treatment with a chance of cure but the majority of cases are inoperable and die from their disease. Palliative radiotherapy may be worthwhile in some cases, but not, as of present, cytotoxic chemotherapy.

BRONCHIAL TUMOURS

Bronchial adenomas are of two types – both atypical in that they tend to be locally infiltrative, unlike a classic adenoma or benign tumour. Both the bronchial carcinoid (an apudoma similar to carcinoids elsewhere in the body) and the cylindroma (or adenoid cystic carcinoma arising from mucous glands) tend to arise

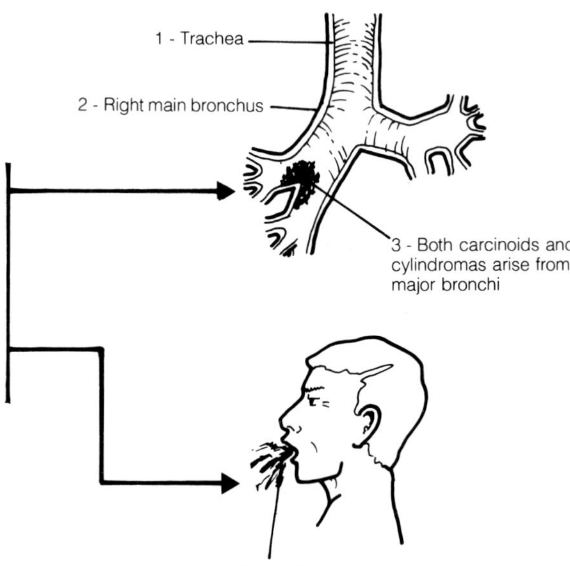

from the more major bronchi. The clinical **presentation is usually with haemoptysis** and bronchoscopic biopsy gives the diagnosis. The majority are curable by surgery but malignant change with metastases may occur.

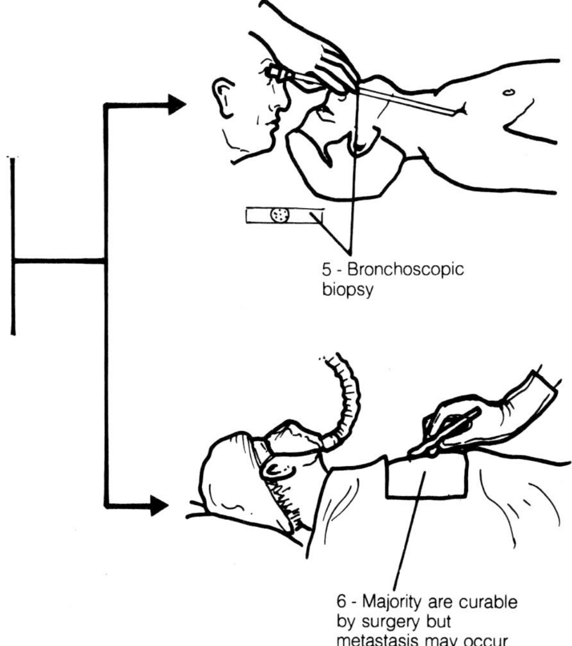

5 - Bronchoscopic biopsy

6 - Majority are curable by surgery but metastasis may occur

Bronchial carcinoma is the commonest adult, solid, malignancy in the U.K. causing over 30,000 deaths annually. Bronchial carcinoma incidence rises steeply in the fifth and subsequent decades, is commoner in males, and shows a strong association with cigarette smoking: the death·rate from this disease amongst heavy smokers is twenty-fold

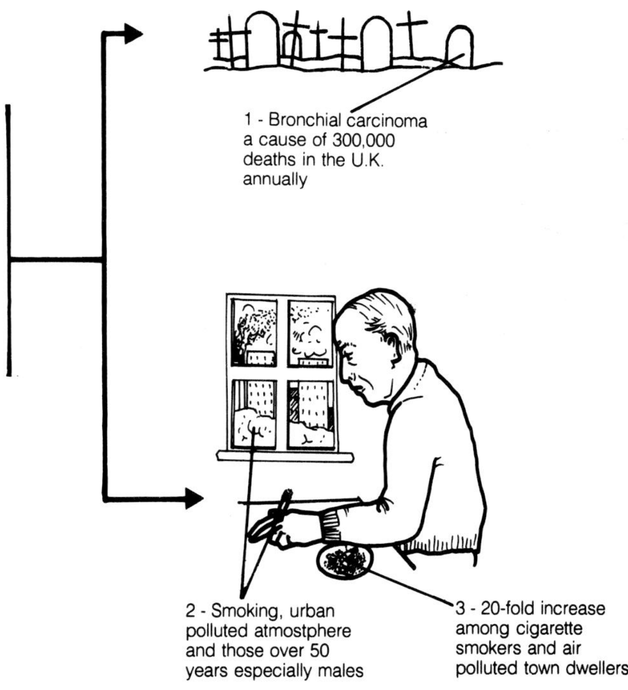

1 - Bronchial carcinoma a cause of 300,000 deaths in the U.K. annually

2 - Smoking, urban polluted atmostphere and those over 50 years especially males

3 - 20-fold increase among cigarette smokers and air polluted town dwellers

that of non-smokers. Urban atmospheric pollution is a risk factor for town dwellers. Occupational risks exist particularly for those exposed to asbestos, radioactive mineral dusts, nickel and chromium.

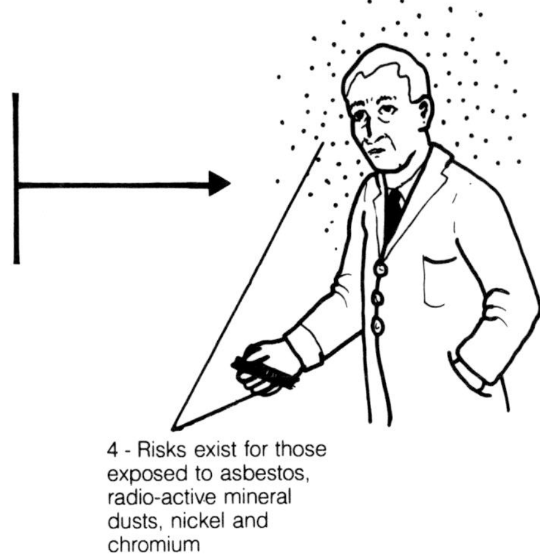

4 - Risks exist for those exposed to asbestos, radio-active mineral dusts, nickel and chromium

Bronchial carcinoma occurs most commonly in the main, lobar and lobular bronchi i.e. in the proximal bronchial tree. Carcinoma of the trachea is rare but peripheral carcinomas are not uncommon and an unusual form of bronchial carcinoma – bronchiolo-alveolar cell carcinoma – always arises peripherally. There is a

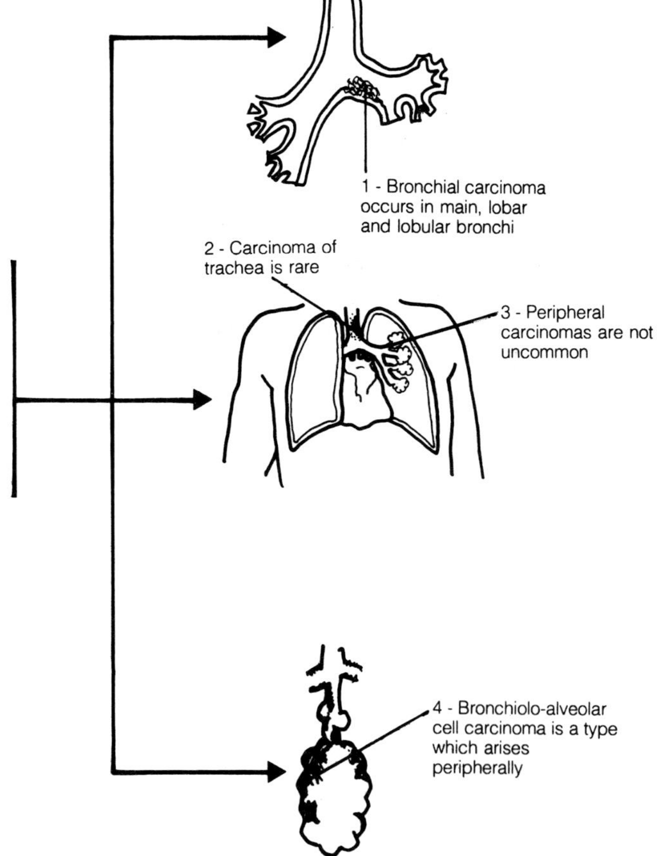

1 - Bronchial carcinoma occurs in main, lobar and lobular bronchi

2 - Carcinoma of trachea is rare

3 - Peripheral carcinomas are not uncommon

4 - Bronchiolo-alveolar cell carcinoma is a type which arises peripherally

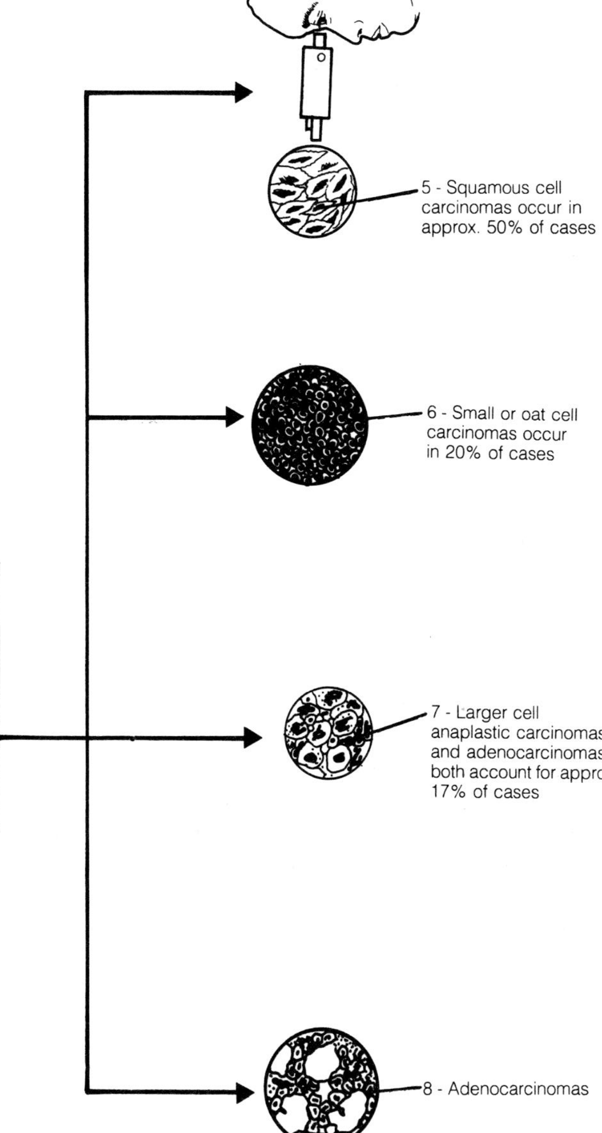

spectrum of histologies such that bronchial carcinoma is not one disease. Approximately 50% of all cases are squamous cell carcinomas, about 20% small round cell carcinomas (small cell carcinoma or oat cell carcinoma) whilst larger cell anaplastic carcinomas and primary adenocarcinomas of the bronchi account for approximately 17% of the total each.

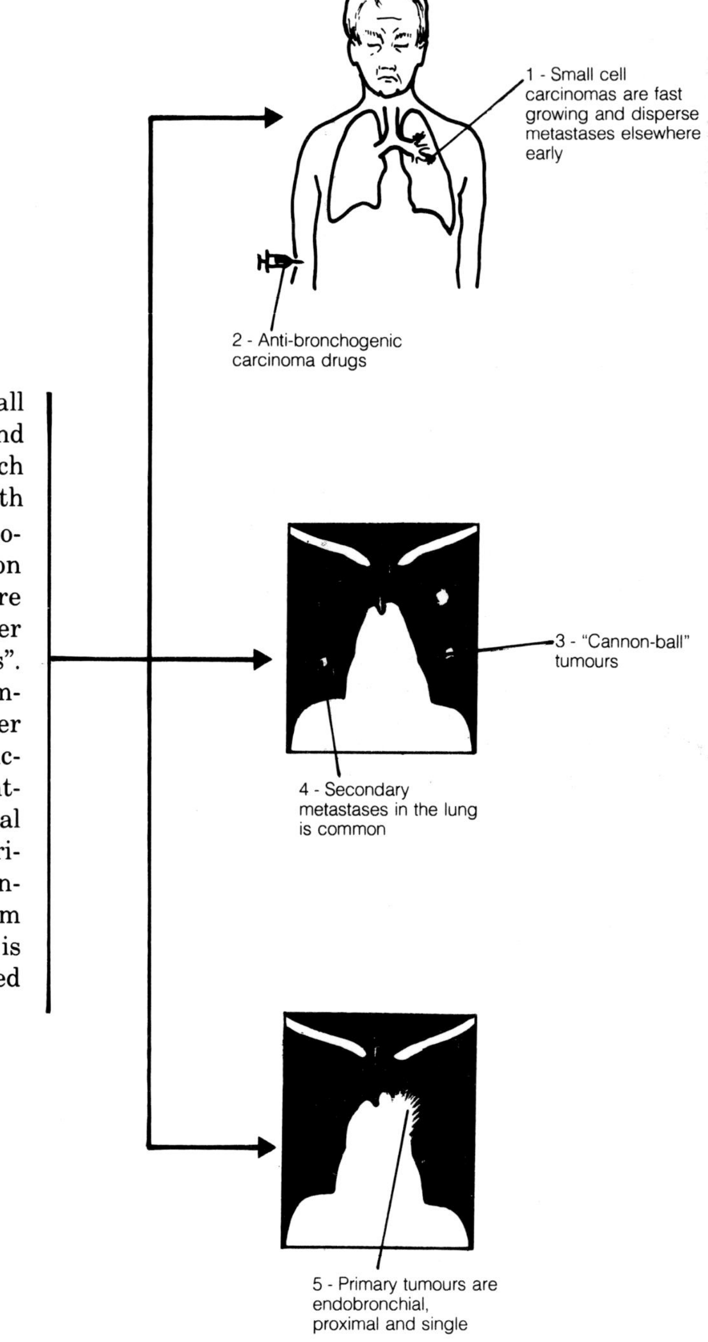

The small cell carcinomas are fast growing and early metastasising growths, for which surgical resection of the primary growth is rarely indicated and for which chemotherapy has made a significant impact on survival. These small cell carcinomas are managed differently from the larger group of "non-small cell carcinomas". The lung is of course one of the commonest sites for metastases from other tumours. They differ from primary bronchial carcinoma in that they are frequently multiple, occurring in the parenchymal lung field and growing at this site spherically. The chest X-ray shows "cannonball" tumours – a different picture from primary bronchial carcinoma which is endobronchial, usually proximally sited and single.

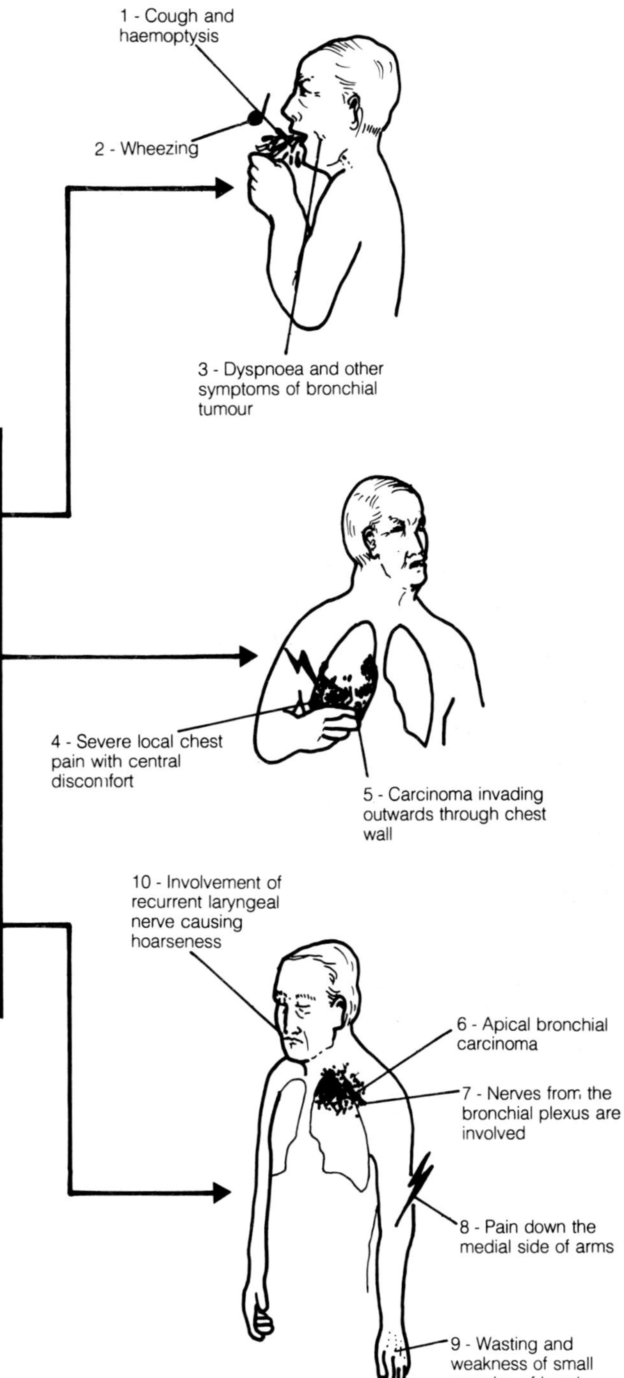

The **clinical presentation** varies and may be due to symptoms from metastatic spread. However, the primary bronchial tumour usually causes the presenting symptoms and cough with haemoptysis is one of the commonest causes of presentation. Dyspnoea, occasionally with localised wheeze, is another common presenting feature. Chest pain may be mild central discomfort or severe pleural and local chest wall pain if a carcinoma is invading outwards through the pleura into the chest wall; and apical bronchial carcinoma (**Pancoast tumour**) may locally infiltrate the inferior fibres of the brachial plexus causing severe pain down the medial aspect of the arm and weakness with wasting of the small muscles of the hand (T1 myotome). These symptoms and signs may progress and the cervical sympathetic may become infiltrated with the development of a **Horner's syndrome.** More centrally placed carcinomas may infiltrate the recurrent laryngeal nerve (causing hoarse-

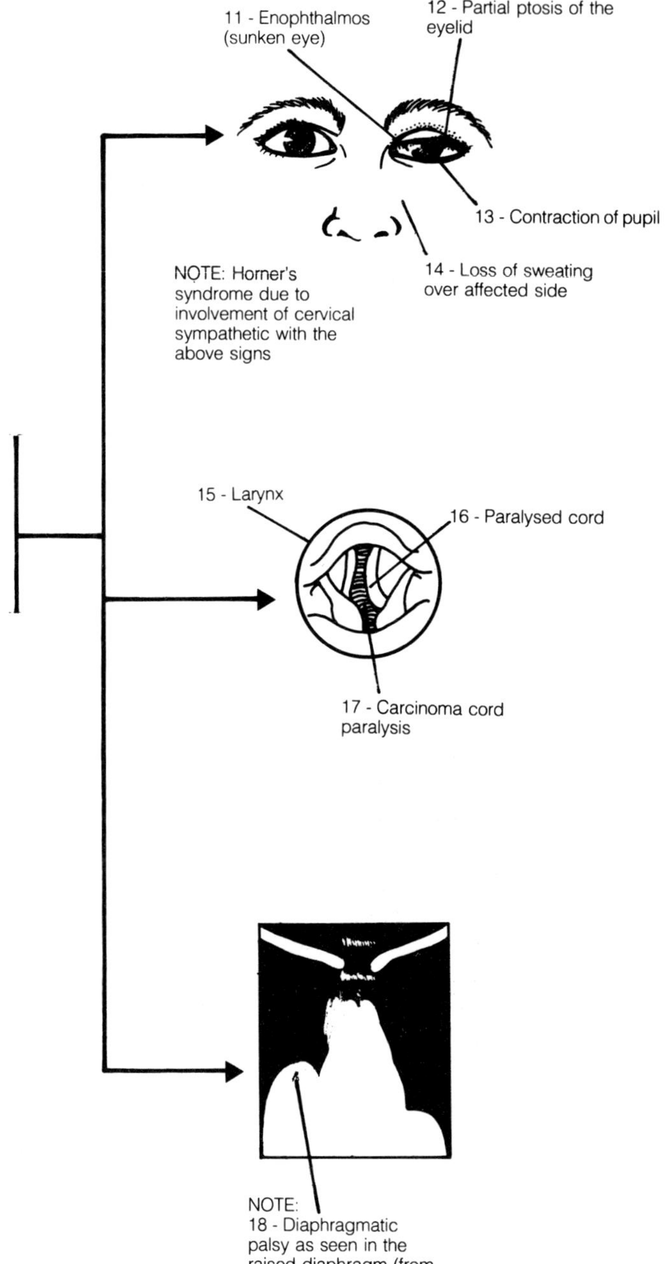

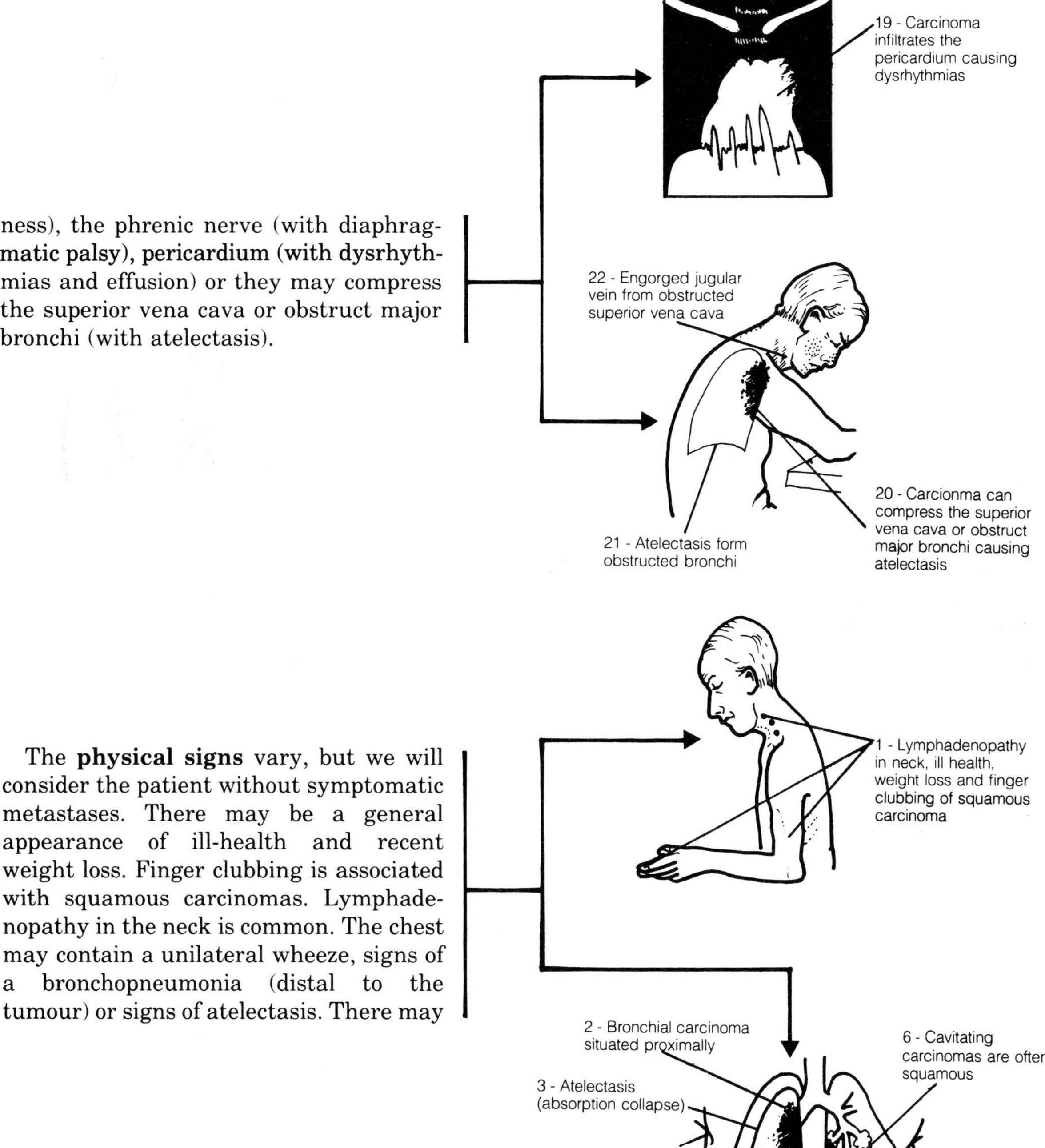

ness), the phrenic nerve (with diaphragmatic palsy), **pericardium (with dysrhythmias and effusion)** or they may compress the superior vena cava or obstruct major bronchi (with atelectasis).

The **physical signs** vary, but we will consider the patient without symptomatic metastases. There may be a general appearance of ill-health and recent weight loss. Finger clubbing is associated with squamous carcinomas. Lymphadenopathy in the neck is common. The chest may contain a unilateral wheeze, signs of a bronchopneumonia (distal to the tumour) or signs of atelectasis. There may be signs of a pleural effusion. Radiologically a mass is usually apparent and usually situated proximally. Cavitating carcinomas are usually squamous; peripheral carcinomas are rarely small cell carcinomas.

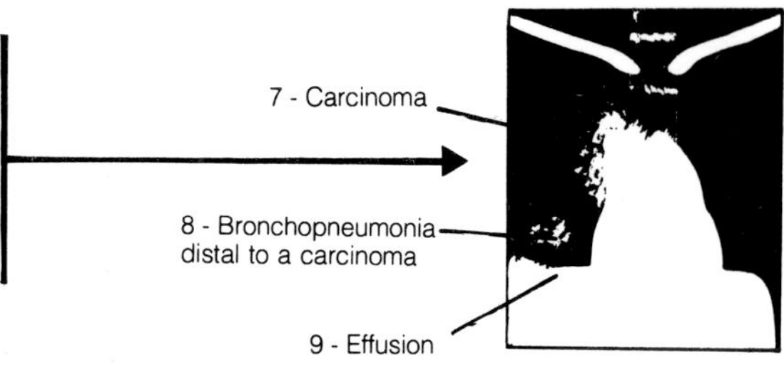

If three sputum specimens are examined by an expert cytologist, the diagnosis of carcinoma of the bronchus is usually obtained and almost always if there is haemoptysis. Salivary specimens must not be sent instead of sputum, which are best collected by the ward physiotherapist. Peripheral carcinomas and secondary deposits are less commonly diagnosable by sputum cytology. A bronchoscopy may be required to make a histological diagnosis (where sputum cytology is negative), to see if the lesion is operable or to stage the disease prior to chemotherapy. The greater range of the flexible fibreoptic bronchoscope makes this preferable for all examinations except testing for operability – here the fixity of mediastinal structures is best assessed by rigid bronchoscopy, and some thoracic surgeons prefer a formal mediastinoscopy preoperatively.

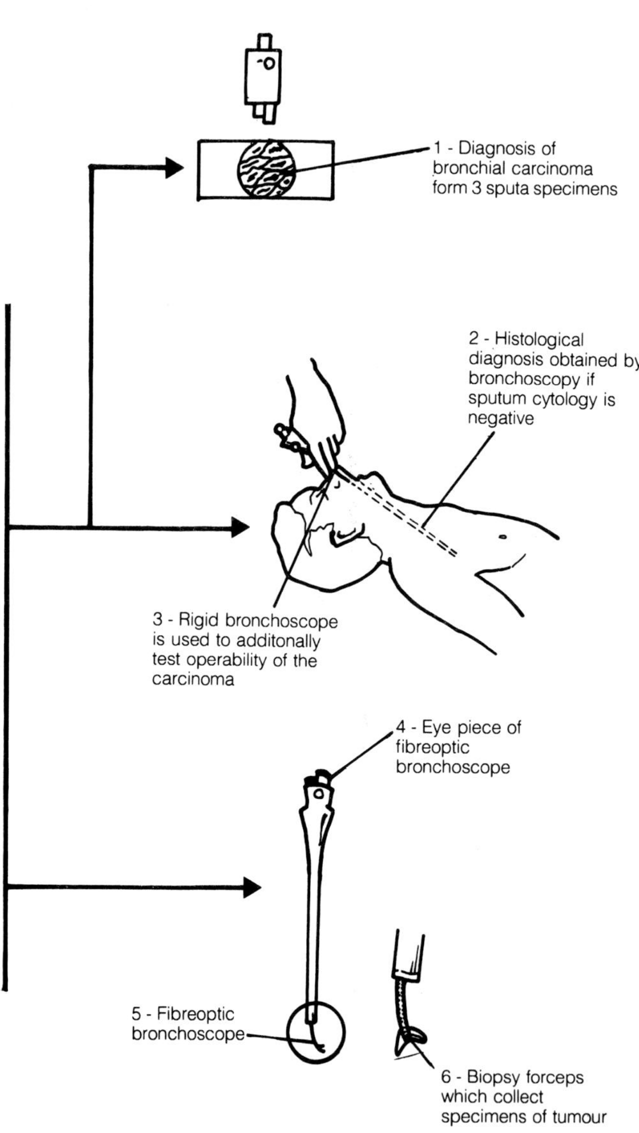

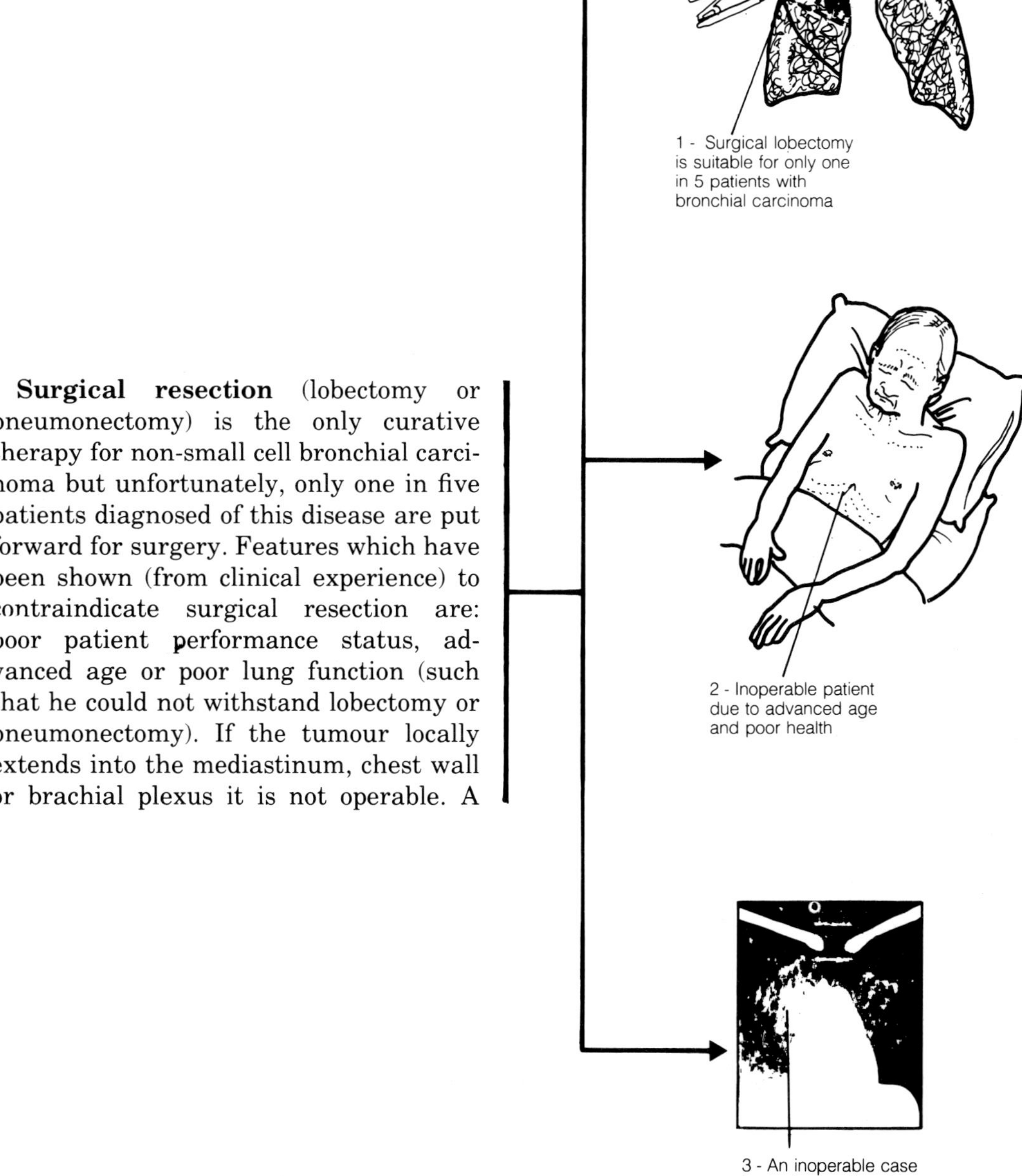

1 - Surgical lobectomy is suitable for only one in 5 patients with bronchial carcinoma

2 - Inoperable patient due to advanced age and poor health

3 - An inoperable case from chest-wall and bilateral involvement

Surgical resection (lobectomy or pneumonectomy) is the only curative therapy for non-small cell bronchial carcinoma but unfortunately, only one in five patients diagnosed of this disease are put forward for surgery. Features which have been shown (from clinical experience) to contraindicate surgical resection are: poor patient performance status, advanced age or poor lung function (such that he could not withstand lobectomy or pneumonectomy). If the tumour locally extends into the mediastinum, chest wall or brachial plexus it is not operable. A

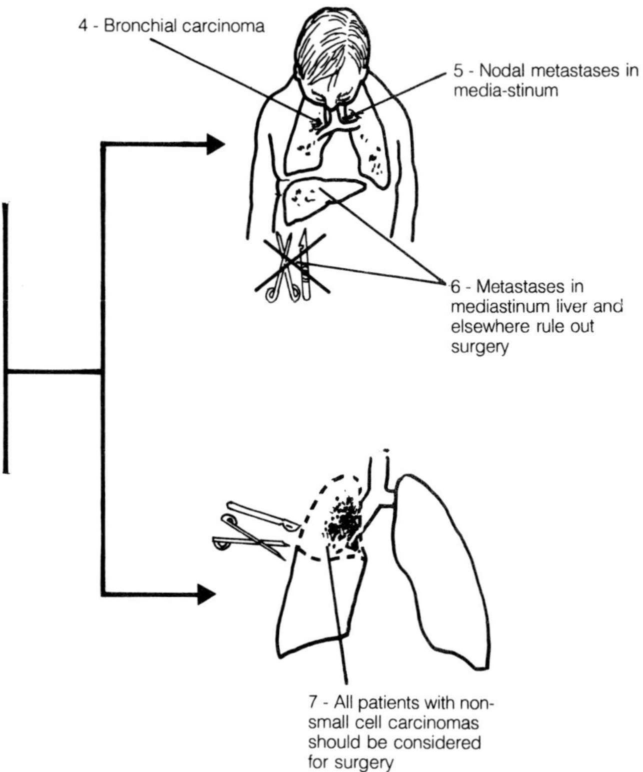

patient with metastases including mediastinal nodal metastases picked up by radiological imaging is not a surgical candidate. Nevertheless, all patients with non-small cell cancer should be considered surgical candidates until clinical or staging considerations rules this out. A minority of surgically resected bronchial carcinoma cases are cured.

The **management** of the majority or the inoperable non-small cell carcinoma patients depends on whether there are symptoms. Palliative radiotherapy is indicated for superior vena cava obstruction (manifested by suffusion of head and arms with dilated veins in these areas and a fixed, raised jugular vein); cough due to major airways involvement;

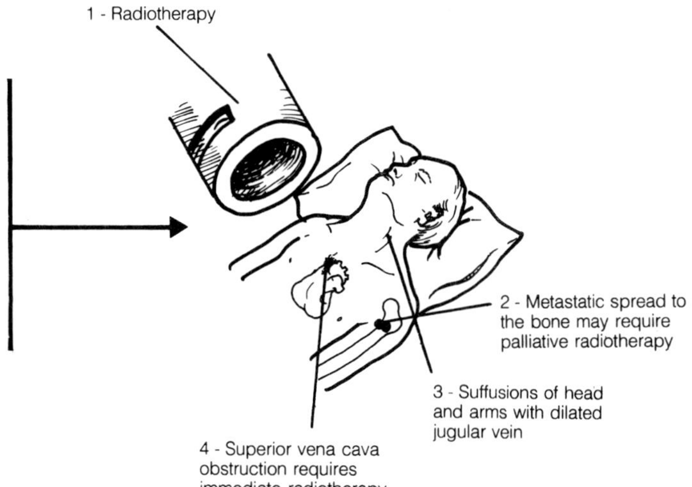

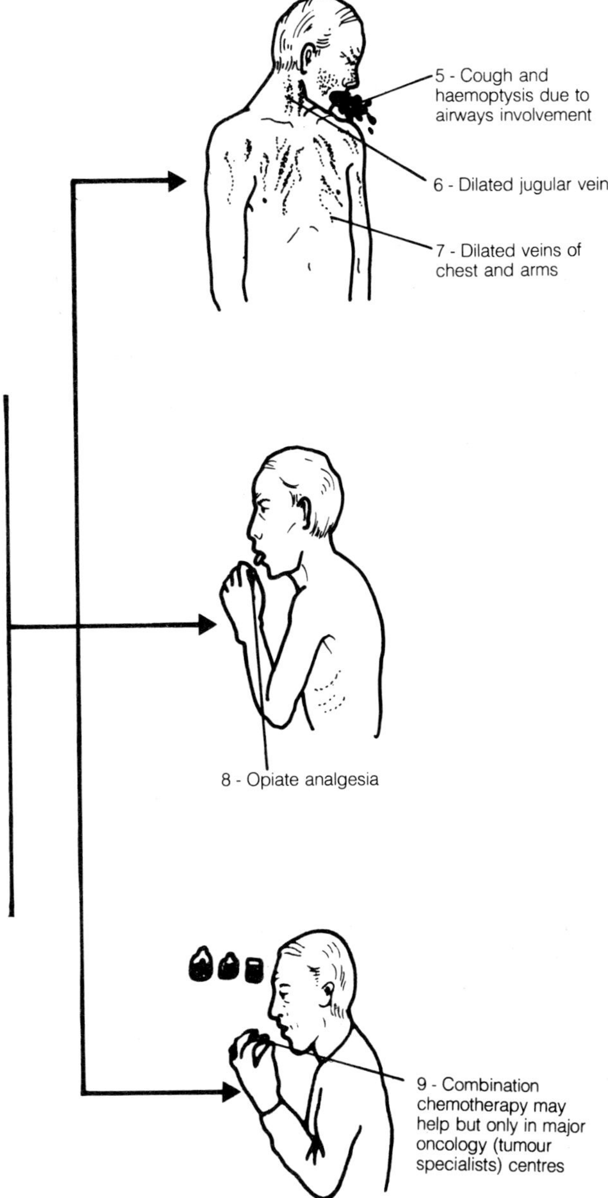

haemoptysis; imminent or recent lobar or lung collapse. Palliative radiotherapy may also be useful for symptomatic metastases particularly in bone, but where the general state of health is declining rapidly, it is preferable to use opiate analgesia to contain such pains. Cytotoxic chemotherapy is not recommended routinely in non-small cell carcinoma, except in carefully conducted clinical trials. It is quite possible to see regressions of non-small cell carcinoma with combination chemotherapy but the regimes to date have not improved the quality or quantity of life and are not to be recommended outside major oncology centres.

Small cell carcinoma of bronchus is chemo- and radiosensitive. Because dissemination is early so chemotherapy is the preferable initial therapy and is commenced with a combination of drugs such as adriamycin, vincristine, cyclophosphamide, or another triple drug regime with cyclophosphamide, metrotrexate and CCNU; a further drug, VP16 also has high activity against small cell carcinoma. A fast response is usual and it is now quite routine to have disease free remissions for longer than a year in this once rapidly fatal disease. Patients with overt metastatic small cell carcinoma at presentation still have a very gloomy outlook and rarely survive 6-12 months: patients who relapse after their chemotherapy-induced remission rarely achieve a second remission and soon die. The indications for palliative radiotherapy are as before, but whole brain radiotherapy for cerebral metastases has an established useful role in good performance status patients.

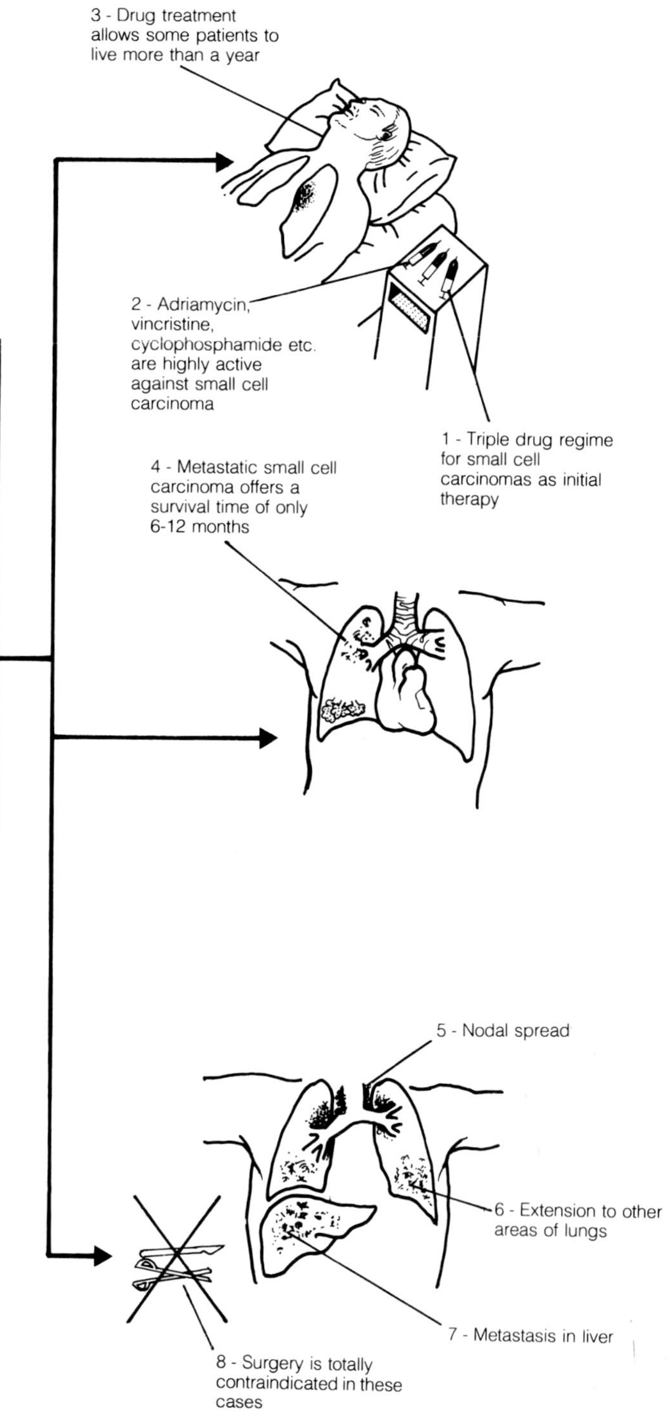

Index